Health Care Informatics:
A Skills-Based Resource

Notice

The authors, editors, and publisher have made every effort to ensure the accuracy and completeness of the information presented in this book. However, the authors, editors, and publisher cannot be held responsible for the continued currency of the information, any inadvertent errors or omissions, or the application of this information. Therefore, the authors, editors, and publisher shall have no liability to any person or entity with regard to claims, loss, or damage caused or alleged to be caused, directly or indirectly, by the use of information contained herein.

Health Care Informatics:
A Skills-Based Resource

Bill G. Felkey, Brent I. Fox,
and Margaret R. Thrower

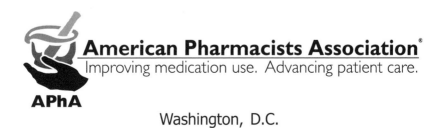

American Pharmacists Association®
Improving medication use. Advancing patient care.

APhA

Washington, D.C.

Managing and Content Editor: Vicki Meade, Meade Communications
Acquiring Editor: Sandra J. Cannon
Copy Editors: Mary De Angelo, Lucy Oppenheim
Proofreaders: L. Luan Corrigan, Corrigan Editorial Services; Suzanne Peake
Indexer: Mary Coe
Book Design and Layout: Michele A. Danoff, Graphics by Design
Cover Design: Tanaquil Baker, Groff Creative Inc.
Editorial Assistant: Kellie Burton

© 2006 by the American Pharmacists Association
Published by the American Pharmacists Association
2215 Constitution Avenue, N.W.
Washington, DC 20037-2985
www.aphanet.org

APhA was founded in 1852 as the American Pharmaceutical Association.

To comment on this book via e-mail, send your message to the publisher at aphabooks@aphanet.org

Library of Congress Cataloging-in-Publication Data

Felkey, Bill G.
    Health care informatics : a skills-based resource / Bill G. Felkey,
Brent I. Fox, and Margaret R. Thrower.
        p. ; cm.
    Includes bibliographical references and index.
    ISBN 1-58212-060-9
    1. Medical informatics. I. Fox, Brent I. II. Thrower, Margaret R.
III. Title.
    [DNLM: 1. Medical Informatics Applications. 2. Computer Systems.
W 26.5 F316h 2005]
R858.F47 2005
610'.28—dc22

                2005023222

How to Order This Book

Online: www.pharmacist.com
By phone: 800-878-0729
VISA®, MasterCard®, and American Express® cards accepted

Dedication

To Judy, who possesses, appreciates,
and supports having a servant heart.

To Georgia for your patience,
encouragement, and laughter.

To Greg Thrower, Anne Cancelosi,
Carol and Richard Ryman,
and Kohler and Licorice:
thanks for your love and support.

Table of Contents

Preface

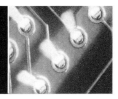

Through many years of teaching health care professionals, we have watched them struggle with technology. Some limp along, satisfied to reap only 10% of its capacity. Others are computer illiterate—at times to the point of phobia. We have seen health care leaders shun technology that would help their organizations deliver patient care more effectively and efficiently.

People often resist technology simply because they do not understand how to use it and integrate it into their workflow. That is why we wrote this book. Our goal is to help busy professionals learn the skills necessary to make good use of computers and information tools. Although this book does not teach everything necessary to transform you into a "power user," it gives basics on which to build.

We created a multidisciplinary book because the need to use and evaluate information is a common denominator in all areas of health care, regardless of specialty or job definition. Physicians, pharmacists, nurses, physician assistants, nurse practitioners, dentists, and other providers can benefit from this work.

Tools for Better Decisions

Health care today is so complex that it surpasses the human mind's capacity to operate without technology. Practitioners need tools that reduce uncertainty in decision making, promote efficient patient care, and help bring about the best outcomes possible. Compared with other key industries, health care has been slow to accept technology support. We believe that health care informatics is likely to follow a path similar to banking and finance, which long ago realized the importance of investing in information technology. Although health care organizations are becoming more willing to allocate funds for technology, they remain fearful of spending scarce dollars unwisely.

The patient should be at the center of all technology decisions in health care systems. Although health care is a business and has to remain profitable, it is also a service industry that must balance access, quality, and cost. Technology is a tool for achieving organizational objectives, not an end unto itself. Patients will ultimately judge whether a health care organization has fulfilled its vision and mission. Thus, a patient-centered focus will drive technology forward in a way that best serves a health care organization's goals.

Here's an example of what can be done. The chief information officer of Baylor Health Systems in Dallas, Robert Pickton, believes so heavily in the power of the Internet's ubiquity that many years ago he decided to build Baylor's information system so it would eventually operate completely on the Internet. At Baylor they have gone so far as to create a "Webtop"—a workstation that uses an Internet browser to perform all tasks in the health system. Each user can log in to any workstation and access a customized view of all the most-used applications and other icons. This Web browser interface looks and operates the same way no matter where the user is located in the system, from the pharmacy to the physicians' lounge to the nurses' station, an approach that benefits patients because it reduces the potential for errors from unfamiliarity with computer screens.

Quick Learning for Busy Professionals

We know that health care professionals do not have a lot of free time. In writing this book, we've tried to use the same sensitivity we invest in our bootcamps, which we've offered for years to teach people how to quickly integrate technology into personal and professional life. For these intensive, one- to two-day bootcamps, each participant is given a personal computer, Internet connectivity, productivity software, and personal digital assistant. As compared with courses that take three months to teach how to operate Microsoft Windows XP, our bootcamps cover everything health care professionals really need to understand about their operating system within three to four hours. In this book, our approach includes:

- Focusing on practical skills that will make you more effective and efficient.
- Explaining why investing your time in learning a particular skill will benefit your practice.
- Teaching you ways to assess whether studies, information in electronic databases, and material on the Internet is relevant and applicable to your patients and practice.
- Presenting information to enhance your literature retrieval skills and your ability to make evidence-based health care decisions.

- Providing lists of resources, such as online glossaries and Web site addresses, so you can expand your learning online.
- Including activities that allow you to apply material to your particular practice area and internalize key concepts and skills.
- Writing succinctly to convey what you need to know, and no more.

When new studies are published, practitioners often ask us, "Does this apply to my patients?" "Is this going to change my standard of practice?" and "Which patients will I apply these results to?" Other common questions we hear are, "Can you tell me a good Internet site where I can refer patients to learn about their diseases and medicines?" or "What's a good Web site I can use on the spot to help me answer questions when a patient asks?" After reading this book, you'll be able to answer these questions for yourself.

Bill G. Felkey
Brent I. Fox
Margaret R. Thrower
August 2005

About the Authors

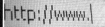

Bill G. Felkey, MS, professor of pharmacy care systems at Auburn University School of Pharmacy, is a well-known expert in pharmacy and health-system technology who has given more than 800 presentations on computers, informatics, and management issues in health care.

Brent I. Fox, PharmD, PhD, is assistant professor and director of the Center for Pharmacy Informatics at Shenandoah University and a consultant on integrating information technology into health care.

Margaret R. Thrower, PharmD, director of clinical services at HospiScript Services, LLC, maintains an affiliate faculty position at Auburn University School of Pharmacy, where she was formerly assistant professor and drug information specialist.

What Is Informatics? 1

Brent I. Fox

Chapter Objectives

After completing this chapter, you should be able to:

- Understand the role of information and technology in health care.
- Formulate a clear, practical definition of health care informatics.
- Briefly describe the history of health care informatics.
- Discuss subdisciplines of health care informatics.
- Identify and discuss obstacles to developing a practice heavily supported by health care informatics.
- Identify Internet-based resources for more health care informatics information.
- Identify health care informatics educational programs in the United States.

ACTIVITY 1-1

Defining Informatics

In keeping with our skills-based approach to teaching health care informatics, we give you activities and readings throughout this book to expand your abilities and help you retain key concepts. Your first activity, before reading further, is to:

1. Stop and draft your own definition of informatics.
2. Check it with at least one online resource to compare your understanding of the term with other published definitions on the Internet.

Completing this exercise will help you define your starting point and your objectives for learning about health care informatics.

Do you know what information is? Like many words in health care practice, "information" is often used with little thought to its true definition, yet we rely on it tremendously. Information may be the latest results from a literature article, something we learned from a colleague, or a series of hemoglobin A1c results indicating a patient's blood sugar control over the last 12 months.

To define information, it helps to understand the meaning of the word "data": a representation of facts or concepts. For example, patients with diabetes record their blood sugar levels several times a day and create a daily log showing individual facts about their blood sugar levels. Each blood sugar reading represents individual data points, or facts. A health care practitioner then uses this collection of data points to determine the effectiveness of the patient's lifestyle modifications and medication therapy. Together, these data points provide information.

"Information" is data that have meaning. It can be presented in any medium, such as prose, lists, or graphics—but the best way is in the manner that the end user prefers.

Information is data that have meaning for the ultimate user.[1] For example, a patient's individual blood sugar readings do not have much meaning without context—details about the person's health and circumstances.

Information can be presented in any medium, such as prose, lists, or graphics.[2] Which medium you use most may depend on your practice setting or learning style. The ultimate users of information can best determine what information format most closely meets their needs.

Technology, the other key component of informatics, is another word we often use without defining its true meaning. Most people associate the personal computer and cell phone with the term technology. But what about the common ballpoint pen? Or a book bag your child uses to tote around reading materials? These very different objects are technologies. By our definition, technology is any tool that extends the capabilities of the user or performs tasks the user finds repetitive or tedious. Thus a computer is a technology because it allows you to manipulate information. A ballpoint pen allows you to transfer data or information from a source to paper. Even a book bag is a technology because it allows you to carry things more easily. From these examples, we see that some technologies are more complex and powerful than others.

As a whole, health care is increasingly focused on using technologies to improve patient care. One of the greatest challenges for health care practitioners is to take the appropriate information and apply it to individual patients who can benefit from it. At the same time, practitioners must consider patient safety issues and provide care in a way that minimizes risks while improving patient outcomes.

One of the most talked-about technologies today for improving patient outcomes by reducing medication errors is computerized prescriber order entry (CPOE).[3,4] Computerized prescriber order entry systems allow prescribers to create electronic versions of paper-based medical orders, giving them access to information when and how they need it. Bar codes and the electronic health record (EHR) are also ways to increase the efficiency of health care delivery while simultaneously improving patient outcomes.

What, then, is the true role of information and technology to the health care professional? Practitioners are finding it increasingly important to find, select, and apply valid, appropriate clinical information when making decisions about the care of their patients—an approach known as evidence-based health care.[5,6] In the evidence-based approach to practice, information is the key to improving health care.

But how is the information best delivered? The answer to this question is always the same: in the manner the end user prefers. This is where technology—or more specifically, information technology—enters the equation. Information technology refers to the activities and tools used to locate, manipulate, store, and disseminate information. An obvious example of information technology in institutional settings is the clinical information system that all departments of the facility connect with so they can locate, manipulate, store, and disseminate information related to providing care.

Three key technologies in health care today are computerized prescriber order entry (CPOE), bar codes, and electronic health records (EHR), which increase efficiency and help improve patient outcomes.

Defining Health Care Informatics

Informatics can be a standalone term, but in many cases it is combined with words such as medical, biomedical, nursing, pharmacy, or dental. In this book we use the phrase "health care informatics" to embody the multidisciplinary nature of informatics as it relates to patient care.

In simplest terms, health care informatics is the science that uses information to improve health care.[7] On a more complex level, health care informatics acquires, structures, and uses data and information in the patient care decision-making process.[8]

People in many roles make up the health care informatics spectrum, including information technology professionals, researchers, clinicians, educators, administrators, and theorists. This book focuses on the clinical side of health care informatics and how clinicians can apply information technology to their daily patient care practice.

Health care informatics is an interdisciplinary field that applies technology and information to enhance health care delivery, support biomedical research, and foster education of health professionals and the public. The study of health care informatics leads to new problem-solving techniques, analytic methods, technology, and tools. You can think of informatics as a crossroads where data, information, and knowledge meet.

Health care informatics involves people with diverse backgrounds and training. For example, both clinical and nonclinical researchers generate much of the information used in practice. Researchers may not apply the information at the bedside, but through their activities they explore and discover the information others use to provide care.

Health care informatics also encompasses people from the information science field. These "information technology" professionals use computing technologies to manage information within an organization.

Clinicians are an obvious piece to the health care informatics puzzle because they usually put health care informatics activities to work in caring for patients. Often viewed as the end users of health care informatics, clinicians evaluate information and apply it in the appropriate situations. People in many other roles, including educators, administrators, and theorists, are also part of the health care informatics spectrum.

Health care informatics is an extremely broad discipline. Many times, people take on several roles as they try to apply health care informatics practices to patient care. In this book, we will primarily focus on the clinical side of health care informatics, discussing ways you can use information technology in daily practice.

A Brief History of Health Care Informatics

Informatics began in Europe in the mid-1900s. In 1949, Gustav Wagner founded the first professional organization for informatics in Germany, currently known as the Deutsche Gesellschaft für Medizinische Dokumentation, Informatik und Statistik. The term "medical informatics" first appeared in France in the 1960s. During that same decade, the first organized training programs in informatics began appearing in France, Germany, Belgium, and the Netherlands. Similar programs began appearing in Poland and the United States in the 1970s.[8]

Health care informatics has been linked to development of the modern computer. Information gained from a punch-card data-processing system in the 1890 U.S. Census was used in the 1920s and 1930s in several types of national surveys. This technology laid the groundwork for the completely electronic digital computer of the 1940s.[9]

The years between 1950 and 1970 brought big changes as technological advances helped shape the role of computers in

---

BOX 1-1

Five Ways You Benefit from Knowing About Health Care Informatics

1. Information technology is here to stay, yet many clinicians are uncomfortable with it. Increasing your comfort level will enhance your ability to use the latest tools for finding, evaluating, and applying information.

2. The good news is that there is a wealth of medical, scientific, and practice information available to clinicians. The bad news is that there is so much medical, scientific, and practice information in the world today, and this information is changing so fast, no single person can manage it alone. Health care informatics skills give you quick, efficient access to what you need to know to make the best decisions for patients.

3. Patients are increasingly relying on information technologies to obtain health-related information, connect with communities of others with similar interests and needs, and communicate with caregivers. Clinicians who are able to efficiently and effectively use information technology will be better able to meet patients' needs.

4. Health care institutions are under increasing pressure from patients, regulatory bodies, and the public to use information technologies that improve care delivery and patient outcomes. Clinicians knowledgeable in the practical application of health care informatics will be an asset to the health care team.

5. Research has consistently shown that information technologies can improve many facets of health care delivery. The U.S. government has firmly indicated its desire to replace outdated and ineffective processes and technologies with those that have demonstrated a positive impact on patient care. If you don't develop health care informatics skills, you may soon be considered outdated and ineffective.

institutional settings and people started investigating the potential of a total hospital information system. The Medinet project at General Electric in the mid-1960s was probably the earliest work on a hospital information system in the United States. Similar projects were later conducted at Massachusetts General Hospital in Boston, Latter Day Saints Hospital in Salt Lake City, Kaiser Permanente in Oakland, and Stanford University.[9]

In the 1970s, two approaches to hospital information systems emerged. The first relied on a single mainframe, time-share computer to support all applications. Several leading academic institutions developed large-scale clinical information systems that included prototypical artificial intelligence methods.[8,9] The second favored using individual minicomputers within specific application areas, all sharing a single patient database. However, networking technologies of the time did not support this approach to hospital information systems.[9]

The early 1980s to 1994 was a very important time on both technological and professional levels. The modern personal computer was introduced, enabling individual practitioners to buy their own computers and software, and personal computers became smaller and increasingly powerful, launching their use as a clinical tool.[9] Leading research centers further developed sophisticated clinical information systems, and hundreds of commercial vendors began offering products to support health care informatics. Health Level 7 (see discussion on page 15) and other standards-setting organizations began developing protocols for transmitting health care information.[8]

At this time, informatics training, research, and development were recognized as high-priority strategic goals for the United States and the European Union. The American Medical Informatics Association was formed in 1990 by the merger of the American Association for Medical Systems and Informatics (AAMSI), the American College of Medical Informatics (ACMI), and the Symposium on Computer Applications in Medical Care (SCAMC). This 3200-member organization focuses on using information technologies to improve health care.[10]

The current era of health care informatics, which began around 1995, is characterized by extensive, highly connected network environments where clinical information flows freely.[8] Ubiquitous computing and the Internet give clinicians access to information anytime from any Internet-connected device. Broadband wireless connectivity is also becoming widespread.

The American Medical Informatics Association, formed in 1990, focuses on using information technologies to improve health care (Web site: www.amia.org).

Health Care Informatics Subdisciplines

Many terms describe health care informatics—dentistry informatics, medical informatics, nursing informatics, and pharmacy informatics. Why? Are they describing similar or distinct fields? Actually, they are all subdisciplines of health care informatics.

If you compare our definition of health care informatics, "the science that uses information to improve health care," to leading definitions of medical informatics, you will see they are virtually the same.[7,11] Despite the similarities in definition, we use the term "health care informatics" because it appeals to the most people. Throughout this book, as we use the term "health care," you can substitute the word "medical" without changing the meaning of the material.

Regardless of the adjective used, informatics is not just a provider-focused discipline. Health care informatics focuses on the methods, techniques, and theories that support the use of information in health care.[12] Why, then, are adjectives placed in front of the term "informatics"?

Health care informatics is an emerging field in which people are exploring new domains and making connections between existing ones. One way to define these new domains is to identify them by the health care practitioners using an informatics approach, such as "nursing informatics" for applications related to the practice of nursing. Figure 1-1 on page 8 illustrates subdisciplines of health care (medical) informatics.

Figure 1-1 also shows the relationship between research and research applications. The research component comprises the "roots" of informatics and includes the study of methods, techniques, and theories that underlie health care informatics. The four primary branches in the top of the figure are applications of the basic research components—applications that target the leafy areas of the tree, such as society or body organs.

The clinical component of health care informatics (that is, nursing informatics and the other terms mentioned above) exists on a continuum starting with bioinformatics, where informatics methods are applied to molecular and cellular processes, and continuing to the other end of the spectrum, public health informatics, which addresses the problems of complete populations and society as a whole.[12] Think of the clinical informatics "limb" depicted in Figure 1-1 as health care informatics applied to the care of individual patients. This book focuses on that limb

Health care informatics focuses on the methods, techniques, and theories that support the use of information in health care. It is an emerging field in which people are exploring new domains and making connections between existing ones.

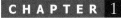

CHAPTER 1

because it's where you can use information technology to improve patient care. At the base of the tree are component sciences striving to understand "how" and "why" things exist.

Box 1-2 gives definitions for specific component sciences of health care informatics.

FIGURE 1-1

Basic and applied research components of health care (or medical) informatics.

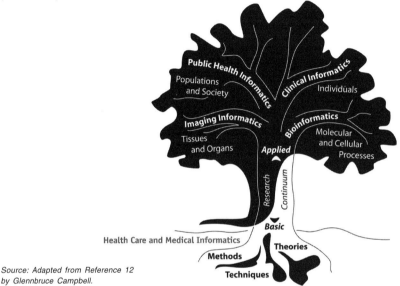

Source: Adapted from Reference 12 by Glennbruce Campbell.

BOX 1-2

Core Scientific Components of Heath Care Informatics

Cognitive Science: The study of how people think and learn, rather than what they learn.

Computer Science: Broad area describing the study of computing systems; includes theories, methods, design issues, and implementation.

Decision Science: The application of mathematical modeling and analysis to the decision-making process.

Information Science: The study of information in terms of its creation, use, and management.

Management Science: The study of decision making and planning within an organizational setting.

Source: Reference 12.

As suggested earlier, health care informatics is not solely a field for health care practitioners. Figure 1-2 depicts the relationships between health care (medical) informatics, other component sciences, and public health domains. This image of gears interconnecting shows you the close relationships between domains, with information sharing as the common theme.

New information in one gear can affect all other gears. For example, medical informatics draws on information learned from the component sciences in the leftmost gear, the domain where non–health care professionals can most often be found. Information learned from the component sciences is incorporated into health care informatics and is then applied to the care of individuals and, ultimately, populations.

Alternatively, when problems are identified in the public health domain, the gear to the far right, they spur new research in the health care informatics domain. Health care informatics is the largest and central gear because it unifies all the domains in the other three gears.

FIGURE 1-2

The role of component sciences in health care informatics.

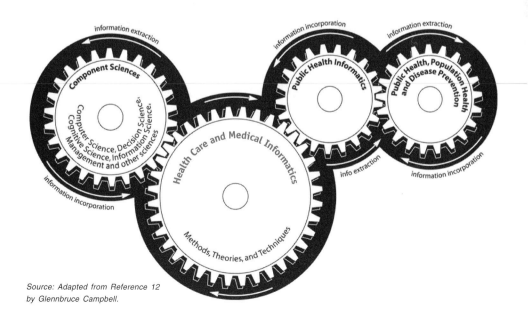

Source: Adapted from Reference 12 by Glennbruce Campbell.

Health Care Informatics Today

Because health care informatics is relatively new, you'll find disagreements on its basic terminology. Some people define health care informatics in terms of the technology used, while others define it in terms of the health care practitioner.

Today, the U.S. health care system is caring for a population that is increasing and aging. Older patients generally consume more clinician time and health care dollars, use more prescription medications, and are more frequently hospitalized due to chronic diseases than any other age group—which translates into increased health care expenditures for both patients and payers. In addition, medication errors continue to harm significant numbers of patients each year and are very costly in terms of patient care dollars and legal expenditures.

According to the Centers for Medicare and Medicaid Services (CMS), the United States spent $1.6 trillion on health care in 2002, a 9.3% increase from 2001. This increase followed a then-record year in 2001 when health care spending increased 8.5% from 2000. Overall in 2002, health care spending consumed almost 15% of the United States' gross domestic product, the largest figure for any country in the world.[13]

The health care system is obviously facing a crisis in which expenses keep going up and patients continue having negative outcomes. Information technology, a key infrastructure component of health care informatics, can alleviate some of these problems. While health care informatics cannot change the demographic shift that we currently see in the United States, it can help deliver health care more efficiently and safely.[13]

Applications on the Institutional Level

Research in an institutional setting has indicated that nearly 80% of medication errors result from lack of access to medication information or information about the patient.[14] The authors of the study that reported this statistic concluded that to increase positive patient outcomes, health care practitioners should have information available to them whenever and however they need it. MercuryMD (www.mercurymd.com), a software company whose focus is in line with the study's recommendation, provides a good example of an applied approach to clinical informatics. Using a wireless infrastructure, the company's MData system gives clinicians mobile access to clinical and medication information anywhere in their institution by way of handheld computers, such as Palm or Pocket PC devices.

Health care informatics can help deliver health care more efficiently and safely as the population ages, which should reduce expenses and improve outcomes. Health care spending in the United States increased 8.5% from 2000 to 2001 and 9.3% from 2001 to 2002, a trend that will lead to a crisis if expenses keep going up.

For an example of how using information technology in basic research can improve patient care, look no further than the famous Human Genome Project, in which scientists used fundamental research methods and techniques to map the complete human genome—providing an enormous opportunity to understand the human body in ways not previously possible. Coordinated by the U.S. Department of Energy and the National Institutes of Health, the 13-year project was completed in 2003, allowing researchers to better identify the cellular processes underlying diseases and, it is hoped, develop completely new diagnostic and treatment methods.

The project relied heavily on information technology to sort and manage the data necessary to map the human genome. Massive amounts of data were generated for scientists and medical researchers to use as they seek to understand human life. In all, information learned from the Human Genome Project is expected to be applied across boundaries between medicine, food, energy, life sciences, and environmental resources.[15] Arguably, this project—which could not have been accomplished without information technology—is the single most important development in our lifetime for furthering our ability to identify and treat human diseases.

The authors of an important study on medication errors concluded that to increase positive patient outcomes, health care practitioners should have information available to them whenever and however they need it.

Applications at the Practitioner Level

What activities must you, as a health care practitioner, perform to be considered someone who uses a health care informatics approach? Perhaps, in the course of treating patients, you draw conclusions from large amounts of clinical data, are engaged in clinical research, or manage databases of health care information. Essentially, using a health care informatics approach means having skills that allow you to apply information in caring for patients and making clinical decisions.

For example, you use informatics skills to formulate the steps to solve a clinical problem. Next, you select appropriate resources to answer questions the problem generates. Then you critically evaluate potential solutions and choose the best one for your patient. Finally, you evaluate the patient's outcome and record your observations to share with other clinicians.

Box 1-3 lists a proposed set of informatics-related skills for medical education, which was developed by Enrico Coiera, a senior project manager with Hewlett-Packard Laboratories.[16] This skill set focuses on general ways that clinicians should be able to find clinical data, assess validity and applicability, apply data to practice, record new information developed from the data, and communicate the information to other colleagues. The 10 skills represent broad abilities. Clinicians must also develop rudimentary skills—building blocks to be set in place before attempting to develop higher-level skills. One such building block is the ability to efficiently navigate an electronic information system.

Nontechnological Barriers to Health Care Informatics

Lack of Knowledge

One obvious and important reason that practitioners do not use a health care informatics approach is simply a lack of knowledge. As a relatively new field in health care, few professional schools include health care informatics as a core component of

---

BOX 1-3

Ten Essential Clinical Informatics Skills

1. Understand the dynamic and uncertain nature of medical knowledge, and be able to keep personal knowledge and skills up-to-date.
2. Know how to search for and assess knowledge according to the statistical bases of scientific evidence.
3. Understand some of the logical and statistical models of the diagnostic process.
4. Interpret uncertain clinical data and deal with artifacts and errors.
5. Structure and analyze clinical decisions in terms of risk and benefits.
6. Apply and adapt clinical knowledge to the individual circumstances of patients.
7. Access, assess, select, and apply treatment guidelines; adapt to the local circumstances; and communicate and record variations in treatment plans and outcomes.
8. Structure and record clinical data in a form appropriate for the immediate clinical task, communication with colleagues, or epidemiological purposes.
9. Select and operate the most appropriate communication method for a given task (e.g., face-to-face conversation, telephone, e-mail, video, voice mail, or letter).
10. Choose communication media, and structure and communicate messages in a manner most suited to the recipient and task.

Source: Reference 16.

---

their curricula. Although this pattern is slowly changing, many of today's practitioners have not been exposed to health care informatics as part of their education.

Fortunately, practitioners who focus on health care informatics have helped to establish and strengthen professional organizations that promote this field. As shown in Box 1-4, both national and international organizations are promoting health care informatics. In addition, individuals can develop their own informatics skills and teach others about this exciting area of health care.

BOX 1-4

Health Care Informatics Professional Associations

American Health Information Management Association: www.ahima.org
An association of health information management professionals focusing on delivering quality health care, advocacy, education, certification, and lifelong learning.

American Medical Informatics Association: www.amia.org
An organization dedicated to developing and using information technologies to improve health care.

American Nursing Informatics Association: www.ania.org
Provides networking, education, and information resources to strengthen the roles of nurses in informatics, including clinical information, education, and administrative decision support.

Canada's Health Informatics Association: www.coachorg.com
Promotes a clear understanding of health informatics within the Canadian health system through education, information, networking, and communication.

European Federation for Medical Informatics: www.efmi.org
Concerned with the theory and practice of information science and technology within the health sciences in a European context.

Healthcare Information and Management Systems Society: www.himss.org
Provides leadership for the optimal use of health care information technology and management systems for the betterment of human health.

International Medical Informatics Association: www.imia.org
Applies information science and technology to the fields of health care and research in medical, health, and bioinformatics.

UK Health Informatics Society: www.bmis.org
Advances the knowledge and application of medical and health informatics to deliver health care and promote health.

However, many clinicians who believe they are applying the principles and practices of health care informatics to their daily activities are actually operating under misconceptions about the field. Health care informatics is more than using a personal digital assistant (PDA) to look up a patient's most recent laboratory value. It's more than the ability to understand and interpret a statistical test used in a primary literature article. Health care informatics applies appropriate information in the patient care decision-making process. Although a PDA search and statistical analysis may be part of the process, these activities alone do not make up health care informatics.

Fear of Change

Psychological factors—especially fear of the unknown—may also prevent clinicians from adopting health care informatics. When faced with change, clinicians are no different from any other professionals in society—they meet it with resistance and anxiety. However, health care providers do not have the luxury of avoiding changes that will clearly have a positive impact on patients.

Complacency

Complacency, another barrier, comes into play when clinicians ignore a critical piece of information because they don't want it to disrupt their workflow or they believe that the information is not important. For example, clinical decision support systems (CDSSs) are designed to help practitioners make informed patient care decisions based on both patient-specific information and the latest research findings. Pharmacists and prescribers using computerized order entry receive drug use review (DUR) messages when their clinical information systems detect potential problems in a patient's medication therapy, such as drug interactions or allergies. Providers can choose sensitivity settings in the CDSS to indicate the level of DUR warnings they want to receive. When they elect to receive messages for only well-established, clinically significant medication-related problems, they may inadvertently miss a problem that is not well documented but is pertinent to the situation.

Providers who choose to see messages for virtually all potential medication-related problems can quickly become overwhelmed by the sheer volume. Because DUR systems generally require action on all DUR messages—even those not important for the patient in question—providers may eventually turn off the system or automatically override DUR messages without fully considering them. Neither approach is the best model for patient care, but these practices are occurring in health facilities across the country.

Another example of complacency involves nurses using unit-based medication dispensers. They may trust that the medication is correct without checking it, simply because the machine selected it. Instead of using technology as a supplement to extend their capabilities, some health care providers either rely on it too heavily or ignore it.

Technological Barriers to Health Care Informatics

Lack of Standards

One of the most significant technological barriers to health care informatics is a lack of standards across the health care system. There are two types: organizational standards accepted as approved formats by standards-setting organizations and de facto standards accepted because of their widespread use. In this book, the standards we talk about specify how health care computing devices connect and how they send information. We also use the term "standard" to indicate the preferred structure for health care information during transactions and for common health care documents (electronic or paper)—standards that are often set by standards-setting organizations as well as governmental and nongovernmental agencies. Significant standards-setting organizations are listed in Table 1-1.

The current challenge in health care is to define, implement, and bring about widespread adoption of health care–specific standards. Work has already begun in this field, most notable being the efforts of Health Level 7 (HL7), a standards-setting organization accredited by the American National Standards Institute (ANSI). ANSI is a private, nonprofit group that coordinates the voluntary standardization and conformity assessment system in the United States. HL7 (found at www.hl7.org), which operates solely in the health care arena, sets standards for exchanging clinical and administrative data within an entire health care organization, so that information can be shared with different departments.

Health Level 7 (www.hl7.org) is an organization that sets standards for exchanging clinical and administrative data within an entire health care organization, so that information can be shared beyond separate departments.

TABLE 1-1

Standards-Setting Organizations and Their Functions

Name	Acronym	Purpose
American National Standards Institute	ANSI	Administers voluntary programs to set standards for devices and procedures in the United States
International Telecommunication Union	ITU	Sets international communication protocols
Institute of Electrical and Electronics Engineers	IEEE	Sets standards for electrical interfaces
International Organization for Standardization	ISO	An umbrella organization composed of other standards-setting groups, such as ANSI; most important standard is OSI (Open Systems Interconnection), which defines networking architecture
Video Electronics Standards Association	VESA	Sets standards for video

Most other organizations working to develop health care standards focus only on individual domains, such as pharmacy or medical devices. Like other standards-setting organizations, HL7 does not develop software, but instead develops software specifications to allow the free flow of health care information for different applications. The standards presented in Table 1-2 have generally been adopted and implemented in health care organizations and information systems.

One exciting way that we are beginning to move health care information between applications, people, and places is through the use of wireless communication standards. Unfortunately, materials and designs that have been used in constructing hospitals are not "wireless-friendly." If physical obstacles are not carefully considered during the planning stages, a wireless installation can be extremely challenging, demanding, and costly. Improved wireless technology together with detailed planning and wireless-friendly construction in new facilities will help overcome this barrier.

TABLE 1-2

Common Standards Used in Health Care and Their Functions

Name	Acronym	Function
Accredited Standards Committee X12	ASC X12	An ANSI-accredited organization that develops standards for integrating e-business applications for exchanging electronic information.
National Guideline Clearinghouse	NGC	Extensive database of clinical practice treatment guidelines developed by the Agency for Healthcare Research and Quality (AHRQ) in partnership with the American Medical Association (AMA) and the American Association of Health Plans (AAHP). Goal is to provide users with accepted standards for treating patients.
Script		Standard developed by the National Council for Prescription Drug Programs (NCPDP) for the electronic transfer of prescriptions between prescribers and dispensing pharmacies.
Systematized Nomenclature of Medicine	SNOMED	A leader in standardizing clinical terminology used in the medical record.

Cost

An additional technology-related obstacle is cost. The U.S. health care industry has traditionally lagged behind other industries in terms of dollars spent on information technology. At the same time, spending on actual patient care continues to escalate. Industry experts and government officials suggest that information technology can play a key role in reducing the amount of money the United States spends on health care.[13,17,18] Some suggest that the federal government is the only source that can provide the necessary funding.[19]

Steps are being taken on the federal level. As of this writing, President Bush's budget for fiscal year 2005 proposes more than $150 million for health care information technology initiatives. Of this total, $50 million have been proposed to go toward the Department of Health and Human Services' grants for advancing health care information technology nationwide. The Agency for Healthcare Research and Quality is also slated to receive a portion of the funding.[20]

What remains to be seen is exactly how much of the proposed budget will make it through Congress.[21]

Will this be enough? With the budgetary limitations throughout the health care system, new technologies must be evaluated for the return on investment related to financial, humanistic, and therapeutic outcomes. Actions taken by the federal government and patient safety groups such as the Leapfrog Group (www.leapfroggroup.org), which is made up of 160 organizations that buy health care, will continue to draw attention to the importance of information technology in health care while simultaneously stirring up funds to implement new technologies.

Health Care Informatics Resources

The Internet's nonproprietary nature and widespread use make it an invaluable resource for locating information on any topic—including health care informatics. Employing that term, a cursory search of the Internet via the Google search engine returns over 22,000 hits in less than 0.12 seconds. A search for "medical informatics" returns 1,890,000 hits. The number of hits increases to 2.1 million if you change the search term to only "informatics."

Obviously, the Internet is a great supplemental resource to this book, but as with any Internet search, sites that truly focus on health care informatics are mixed in with those that only mention the topic. In subsequent chapters you will learn more about how to improve the accuracy and efficiency of your Internet searches.

As a starting point for excellent information on health care informatics, see Box 1-4 on page 13, which gives Web site addresses for some popular informatics-related organizations, and Box 1-5 on page 19, which lists Web sites for informatics publications, organizations, and resources. These Web sites often contain links to coming meetings, recent journal articles, and other publications containing health care informatics materials. You can also sign up on organizational Web sites to have e-mails sent directly to your inbox when new information becomes available. For readers interested in pursuing formalized education in health care informatics, Box 1-6 on page 20 contains the names and Web site addresses of programs in the United States.

BOX 1-5

General Health Care Informatics Sites

Agency for Healthcare Research and Quality (AHRQ) National Resource Center for Health Information Technology: http://healthit.ahrq.gov/home/index.html
Part of AHRQ's initiative to advance the use of information technology in health care, the center provides knowledge, funding, and technical assistance to help transform everyday clinical practice.

Healthcare Informatics Online: www.healthcare-informatics.com
A monthly business magazine providing high-quality intelligence about information technology for health care facilities and organizations.

Health Data Management: www.healthdatamanagement.com
Provides news and in-depth analysis on using information technology to achieve business goals and improve the quality of care.

Health Informatics World Wide: www.hiww.org
A regularly updated index of the most relevant links to Web sites on health, medical, and nursing informatics.

Health Information Management Journal: www.himaa.org.au/HIMJ/journal.html
Promotes the discipline of health information management through a forum of presentations, short communications, reviews, and commentaries.

Health Management Technology: www.healthmgttech.com
A magazine that is a leading source of technology information in health care, useful for senior executives and others.

The Informatics Review: www.informatics-review.com
Designed to help busy medical and information system professionals stay abreast of the latest academic developments in clinical informatics and computing.

International Journal of Medical Informatics: www.harcourt-international.com/journals/ijmi
An international medium for disseminating original results and interpretive reviews concerning the field of medical informatics.

Journal of the American Medical Informatics Association: www.jamia.org
Presents peer-reviewed articles that help health care professionals develop and apply medical informatics to patient care, teaching, research, and health care administration.

Online Journal of Nursing Informatics: www.eaa-knowledge.com/ojni
For health care professionals interested in the theoretical and practical aspects of nursing informatics as they relate to the art of nursing.

BOX 1-6

Informatics Education Programs in the United States

Auburn University Harrison School of Pharmacy, Department of Pharmacy Care Systems: http://pharmacy.auburn.edu/pcs/pcs.htm
Undergraduate and graduate education focusing on pharmacy informatics, including traditional coverage of computer concepts and software applications relevant to the practice of pharmacy.

Clinical Decision Making Group at the Massachusetts Institute of Technology Laboratory for Computer Science: http://medg.lcs.mit.edu
A research group dedicated to exploring and furthering the application of technology and artificial intelligence to clinical situations.

College of St. Scholastica Department of Health Care Informatics and Information Management: http://grad.css.edu/him
Focuses on ensuring the integrity of information resources within the computer-based world of health care and assuring the confidentiality of that information.

Columbia University Department of Biomedical Informatics: www.dbmi.columbia.edu
Explores the scientific field that deals with the storage, retrieval, sharing, and optimal use of biomedical information, data, and knowledge for problem solving and decision making.

Harvard Medical School and Brigham and Women's Hospital, Decision Systems Group: http://dsg.harvard.edu
Creates software environments that facilitate problem-based, integrative access to information to aid decision making for health care professionals and the public.

Johns Hopkins Division of Health Sciences Informatics: http://dhsi.med.jhmi.edu
Seeks to advance the development and use of information technology for decision making, research, and health care delivery in the health sciences community.

Mount Sinai School of Medicine Center for Medical Informatics: www.mssm.edu/medicine/medical-informatics
Focuses on improving patient care, supporting research, and expanding the boundaries of education through the scientific application of information management.

Oregon Health and Science University Department of Medical Informatics and Clinical Epidemiology: www.ohsu.edu/dmice
Provides an academic environment for teaching, research, and service in the areas of medical informatics and clinical epidemiology.

continued on page 21

BOX 1-6 *continued*

Shenandoah University Bernard J. Dunn School of Pharmacy, Center for Pharmacy Informatics: http://pharmacy.su.edu
Focuses on education, research, and service related to the use of information technology in pharmacy.

Stanford University Department of Medicine, Medical Informatics:
www.smi.stanford.edu
Home to scientists and trainees who develop and evaluate new methodologies for acquiring, representing, processing, and managing data related to health care.

University of Alabama at Birmingham School of Health Related Professions, Health Informatics Program: http://main.uab.edu/show.asp?durki=33489
Prepares senior- and executive-level managers through the planning, management, design, integration, implementation, and evaluation of enterprise-wide health care information systems.

University of California, Davis, Medical Informatics: http://informatics.ucdavis.edu
Provides training and research opportunities for individuals to assess, develop, and implement new technologies that will provide decision support to health care professionals.

University of California, San Francisco, Graduate Program in Biological and Medical Informatics: www.bmi.ucsf.edu
Promotes study, use, and development of informatics technologies for conducting biological and clinical research and for promoting more effective patient care.

University of Illinois at Chicago College of Applied Health Sciences, Department of Biomedical and Health Information Sciences:
www.ahs.uic.edu/ahs/php/?sitename=bhis
Focuses on the study, practice, and facilitation of health information technology, education, research, and bioscience.

University of Maryland School of Nursing, Informatics Graduate Program:
http://nursing.umaryland.edu/users/eahpi/web/index.htm
Prepares graduates to analyze, design, manage, identify, and implement management information systems in patient care.

University of Missouri School of Medicine, Department of Health Management and Informatics: www.hmi.missouri.edu
Trains professionals to develop, apply, and evaluate the use of information technology in the health care arena.

continued on page 22

BOX 1-6 *continued*

University of Minnesota Medical School Health Informatics Division:
www.hinf.umn.edu
Trains students to apply computer and information sciences to the quantitative aspects and decision needs of the health and life sciences.

University of Pittsburgh Center for Biomedical Informatics: www.cbmi.pitt.edu
Promotes research addressing the use of informatics in health care and health education and its direct application to ongoing care and education programs.

University of Texas School of Health Information Sciences: www.shis.uth.tmc.edu
Provides educational and research opportunities in informatics to health care professionals, biomedical scientists, and computer scientists committed to collaboration.

University of Utah Department of Medical Informatics: www.med.utah.edu/medinfo
Internationally recognized for its contributions to biomedical informatics research and training in medical informatics

University of Washington Department of Medical Education and Biomedical Informatics: www.bhi.washington.edu
Prepares students for careers in research, teaching, health care information technology, and the health care computing industry.

Vanderbilt Medical Center Department of Biomedical Informatics:
www.mc.vanderbilt.edu/dbmi
Focuses on education and research that addresses the storage, retrieval, dissemination, and application of biomedical information.

Yale University School of Medicine Center for Medical Informatics:
http://ycmi.med.yale.edu
Focuses on creative use of computers in clinical medicine, molecular biology, neuroscience, and other areas of biomedical research.

ACTIVITY 1-2

Becoming Familiar with Health Care Informatics

1. Based on what you've read in Chapter 1, revise your definition of health care informatics, if necessary.

2. Locate the earliest mention of health care informatics in your specific discipline or specialty. You may not find the very first complete reference to the field, but spend some time searching to discover how long ago the first mention occurred. Look ahead to Chapter 9 for search tips.

3. Identify 10 health care informatics publications and professional organizations beyond those identified in Boxes 1-4 and 1-5.

4. Use the information in Box 1-6 to compare several degree or residency programs in terms of training, research, outreach, and clinical practice opportunities.

5. Locate and read a recent health care informatics article published in your discipline or specialty.

6. List three learning objectives you have for expanding your knowledge of heath care informatics and applying your knowledge in your health care setting.

References

1. HIPAA Basics. HIPAA glossaries on the Web 2001. Available at: www.hipaabasics.com/glossary.htm. Accessed January 18, 2004.

2. Office of Management and Budget. Management of federal information resources 2000. Available at: www.whitehouse.gov/omb/circulars/a130/a130trans4.html#6. Accessed January 18, 2004.

3. Bates DW, Leape LL, Cullen DJ, et al. Effect of computerized physician order entry and a team intervention on prevention of serious medication errors. *JAMA*. 1998;280:1311-6.

4. Bates DW, Teich JM, Lee J, et al. The impact of computerized physician order entry on medication error prevention. *JAMA*. 1999;6:313-21.

5. Sackett DL, Rosenberg WM, Gray JAM, et al. Evidence based medicine: What it is and what it isn't. *BMJ*. 1996;312(7023):71-2.

6. Chueh H, Banett GO. "Just in time" clinical information. *Acad Med*. 1997;72:512-7.

7. Hersh, WR. Medical informatics: Improving health care through information. *JAMA*. 2002;288(16):1955-8.

8. Vanderbilt University Department of Biomedical Informatics. What is biomedical informatics? Available at: www.mc.vanderbilt.edu/dbmi/informatics.html. Accessed January 18, 2004.

9. Blois MS, Shortliffe EH. The computer meets medicine: Emergence of a discipline. In: Shortliffe EH, Perreault LE, Wiederhold G, et al., eds. *Medical Informatics: Computer Applications in Health Care*. Reading, MA: Addison-Wesley; 1990:20-6.

10. American Medical Informatics Association. About AMIA. Available at: www.amia.org/about/fabout.html. Accessed January 18, 2004.

11. American Medical Informatics Association. What is medical informatics? Available at: www.amia.org/about/faqs/f7.html. Accessed January 27, 2004.

12. Kukafka R, O'Carrollet PW, Gerberding JL, et al. Issues and opportunities in public health informatics: A panel discussion. *J Public Health Manag Pract.* 2001;7(6):31-42.

13. Reid B. Healthcare spending growth near double digits. [Health-IT World]. January 13, 2004. Available at: www.imakenews.com/health-itworld/e_article000216773.cfm. Accessed February 1, 2004.

14. Leape LL, Bates DW, Cullen DJ, et al. Systems analysis of adverse drug events. *JAMA.* 1995;274(1):35-43.

15. U.S. Department of Energy Office of Science. On the shoulders of giants: Private sector leverages HGP successes. Available at: www.ornl.gov/sci/techresources/Human_Genome/project/privatesector.shtml. Accessed February 1, 2004.

16. Coiera E. Medical informatics meets medical education: There's more to understanding information and technology. Available at: www.mja.com.au/public/issues/apr6/coiera/coierbox.html. Accessed February 1, 2004.

17. Reid B. Healthcare needs its own "Industrial Revolution." [Health-IT World]. January 27, 2004. Available at: www.imakenews.com/health-itworld/e_article000221241.cfm?x=a2wNfjF,a1blVMVB. Accessed February 3, 2004.

18. Berman J. Survey indicates IT key in controlling rising price of healthcare. [Health-IT World]. February 18, 2004. Available at: http://app2.topiksolutions.com/readmore.ts?c=7650&a=296&m=2284&p=907702&t=164. Accessed March 16, 2004.

19. Reid B. Report: Only the Feds can save US healthcare. [Health-IT World]. May 29, 2003. Available at: www.imakenews.com/health-itworld/e_article000154421.cfm. Accessed March 8, 2004.

20. Reid B. Bush budget contains $50 million for HHS Health-IT efforts. [Health-IT World]. February 25, 2004. Available at: http://app2.topiksolutions.com/readmore.ts?c=7649&a=296&m=2284&p=907702&t=164. Accessed March 8, 2004.

21. Reid B. Details lacking on federal aid proposals for health-IT. [Health-IT World]. January 27, 2004. Available at: www.imakenews.com/health-itworld/e_article000221243.cfm?x=a2wNfjF,a1blVMVB. Accessed February 29, 2004.

CHAPTER

Computer and Network Basics

Brent I. Fox

Chapter Objectives

After completing this chapter, you should be able to:

■ Identify the basic components of computer hardware.

■ Determine the speed of your CPU, the amount of RAM on your computer, and the capacity of your hard drive.

■ Assess when to upgrade your computer.

■ Explain the basic difference between operating systems and application software.

■ Be familiar with fundamental skills for managing your computer.

■ Understand the basics of computer networks and their value in health care.

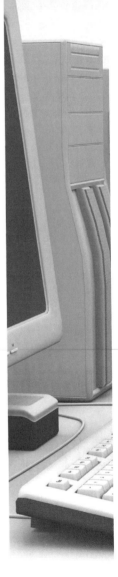

Health care professionals are increasingly reliant on computer systems to store, manipulate, and retrieve information. Understanding computer operations helps us better serve patients— and we can communicate better with support technicians when we encounter a glitch.

The mid-1990s was an important point in the history of the personal computer. The Windows 95 operating system was introduced and major barriers to Internet access were removed. No longer was computer use based on knowledge of computing commands. Windows 95 was also a significant advancement over the 3.x series of the Windows operating system. The graphical user interface (GUI) was introduced during this time frame—presenting information in a user-friendly way with pictures and icons—opening up the Internet to anyone who had a computer.

These two events have had a profound impact on health care. Information management has been streamlined with the connectivity offered by networks, including the Internet. The Windows-based computer has been adopted as a means to give health care professionals tools to vastly increase efficiency and effectiveness.

As health care professionals, our top responsibility is patient care, not computer maintenance, right? We are not expected to design, build, or troubleshoot computer systems. We are, however, increasingly reliant on these systems to store, manipulate, and retrieve information. Just today, as I write this, the newspaper ran a story about a nutrition service in which people can e-mail photos of their daily meals to dietitians for advice. Another article reported on pediatricians using e-mail for patient consultations. These examples give a sense of why you need basic computer knowledge: to help you better serve patients and increase the quality of care.

ACTIVITY 2-1

Assess Your Skills Electronically

Many people aren't sure how complete or sophisticated their knowledge is about computers and informatics. Even if you use computers daily, you may not know where your weaknesses are or what additional information would benefit you.

To assess your current skills, go to www.pharmacy.auburn.edu/informatics_survey/ selfassessment_form/submission_form.asp for a 20-minute online assessment tool that will score your knowledge and give you feedback about areas for improvement.

Understanding computer system operations also decreases our time on the phone receiving technical help. It may seem trivial, but the truth is that being able to speak the language of computer technicians allows you to describe problems precisely, better understand responses, and carry out instructions more efficiently. If to you everything on a computer is a "doohickey," you're set up for frustration whenever you have even a minor technical glitch.

As federal legislation, patient demands, and other pressures push health care down the road to a digital world, it's hard to deny the importance of understanding computer systems. This chapter provides basic knowledge about the personal computer, computer networks, and computer operations. Activity 2-1 on page 26 helps you assess your computer skills.

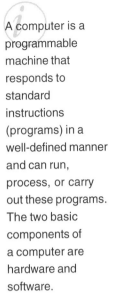

A computer is a programmable machine that responds to standard instructions (programs) in a well-defined manner and can run, process, or carry out these programs. The two basic components of a computer are hardware and software.

Components of Computing Systems

Although you probably know what we are referring to when we use the term "computer" throughout this book, we'd like to present a formal definition. A computer is a programmable machine with two basic characteristics:

1. It responds to a system of standard instructions (program) in a well-defined manner.
2. It can run, process, or carry out these programs.[1]

Computers have two basic components: hardware and software. The physical, mechanical, and tangible items are the hardware components. Software consists of the data and instructions that control the computer. Figure 2-1 provides a diagram of a basic computer system. Computer hardware components can be divided into five general classes:

1. Input devices
2. Output devices
3. Memory
4. Permanent storage devices
5. Central processing units (CPUs)

FIGURE 2-1

A general depiction of computer system components.

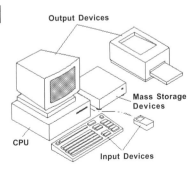

Output Devices

Mass Storage Devices

CPU

Input Devices

Computer Hardware

As a health care professional, you're probably no computer technician—but you do rely on computers every day and need a basic familiarity. You may even be consulted for the next purchase decision when an existing system is being upgraded. Or you may perform the upgrade yourself and must have enough knowledge to ensure that you get what you need. Sometimes you may have to troubleshoot when problems arise. Here are some hardware aspects you may find yourself dealing with.

Input Devices

You use computer system input components to enter information and data into the computer. The most recognizable input devices are the mouse and keyboard. Today's keyboard is known as the QWERTY keyboard, signifying the first six letters read left to right on the top row of keys. There are numerous iterations of this standard keyboard, some with quick-launch keys to open commonly used applications with a single touch, some with keys angled to more closely align with the natural contour of the wrists, and some with wireless connectivity to the computer.

The QWERTY arrangement was developed in the 1870s by Christopher Sholes to actually slow down typists. Early typewriters would jam because typists could type faster than the original typewriters' hammers could move.[2]

Mice (pointing devices) come in many forms as well. The standard mouse usually has two buttons on the top. The left mouse button is for most user activities, and the right button performs more advanced functions, like opening program menus. As mice have advanced over the years, buttons and features have been added. Some of the most advanced mice have up to five buttons, including a wheel for scrolling, and can wirelessly connect to your computer. Regardless of the keyboard and mouse you use, they serve as the primary means of data input. Other inputs include microphones, data gloves, joysticks, light pens, and styli.

Computer system outputs, such as monitors and printers, allow you to see the results of your interaction with the computer.

Output Devices

Computer system outputs allow you to see the results of your interaction with the computer. Monitors are the most obvious example of computer outputs. Printers provide the user with a hardcopy output. There are literally thousands of printers and monitor options to choose from. Decision points for selecting a monitor include the size, intended primary use of the computer, and price. Printers are often selected based on the type of printing to be done, quality of print output desired, space availability, and price. Other examples of outputs include speakers and fax machines.

Memory

A computer's memory is one of the most important components of the computer system because it allows the computer to store and manipulate data and programs during a user's interaction. Memory consists of the physical chips on which data and programs are temporarily stored. Although there are many types of memory, you will most often encounter "RAM," which stands for random access memory. RAM is where programs and data are stored while you interact with the computer. Because RAM is a temporary memory, if the computer is unexpectedly turned off, anything that was in RAM is lost. As you increase the amount of RAM in your computer your programs operate more quickly and you can run more programs at once without seeing any appreciable change in speed.

RAM is commonly measured in megabytes (MB). Personal computers from the early 1990s usually had 8-16 MB of RAM. By 2003, personal computers were commonly shipping with 256-512 MB of RAM. Table 2-1 depicts the relationships between the various sizes of computer memory.

ROM (read-only memory) is the other common type of memory. Unlike RAM, ROM is permanent in nature and cannot usually be modified by the user. ROM normally stores the instructions used for booting up or starting a computer.

RAM, or random access memory, is temporary memory that stores programs and data while you interact with the computer. As you increase RAM, commonly measured in megabytes (MB), programs operate more quickly and you can run more at once. If the computer is unexpectedly turned off without saving your work, anything that was in RAM is lost. ROM, or read-only memory, is permanent and normally stores the instructions used for booting up a computer.

TABLE 2-1

Computer System Memory Relationships

Term	Abbreviation	Definition
Bit		The smallest unit of information on a computer; holds the value of 0 or 1 only
Byte		8 bits; holds the value of a single character
Kilobyte	KB	1024 bytes
Megabyte	MB	1,048,576 bytes
Gigabyte	GB	1,073,741,824 bytes
Terabyte	TB	1,099,511,627,776 bytes

Source: Reference 3.

The capacity of hard drives and tape drives, popular permanent storage devices, is measured in gigabytes (GB).

Permanent Storage Devices

As indicated by their name, these devices permanently store data and software on a computer. Permanent storage devices retain their stored data even when the computer is turned on and off. In the modern personal computer, hard drives and tape drives are popular permanent storage devices. Other types include floppy disks and optical disks such as CD-ROMs and DVD-ROMs.

Permanent storage devices come in many sizes, with capacity usually measured in gigabytes (GB). Currently, laptop computers' hard drives are typically in the 20-60 GB range, while desktop computers generally come with hard drives in the 40-120 GB range. CD-ROMs can hold about 700 MB of data, and current DVD-ROMs hold about 5 GB of data. Notably, recent advancements promise to push DVD capacity in excess of 25 GB. Obviously, your intended use of the computer will dictate what size hard drive (or optical drive) best fits your needs.

As already noted, the amount of RAM a computer has plays a key role in the overall speed of the computer. But the capabilities of a computer's hard drive also can dictate the computer's speed. Data rate and seek time are often used to measure hard drive performance. Data rate is the speed at which the hard drive can return data to the central processing unit (CPU), the computer's main processing chip. Current industry standards for data rates are 5 to 40 MB/second. Seek time indicates how long the CPU has to wait for data to be returned when requested from the hard drive. Current industry standards for seek times range from 10 to 20 milliseconds.[4]

Another closely related measure of a hard drive's speed is the spinning speed of the storage media. Analogous to your automobile's engine, a computer hard drive's spinning speed is measured in revolutions per minute (RPM). This spin rate often affects the computer's overall data access speed, with 7200 RPM generally being the fastest spinning speed for personal computer hard drives.

Central Processing Units

The final piece of the computer system puzzle is the "brains" of the computer—the CPU. Also known as the processor, microprocessor, chip, or central processor, the CPU executes all instructions and has a significant influence on the computer's overall speed.

The first CPU was produced in 1971 by the Intel Corporation. Since then, the processing power of these chips has grown exponentially. As shown in Figure 2-2, Moore's Law (named for Gordon Moore, one of the founders of Intel) states that, generally, CPU processing power doubles every couple of years. Without getting too technical, this increase is due to a rise in the number of transistors on the processor. As the number of transistors increases, the CPU speed (or clock speed) also increases. Central processing unit clock speeds are measured in megahertz (MHz) and gigahertz (GHz), with higher numbers indicating faster speeds.

The brains of the computer, the CPU, executes all instructions and has a significant influence on the computer's overall speed.

Many companies manufacture CPUs, including AMD, but because of Intel's dominance in the current marketplace, we will use them for the following example. Intel's Pentium line of processors began with the original Pentium in 1993 and led to the current chip family of processors, the Pentium 4. Each iteration of the chip, beginning with the Pentium and continuing through to the Pentium 4, signifies a significant increase in processing power—usually 1.5 to 2 times greater than the previous chip.

FIGURE 2-2

Moore's Law of processing power.

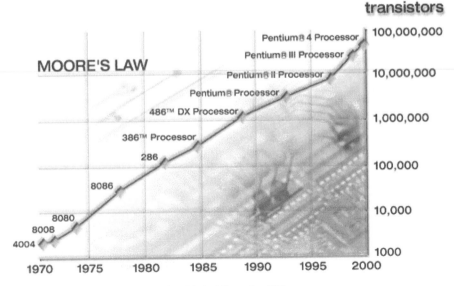

Understanding the functions of a computer system allows you to evaluate and select information technologies that apply directly to your patient care activities.

Pulling It All Together

As CPU technology advances, chip size and power requirements decrease while processing power and speed increase. Accordingly, new input and output devices are being developed that will increase both temporary and permanent storage capabilities. We use the phrase "weighs less, does more" to describe the general trend in computing technology. This means that when existing devices are improved and completely new ones introduced, they are lighter but accomplish more than previous devices.

You, as a health care professional, undoubtedly rely on technology already to perform some of your most important activities, such as documenting patient care, videoconferencing with colleagues, or accessing the most recent medication information through your handheld computer. Health care's reliance on technology will only increase as governmental and nongovernmental agencies require the health care industry to use information technology to increase patient safety and minimize costs.[5]

Activity 2-2 helps you identify your computer's basic components. Understanding the functions of a computer system allows you to evaluate and select information technologies that apply directly to your patient care activities.

ACTIVITY 2-2

Reviewing Basic Computer Hardware

1. Identify the five basic hardware components of the computer you use most frequently.
2. Determine the following on the computer you use most frequently:
   a. RAM.
   b. CPU speed.
   c. Hard drive capacity and available space.
3. Based on the answers to number 2 above, determine which components you should consider for immediate upgrade.
4. Visit an online computer vendor, such as Hewlett-Packard, IBM, Gateway, or Dell, and construct a customized desktop and notebook computer.

Computer input and output devices are easy to identify. You can also easily see permanent storage drives, such as CD-ROMs, DVD-ROMs, and floppy disks. Other permanent drives, such as the hard drive, cannot be identified without taking the computer apart. Unless you are familiar with the process, this is probably something you don't want to do. At this point, it's sufficient for you to know that the CPU, memory, and some permanent storage drives are located within the computer's case. The case can take many shapes, from the base of a laptop computer to the back of a flat screen liquid crystal display (LCD).

If you want to upgrade your computer, check Web sites of major computer vendors and select components based on your specific needs.

There are many ways to determine the answers for items under number 2 in Activity 2-2, the basic properties of a computer system. One of the easiest is to use the computer's operating system. To determine your RAM and CPU speed, go to the Control Panel. (In Windows XP Category View, to find the Control Panel, click the Start button, click Control Panel, then click Performance and Maintenance. In Windows XP Classic View, to find the Control Panel, click the Start button, click Settings, and then select Control Panel.) Then click on the System button to display the computer's properties. You can find your computer's hard drive capacity by clicking the Start button and going to the My Computer menu, where you click on Local Disk.

Should you determine that your computer needs upgrading (see Box 2-1) you can visit Web sites of major computer vendors such as Hewlett-Packard, IBM, Gateway, or Dell, which allow you to construct a customized computer and select the CPU, RAM, hard drive, and other components of your new machine. They will often sort the base machines according to intended use—office, home, gaming, etc. You can then configure the system according to your needs. For example, if you know that you will be configuring for business purposes, you may opt for the largest hard drive available. Or, if you anticipate simultaneously running application programs that require significant memory resources, such as videoconferencing, you might select a larger RAM configuration. And you gain several benefits from this approach—you can configure a computer to your needs and have it assembled and tested and shipped to you ready to go (complete with a manufacturer's warranty).

When Should You Upgrade?

Because technology changes so fast, people are often tempted to upgrade their computer systems. When you find yourself wondering about upgrading, ask yourself what you plan to do with the computer and if it currently meets your needs. If your hard drive capacity is close to three-quarters full, then you may need an upgrade. If you frequently wait more than 1 to 2 seconds for programs to open, carry out an action, or close, then you may need to invest in more RAM.

If your CPU is more than two generations old (which means that your hard drive is probably also close to capacity), then an upgrade may be in order as well, depending on your individual demand and budgetary considerations. When deciding whether to upgrade a CPU, it may be wiser to invest in a completely new computer. You will benefit from advancements in hard drives, RAM, and all the other components of a computer system, such as motherboards, peripheral device connections, and video/audio capabilities.

Application Software and Operating Systems

Application software can be thought of as the software programs we use to solve a specific problem or carry out a specific activity. The operating system (OS) application is the functional software that "controls" a computer system.

Operating systems are part of a larger class of software known as systems software. Operating systems control the activity of the computer hardware and various other software applications. They also provide you with a means for interacting with the computer system, commonly known as the user interface.

Microsoft Windows is the dominant operating system in the

BOX 2-2

Abbreviated Listing of Operating Systems

Linux	Microsoft Tablet PC	OS/2 400	Unix
Mac OS	Microsoft Windows	OS 400	VMS
Mac OS X	MS-DOS	Palm	Xenix
Microsoft Pocket PC	Novel NetWare	Solaris	

United States. As shown in Box 2-2, however, many other operating systems exist. Throughout this book, we will use the Microsoft Windows family of operating systems in examples; many of the functions described are similar across operating systems.

As the "controller" of all activities, the operating system is the most important program running on a computer system. Box 2-3 details the functions performed by an operating system. Figure 2-3 depicts the general relationship between the operating system and the other components of a computer system.

BOX 2-3

What Operating Systems Do: A Sampling

- Recognize and translate input, such as keyboard commands, mouse movements, and stylus touches to a touch screen.
- Manage and control output, such as the monitor images, sound, and printed pages.
- Serve as the user interface—the link between you and the computer's workings.
- Manage files.
- Manage system resources, such as disk space and power.
- Manage system memory.
- Manage external devices, such as printers and mice.
- Control user access via usernames and passwords.
- Control hardware interactions with the other computer components.
- Serve as a platform for application software.

Source: Reference 5.

FIGURE 2-3

Relationships between an operating system and the other components of a computer system.

Copyright 2003 Jupitermedia Corporation.
All Rights Reserved.
Reprinted with permission.
www.webopedia.com/TERM/
o/operating_system.html

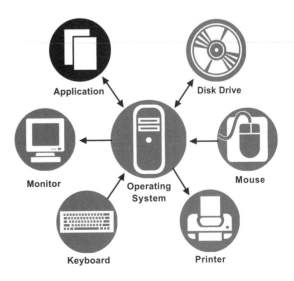

Application

Disk Drive

Monitor

Operating System

Mouse

Keyboard

Printer

Any specific task you complete at a computer is carried out with application software, which falls into three general classes: personal software (e.g., word processors, Web browsers, e-mail, spreadsheets, database programs), enterprise software (e.g., order entry, billing), and workgroup software (e.g., videoconferencing).

There are literally tens of thousands of application software packages available. They fall into a broad range of categories, but all function "on top of" the operating system and perform a specific user function. Application software cannot do its job without an operating system. Any specific task you complete at a computer is carried out using application software.

Application software can be divided into three classes based on the users served. Personal software is designed for use by a single person to support individual needs. Examples include word processors, Web browsers, e-mail, spreadsheets, and database programs. Enterprise software is intended for a larger user base and serves individuals across a complete enterprise. Examples include order entry and billing applications. The final category, workgroup software, meets the needs of groups of people working together on a specific task. Videoconferencing software is a good example.[6]

Computerized prescriber order entry (CPOE), becoming more prevalent in health care, is both hardware and software technology. On the software side, CPOE consists of applications that capture medical orders, format the orders, and transmit them to the appropriate provider. In fitting with the definition above of application software, CPOE was designed to solve a specific problem. It is intended to prevent medical errors, increase efficiency, and decrease costs.

Other examples of application software in health care include physician charge capture software, nursing software for documenting patient progress notes, laboratory software for analyzing and reporting results, and pharmacy software for medication management. The important point to remember about application software is that applications exist for virtually every need you have as a health care provider.

Using Computer Parts and Features

You probably hear computer terminology all the time, but may wonder what the words relate to. Even if you know what the terms mean, do you know how best to manage basic functions on your computer? These topics are discussed below. For a checklist of basic skills for managing your computer, see Box 2-4.

BOX 2-4

Checklist of Basic Skills for Managing Your Computer

Health care professionals should be able to do the following on their computers:

Desktop Skills
1. Arrange and group software icons on the desktop.
2. Create shortcuts to frequently used software on the desktop and taskbar (the bar across the bottom of the screen in a Windows-based computer. It contains the Start button).
3. Change the desktop background.
4. Change the location and properties of the taskbar.
5. Modify the properties of the Start Menu to fit your computer usage by adding and removing icons.
6. Modify user accounts, controlling who has access to the computer system.

File Management Skills
1. Open the file management application on your computer.
2. Collapse and expand various files.
3. Change the viewing properties for the file management application.
4. Sort files within a folder by specific file attributes, such as date.
5. Create new file locations (folders) in predetermined locations.
6. Copy/cut a file from one folder and paste it in another folder.
7. Delete a file and/or folder.
8. Restore deleted items.

System Administration Skills
1. Add and remove programs from the computer system.
2. Create new user accounts for the computer system.
3. Delete existing user accounts from the computer system.
4. Modify the properties and permissions for an individual user.
5. Add and remove a printer from the computer system.
6. Use the operating system or application software to create a backup copy of the files on your computer system.
7. Use the operating system's disk defragmenter to clean up the hard drive and increase the speed of the computer.

A simple way to find information faster is to organize the program icons on your computer desktop by single-clicking each one and dragging it to the desired location.

Keyboard and Mouse

Computer users usually have a specific way that they interact with the system—the primary means being the mouse and keyboard. When we move our mouse or type on our keyboard, the operating system translates these inputs into our desired actions. For example, if we are searching for the most recent entry in a particular patient's electronic medical record, we would probably use our mouse to open the patient profile software application and then search for the patient in question by using the keyboard to enter his or her last name or identification number. Our actions of clicking the mouse and typing on the keyboard are interpreted by the operating system to produce the actions we desire.

Icons

The operating system also provides the graphical user interface for our patient profile software applications. The term "graphical" describes icons that send commands to the computer system.[1]

As computer system use increases among health care clinicians, efficiency and speed in navigation are critical to locating desired information. One simple way to find information faster is to organize the program icons on your computer desktop. Generally, you can do this by single-clicking on an icon and dragging it to the desired location. If you are using multiple applications, you can reposition these icons and locate them together in a specific region of your desktop. Another tip is to hold down the Control key on your keyboard while single-clicking on desired icons. This allows you to select multiple icons at the same time for repositioning.

Although this simple process can help you quickly locate applications and the information they contain, it assumes that the desired icons are already on your computer's desktop. When adding new software to your computer system, you often need to place application icons on your desktop for speedy access.

Whether applications are previously existing or newly added, the process for adding icons to your desktop is the same. It's impossible to spell out all the ways to add icons, given the many operating systems and versions existing today—not to mention those to be released in the future. Generally, you need to locate the specific application in the computer's listing of all applications, most often found by clicking the Start button and selecting All Programs. Right-clicking on the application name gives you the option to create a shortcut on the desktop. When you do this, an icon for that application appears on your desktop.

Desktop Backgrounds

As you add more icons to your desktop, it gets cluttered. The picture or color scheme on the desktop, known as the background, can be distracting, too. The desktop background is often arbitrarily set when the operating system is installed on the computer. Some health systems have professionally designed logos that serve as the desktop background for computers throughout the organization. If you don't like your background display you can customize it, even when there are multiple user accounts on one computer, because many operating systems, such as Windows XP, allow users to personalize the desktop according to their preferences. These changes appear only for the user who has elected to make these changes.

To change a desktop background, locate the operating system function that allows you to modify the overall appearance of the computer system. In Windows XP, right-click on the desktop and select Properties. Then, select the Desktop tab. Then select the option that enables you to modify the desktop background and change the color or image to suit you.

Taskbar

"Taskbar" is a general term used to describe the starting point of user interaction with a computer system. It contains links to application software, the controls for system maintenance, shortcuts to locations and software within the computer system, the Help feature, and other system functions. Figure 2-4 shows the taskbar on my own computer as I write this chapter.

FIGURE 2-4

A Windows XP Professional taskbar with a Google Deskbar search window.

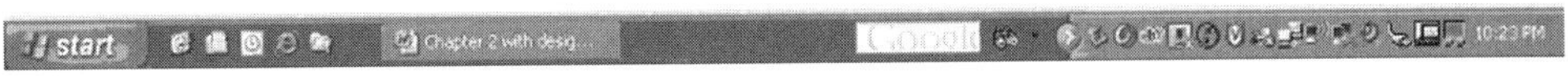

When a single computer is used by many people, multiple user accounts allow each user to customize the desktop, taskbar, and other features for individual preferences and purposes.

The taskbar usually extends left to right across the entire bottom length of the computer display. You can modify the taskbar's properties to fit your needs. For example, some clinicians' eyes naturally focus on the top of the display when they first sit down to a computer. Accordingly, the taskbar can be repositioned to any of the four sides of the computer display by clicking on it and dragging it to the desired side. Depending on the operating system version in use, you may have to first right-click on the taskbar and unlock it.

Other features you can customize include adding quick links (shortcuts) to frequently used applications, making the taskbar appear even when applications are open, or displaying the system clock. You can explore all these features by right-clicking on the taskbar and selecting the feature that allows the taskbar's properties to be modified.

Start Menu

The Start Menu is an operating system feature closely related to the taskbar. The term "Start Menu" is specific for Microsoft Windows, but the general feature is found in most operating systems that use Windows for navigation. This menu is displayed by selecting the primary launching button on the taskbar, which in Windows is the Start button.

Just as shortcuts can be added to the desktop and quick links can be added to the taskbar, clinicians who require quick access to important applications can use the Start Menu to open these applications. Keep in mind, however, that the Start Menu listing of programs is continuously changing as you open new applications. You can specify the number of applications to be displayed, but once this number is reached, recently opened applications will replace less frequently used applications in the list.

The Start Menu also contains links to health care communication technologies we will discuss in subsequent chapters, specifically the Internet and e-mail. You can create quick access points to your favorite Internet browser and e-mail program in the Start Menu.

Multiple User Accounts

In health care environments where a single computer is used by many people, customizing the features can be a big advantage. Just as people have preferences for a favorite Web site, clinicians also prefer to customize computers to suit their needs—which is easily done thanks to today's operating systems, which allow multiple user accounts to be created on a single computer system. Each account can have a customized desktop, taskbar, Start Menu, and other features.

There are many ways to change user accounts. Typically the user must log off first; the two most common methods for this are to simultaneously press the Control, Alt, and Delete keys, which brings up a security window where you can log off, or you can select Start and Log off to perform the same function. After that, any user has the opportunity to log on.

Locating, Viewing, and Managing Information

As you use patient profile software, your operating system is continually running in the background performing its activities. Ethical and legal responsibilities dictate that patients' information be stored in a secure and confidential manner. The operating system plays a key role in this by providing user authentication and verification steps.

Once a user is verified and granted access to the computer system, the operating system is the gateway to all other applications on the system. The operating system's presence may not be apparent, but any application, including patient profile software, is essentially sitting "on top" of the operating system. The operating system is like the frame of an automobile—the foundation on which all other components rest.

The operating system, the gateway to all other applications on the system, is kind of like the frame of an automobile—the foundation on which all other components rest.

When you find patient information you've been seeking and want to send it to other locations, the operating system plays a key role. If you send the information to a storage medium, such as writable CD-ROMs, the operating system manages the process. Likewise, if you print out a patient's most recent complete blood count, the operating system controls the printing process. You may also need to send the information electronically to remote locations—not uncommon as health information becomes more portable. Once again, the operating system plays a key role in managing these transmissions.

The operating system is also instrumental in managing information storage on the computer system as a whole. As clinicians provide care to more patients, the number of patient profiles and bits of associated information increase considerably. Each patient's profile can contain literally thousands of pieces of information. This information is usually arranged in a "filing system" on the computer's hard drive, the main permanent memory storage location. The operating system uses a file management system to oversee the information storage process.

Navigating Through Stored Files

The file management application is a component of the operating system, but it exists as another program on the computer and can be thought of as a tree format, with secondary files extending from core files flowing top to bottom.

File management has as many names as there are operating systems. The Microsoft name for this application is Windows Explorer. In general, there are many ways to access the file management application, but one of the simplest is to select it from the list of programs on the computer. In Windows XP Professional, click the Start button, All Programs, Accessories, and then Windows Explorer.

The file management application is a component of the operating system, but it exists as another program residing on the computer. This is a definite advantage of the current generation of Windows-based operating systems. Previous operating systems required you to type in commands to display a list of files on your computer, but today's have a much more intuitive interface for locating, moving, and deleting files.

The general structure for the file management application can be thought of as a tree format with secondary files extending from core files. The file management structure is actually closely related to a document outline.

The structure gives you several ways to navigate through files such as spreadsheets, presentations, and word-processing documents that are arranged within folders. A simple click on a folder name displays the contents of that folder, including any folders within the folder. Or a folder containing other folders will have an indicator to its left. You can then click on this "expand" indicator (often a + symbol) to display all folders within it. The indicator will change to show that clicking on it again will collapse the subordinate folders into the superior folder. This "collapse" indicator is often a minus (-) symbol.

The benefit of developing navigation skills for file management is obvious: it allows you to find any file or document on the computer. What about when repeated use of a particular software program leaves you with many files of similar names stored in the same folder? For example, when using a patient profile application, new files may be generated for that person each time he or she returns for an office visit. The default view for files within most file management applications displays only a listing of all the file names within the folder. Thus it's helpful to view and sort files using unique characteristics, such as the date the file was modified, created, or last accessed, or perhaps the file size and type. Use the View pulldown menu to see dates and other fields. The detailed view lets you see a large amount of information about files stored in a folder so you can quickly sort through and find the file you need.

You can also sort by clicking on each viewing field. For example, clicking on the Date Modified field will sort the files based on their most recent modification date. The Name field can be used to sort files alphabetically by name.

Creating Folders

As discussed above, application software creates its own folders and filing conventions as defined by the software developers. It's best not to move these folders or change their properties because they store important information the software needs.

File management software, however, allows you to create new folders in any desired location for storing information. Creating new folders is easy. The simplest way is to right-click with the mouse in the location where you want to add the new folder, then select the option to create a new folder.

Moving and Copying Files and Folders

Moving a file, multiple files, or complete folders from one folder to another is very useful. A file can be "copied" and placed in another folder, or it can be "cut" from one folder and moved to another folder. The copy process makes an identical copy of the original file for placement in another location—so it now exists in two places—while the cut feature removes the item from the original location for placement in a new spot. To use either feature, right-click on the item and select either Cut or Copy, depending on which you want to do. Create a new folder or navigate to the one you want, right-click on it, and select Paste.

Deleting Files and Folders

Deleting information, whether a file or entire folder, is one of the simplest tasks in a file management application. Before you delete clinical information, however, be sure you have a backup copy or are certain the information is no longer needed. Most deleted files and folders can be restored, but not always, so when dealing with critical information be safe and create a backup.

File management software allows you to create new folders in any desired location for storing information.

To delete an item, right-click on it and select Delete from the menu. You can also single left-click on the item and select Delete from the File menu. The third alternative is to single-click on the item and then press the Delete key on the keyboard. No matter how you do it, the operating system will give you one last opportunity to not delete the item by asking if you are sure you want to proceed.

Restoring Deleted Items

Even with multiple checks and balances, there will almost always come a time when something is accidentally deleted. Usually, to reverse the process, you can go to the location where deleted files are stored. In the Microsoft family of operating systems, this is the Recycle Bin. Once you find the title of the item, right-click to access the Restore option.

System Administration

Administering System Memory

The computer's temporary memory (RAM) is used by application software. Basically, more RAM means that more applications can be opened simultaneously and still respond to user inputs quickly.

A crucial management function of the operating system is administering system memory. Computer systems have both temporary and permanent memory capabilities. The permanent memory stores information. It also stores application software. The computer's temporary memory (RAM) is used by application software. Basically, more RAM means that more applications can be opened simultaneously and still respond to user inputs quickly. The operating system controls the allocation of RAM to open applications.

For example, you want to check a continuously updated clinical resource through an Internet portal. When you double-click to open the browser and sign in to the secure portion of the Web site, the operating system allocates temporary memory to that application without your realizing it.

It's not necessary to have a technical understanding of computer memory, but a functional understanding of the system administration activities listed at the bottom of Box 2-4 can be very helpful. These are common activities that you can expect to encounter as you increasingly use computing technology in your practice.

Installing and Removing Software Programs

One simple and very useful activity is the ability to add or remove clinical programs. To install a program from a CD-ROM, insert the CD in the appropriate drive and let it install automatically. It's usually safe to accept the default options during installation, but sometimes you may need to change an option, such as the default installation folder.

It is good practice to restart the computer after uninstalling any program.

Operating systems have built-in features for uninstalling programs. The Microsoft Windows family of operating systems allows programs to be removed through the Control Panel. Clicking on the option to remove programs displays a list of all applications on the computer. You can click on the desired program and then on the button to remove this program. Additionally, some programs come with their own uninstall feature, which is usually located in the program's folder in the Program menu. It is good practice to restart the computer after uninstalling any program.

Configuring for Multiple Users

One of the benefits of today's operating systems is that they can be configured for multiple users. You can add, delete, and modify accounts through the Control Panel (or through its comparable feature in other operating systems). The User Accounts option in Windows XP provides information on existing accounts and gives you options for modifying these accounts. Here, new accounts can be added and existing accounts can be deleted by simply clicking on the option to create a new account or to modify existing accounts.

Setting Printer Functions

Printers are essential computer components because they allow the physical sharing of information. Earlier we discussed that printers fall into the "output" category of computer hardware components. Because printers are a core component of the computer system, their administrative functions are most easily accessed under the Start Menu. Here you can add or delete printers and troubleshoot problems. Knowing how to perform printer administrative functions is important, especially in systems with more than one printer. If the default printer isn't working right, you can use a few simple mouse clicks to divert jobs to a functioning printer, saving time and effort.

Backing Up Information and Data

Although subsequent chapters discuss the importance of secure information storage, the role of information/data backup deserves mention here. If information truly is the key to health care, you need to take appropriate backup steps to prevent loss. A simple approach is to write this information to permanent storage media, such as CDs or DVDs. Computers with drives that can "write" to these media come with software that allows you to select the files you want to write and simply point to the drive where you want them written.

Alternatively, there are software packages, such as those listed in Box 2-5, that let you back up information stored on your computer. As detailed in Box 2-6, these software packages come with a wide variety of features. Regardless of the backup method chosen, health care professionals must ensure security and confidentiality of patient information.

BOX 2-5

Abbreviated Listing of Backup Utility Software

- BackUp MyPC
- BrightStor ARCserve Backup
- NovaBackup
- NTI Backup Now!
- Retrospect Backup

BOX 2-6

Features of Backup Utility Software Applications

- Unattended backup scheduling.
- Individual computer and network backup capabilities.
- Variable backup capabilities: full, incremental, and differential.
- Compression capabilities for large backups.
- Multiple media backup capabilities: tape, Zip, CD, DVD, alternate hard drive, etc.
- Disaster recovery capabilities.
- Bootable disk creation.

Defragmenting the Hard Drive

As you access, manipulate, and save information, the "brains" of the computer are continuously managing the storage of this information so it can operate at optimal speeds. Although this is a fairly technical process, you can essentially think of the information being stored in bits and pieces throughout your computer's hard drive. As this occurs continuously over time, you may notice that your computer's speed decreases. Defragmenting your hard drive allows you to reverse this process.

Use the Control Panel to access the Performance and Maintenance menu, where you'll find the option to defragment the hard drive. Depending on the level of fragmentation, this process can take considerable time, up to several hours.

As you access, manipulate, and save information, it is continuously being stored in bits and pieces throughout your computer's hard drive, which over time can decrease its speed. The answer is to defragment your hard drive.

Computer Networks

Engineers design and develop networks, while management information systems (MIS) professionals manage networks. As a health care professional you are a key player in the world of networks as well, because you use them every day to access and store information, send e-mail, share printers and peripheral devices, and perform other common tasks. That's why you need an understanding of networking basics.

Dictionary.com defines a network as "an openwork fabric or structure in which cords, threads, or wires cross at regular intervals."[7] Carr and Snyder's more technical definition states that a network is an "interconnected group of systems or devices that are remote from one another."[8] If you combine these two definitions and think of every computer, cell phone, printer, personal digital assistant (PDA), etc. connected to every other computer, cell phone, printer, and PDA through wired and wireless means, you are imagining a network.

Protocols

When personal computers were introduced, people used them as word processors to replace typewriters. These early computers were generally not connected to anything other than a printer. Today's networks allow devices that are thousands of miles (or a few feet) apart to communicate in real time with voice and data capabilities. One of the most critical aspects that can facilitate or hinder network communications is the communication standard used.

Protocols, also called network communication standards, are predefined, agreed-upon rules for the structure and function of communication across networks. They control the flow of traffic across hardware, serving as both road map and traffic cop.

Network communication standards, also called protocols, are simply predefined, agreed-upon rules for the structure and function of communication across networks. Protocols are important because they control the flow of traffic across computing systems that may or may not be similar. In essence, protocols serve as both the road map and the "traffic cop" for network-based communications.

Table 2-2 lists common networking protocols found in information systems across industries. Chapter 6 provides more details on protocols in health care.

TABLE 2-2
Common Networking Protocols

Name	Acronym
Dynamic Host Configuration Protocol	DHCP
File Transfer Protocol	FTP
Internet Protocol	IP
IP Security	IP Sec
Secure Socket Layer	SSL
Transmission Control Protocol	TCP

Network Topology

Networks can be categorized using two broad characteristics: topology and geography. Topology defines how the individual network nodes (or devices, such as printers and computers) are physically and logically connected to other nodes on the network. Geography refers to the relative size and distribution of networks.

Network topologies have a physical and a logical component. The physical topology describes the actual arrangement of wires and cables connecting network nodes. The logical topology describes the path that data travel along the wires and cables between devices on the network. Network protocols define the logical topology that is used. There are three primary physical network topologies: star, bus, and ring arrangements.[8]

Star Topology

Star topology is distinctive because it contains a central node, known as a hub, through which all data must pass. Reliance on this central node can cause delays or even data transfer failure in times of heavy traffic. All devices connected directly to this particular hub will be affected if the network hub fails.

Multiple star networks can also be connected to each other. When one hub in a multistar network fails, the other hubs are not affected.[8] Star networks, depicted in Figure 2-5, are relatively easy to install.[9]

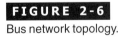
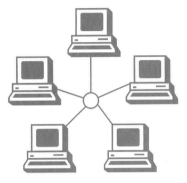

Bus Topology

The bus topology consists of a central channel, or backbone, with many nodes connected to it. The nodes operate independently of each other, and all nodes are of equal status. A failure at one node does not affect the other nodes, and new nodes are easily added.

Ethernet is a common bus network.[8] Bus networks are relatively inexpensive and easy to install.[9] Figure 2-6 shows a sample bus topology.

FIGURE 2-6

Bus network topology.

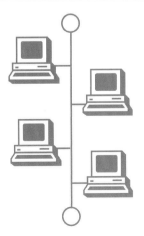

Ring Topology

In ring topology, all data travel through all nodes. Each node analyzes the data it receives and keeps only the data addressed to it. All other data are forwarded to the next node. An obvious limitation of this topology is that failure at one node can affect data transmission to all nodes. However, redundant reverse rings can bypass any node that fails.[8]

Ring networks are relatively expensive to install, but they do offer high bandwidth.[9] Figure 2-7 shows a ring topology.

FIGURE 2-7

Ring network topology.

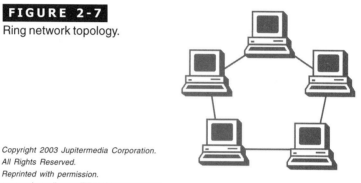

Copyright 2003 Jupitermedia Corporation.
All Rights Reserved.
Reprinted with permission.
www.webopedia.com/TERM/t/topology.html

Other network topologies, usually created by combining the three most common topologies, are the following:

Tree—Combines bus and star topologies.
Mesh—Increases connectivity between nodes to increase reliability.
Hybrid—Any combination of the other networks.

Network Geography

When you or your coworkers talk about connecting to the network in your practice environment, you are more than likely talking about your geographical network. The geographical network describes the area over which a network is dispersed. The four most common network geographies are the following:

Local Area Network (LAN). A LAN consists of nodes connected over a relatively small area, usually spanning the distance of one building or a group of buildings. Many of today's health care facilities are made up of at least one LAN.

Metropolitan Area Network (MAN). A MAN is larger than a LAN, roughly the size of a city, connecting nodes dispersed across many blocks.

Wide Area Network (WAN). A WAN can span a continent or more and is often composed of many LANs and MANs connected together. The most extreme example of a WAN is the global network known as the Internet.

Wireless Local Area Network (WLAN). This is a special class of LAN using radio waves instead of physical wires to connect nodes on the network. You may have heard the term "802.11b," which is a protocol used for wireless communication. There are a variety of 802.11 protocols, primarily differentiated based on their speed. The "a" and "g" versions are faster than the "b" version (54 MBps vs. 11 MBps). The "b" version recently made significant inroads in a variety of health care and educational settings due to its low cost and reliability. Wireless networks in health care will be discussed in more detail in Chapter 6.

 Network infrastructure has become a key factor for some clinicians as they make decisions about where to practice.

Networks in Health Care

Networks are playing an interesting role in health care today. It has reached the point where network infrastructure can be a key factor for clinicians as they make decisions about where to practice.

Financial and clinical demands place health care providers in a crunch to deliver the best, most efficient care possible. A reliable and accessible network infrastructure throughout the organization can make a significant difference in a clinician's ability to meet (and exceed) demands. Box 2-7 lists the essential components of a health care network.

BOX 2-7

Essential Components of a Health Care Network

1. Integrates all appropriate systems and devices, whether internal or external.
2. Provides real-time access to critical patient information.
3. Automatically generates appropriate documentation and billing records in real time.
4. Supports wireless access via multiple platforms, including but not limited to PDAs and tablet PCs.
5. Supports telehealth services.

Evaluating Networks

Although evaluating networks is not necessarily part of your role as a health care professional, you do need to understand which technologies must be in place for you to provide the best care possible. You may also find yourself serving on a committee that is selecting technology or representing your discipline as a liaison to the information technology (IT) department. Many of today's health care facilities are made up of the least one LAN, which may be the size of a single office or may stretch for several buildings.

Activity 2-3 helps you assess the networks in your organization. Rather than get down on your hands and knees to scope out the physical layout of your networks, ask for help from your organization's IT specialist—a professional trained in the ins and outs of information technology. These professionals can answer your questions about the characteristics of your network and any external networks your network is connected to.

Although health care facilities and providers all strive for the same goal—to provide the best care at the best price—they may go about achieving it differently. A good way to assess the capabilities of an existing network, as well as areas of need and potential improvement, is to compare it to other networks. You can explore information system vendors' Web sites to determine the configuration and capabilities of their products, or discuss network features at professional meetings such as the annual conference of the Healthcare Information and Management Systems Society (www.himss.org). Consultation with colleagues at other facilities can also provide valuable insight into the pros and cons of a network.

ACTIVITY 2-3

Computer Networking

1. Within your organization, identify the type(s) of network(s) in use, including protocols and topologies.
2. If your network is connected to a larger MAN or WAN, identify these broader networks.
3. Identify areas within your organization that can benefit from network technologies. Pay special attention to wireless opportunities, as well.
4. Assess your needs as a health care provider, and determine where you feel networking technologies can be put in place to help you provide optimal care.

Think about your workflow and the needs of the users in your organization. Consider the mobility of practitioners, along with their needs for information access as they care for patients. If you don't already have a network, ask yourself if installing one would be beneficial. Discuss your thoughts with other clinicians and solicit their input on what areas of the practice might improve by adding networking technologies.

After compiling a list of networking needs, identify the top five networking functions you'd like to have, such as access within a single room, access within a single building, or access across several buildings. Use this information as the first steps in developing a strategic planning tool for bringing your practice into a fully networked environment. Consider security throughout the process.

In the minds of many patients, who are growing more savvy about networks and technology, having the latest advancements equals better care.

Conclusion

Computer technology is increasingly important for overcoming communication and information access barriers clinicians face in today's health care environment. Not only can technology make your practice more efficient, but it may play a vital role in attracting patients. The Internet has opened up new worlds to patients, allowing them to access nationally endorsed treatment guidelines for any disease. The public is growing more savvy about networking technologies as well, and is likely to choose practitioners and facilities keeping up with recent advancements. In the minds of many patients, newer technology equals better care.

References

1. Jupitermedia. Definition of computer. Webopedia Web site. Available at: www.webopedia.com/TERM/c/computer.html. Accessed August 9, 2003.

2. Bigler J. Early typewriter history. Available at: www.mit.edu~jcb/Dvorak/history.html. Accessed August 10, 2003.

3. Jupitermedia. Data Sizes. Webopedia Web site. Available at: www.webopedia.com/Data/Data_Sizes. Accessed September 30, 2003.

4. Brain M. How hard disks work. How Stuff Works. Available at: http://electronics.howstuffworks.com/hard-disk1.htm. Accessed August 24, 2003.

5. Kohn LT, Corrigan JM, Donaldson MS, eds. *To Err Is Human: Building a Safer Health System*. Washington, DC: National Academy Press; 2000.

6. Stair RM, Reynolds GW. *Principles of Information Systems: A Managerial Approach*. 5th ed. Boston, MA: International Thomson Publishing; 2001:124-36.

7. Lexico Publishing Group. Definition of network. Dictionary.com Web site. Available at: http://dictionary.reference.com/search?q=network. Accessed September 22, 2003.

8. Carr HC, Snyder CA. *The Management of Telecommunications: Business Solutions to Business Problems.* Boston, MA: Irwin McGraw-Hill; 1997:210-312.

9. Jupitermedia. Definition of topology. Webopedia Web site. Available at: www.webopedia.com/TERM/t/topology.html. Accessed September 28, 2003.

Data Processing in Health Care ③

Brent I. Fox

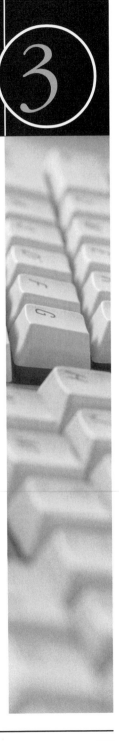

Chapter Objectives

After completing this chapter, you should be able to:

- Discuss problems related to documenting and sharing information in health care.
- Define the four types of data-processing systems.
- Discuss ways to increase efficiency in managing information.
- Describe specific ways that data-processing systems are used in health care.

ealth care professionals rely heavily on the timely flow of accurate, reliable, and secure information to make decisions about patient care. Information is also essential for managing the business of health care. General trends that have emerged regarding information use in health care include the following:

- An increasing number of practitioners is using the Internet as a key way to get health care information.
- The Health Insurance Portability and Accountability Act (HIPAA), passed by Congress in 1996, has profoundly affected how the business of health care is conducted in the United States. Entirely new companies have been created for the sole purpose of helping clinicians and providers comply with HIPAA's guidelines on the flow of health care data and information.
- Mergers and buyouts are decreasing the number of health care information system vendors while increasing the size of surviving companies. These companies are receiving millions of dollars from health systems grappling with how to efficiently manage the flow of data and information throughout their organizations.
- Increasing attention is being placed on evidence-based decision making, giving clinicians access to real-time information, using information technology to decrease medical errors, and increasing the overall efficiency of practice.

The nature of health care requires documenting literally everything that can have an impact on patients.

As noted in Chapter 1, "information" is data that have meaning. Both information and data are critical components of health care informatics. This chapter focuses on issues related to collecting and sharing data in a health care environment and the types of data-processing systems clinicians use as they deliver care.

Moving from Paper to Electronic Systems

In the health care environment, clinicians generate large amounts of data as a byproduct of the work they do. In fact, if you analyze everyday practices in health care you'll find countless critical measurements and data points. Many barriers get in the way of collecting, disseminating, and using these data in caring for patients, however.

The nature of health care requires documenting literally everything that can have an impact on patients. For decades—

What Is a System?

Because we use the word "system" so much in this chapter, let's define our meaning. A system is a group of interrelated parts working toward a common objective. It's not limited to mechanical or electrical equipment, however: when we refer to a system, we include people and procedures.

Source: Reference 1.

even centuries—pen and paper have been used to document health care activities, but this approach, although customary and familiar, has many drawbacks:

- It's a manual process that takes clinicians a lot of time.
- Only one person at a time can have access to paper-based documents, such as the medical chart. This creates "downtime" for other clinicians needing to use the chart.
- Manual, paper-based documentation requires clinicians to physically write on the document. Unfortunately, patients are sometimes harmed because clinicians' illegible handwriting is misinterpreted.
- Paper-based documents are not easily and efficiently transferred from one location to another, which delays sharing important clinical information.

In other words, generating data from paper-based documentation is inefficient, cumbersome, time-consuming—and sometimes even harmful, if it results in errors. Paper is one of the biggest barriers to making the most of data generated in health care environments.

The trend toward electronic data integration in health care—pulling together data from independent sources in a standard format—is a huge step in the right direction. The case example in Box 3-2 reflects the way things are done in many U.S. health care settings and how electronic integration can improve them.

Leading institutions are moving to electronic health records, a transition that governmental action is beginning to support through grants and research funding. When a single, electronic documentation method is used, it's relatively simple to collect data in a standardized format from multiple medical charts so the data can be analyzed and presented to clinicians as a resource in their decision making.

> The trend toward electronic data integration in health care—pulling together data from independent sources in a standard format— is a huge step in the right direction.

Electronic data allow for specialized techniques such as data mining, the purposeful extraction of unknown relationships within large data sets—such as symptom clusters suggesting the emergence of a new infectious disease. And because electronic data are highly portable, clinicians and institutions can easily use them to collaborate on projects or share new knowledge.

BOX 3-2

Case Example: Better Documentation

Imagine a 300-bed hospital, County General, with an average annual census of 160 patients. County General mainly uses paper-based medical charts that are managed manually and follows a model in which each department's information system operates independently. What happens if the clinical administrative staff decides to retrospectively review use of the (fictitious) antibiotic Atekenkel for methicillin-resistant *Staphylococcus aureus* (MRSA) infections to discover how they might improve patient outcomes and save money?

All the pertinent information has been documented in 75 charts from the last 24 months. All the charts are available for review (a situation unlikely in the real world because clinicians would have charts in their possession while they care for patients). However, conducting the analysis means someone must be taken away from regular duties. While this clinician (or group of clinicians) searches the identified charts for information, other clinicians have to "take up the slack." It is feared that responsibilities will be overlooked and clinicians and staff will pay less attention to detail as they hurry to complete newly assigned patient care and administrative tasks.

So County General's clinical administrative staff elects to use an electronic-based medium for data gathering. They create a Microsoft Access database that essentially walks clinicians through a documentation process that, in the past, would have been done using paper forms. Made available to the clinicians in a variety of platforms— notebook computer, tablet PC, personal digital assistant (PDA), etc.—the database contains mandatory fields to fill in by selecting from preset responses, ensuring that all pertinent data are captured and provided in a consistent way across clinicians.

The County General clinicians and staff involved in the project are so impressed with its success that they share their experiences with others in the hospital, who, as a result, begin to use electronic data capture processes. Furthermore, upper-level hospital administration begins to explore the possibilities of implementing a complete, hospital-wide integrated information system, so excited are they by its promise for better information collection and dissemination.

Planning Ahead to Meet Users' Needs

Even when you're able to collect and analyze health care data, how do you determine the best way to get information out to clinical and administrative personnel? Clinicians need current, accurate information to make the best decisions about each patient's care, and administrative personnel need the right information to manage human, technical, and financial resources. It's tempting to quickly identify one way to deliver clinical information to end users, but the best approach considers each user's situation and preferences. For example, physicians may want concise guidelines while administrators want a complete set of data.

Health care information must be disseminated in a format and on a time frame that meets end users' needs. So why not simply *ask* users their preferences? Sounds good, but logistically it's difficult and expensive to identify all end users, learn their requirements, and develop individualized solutions. A better approach uses representatives from specific disciplines on development teams—an approach frequently used in the software development industry. These representatives understand and voice the end users' requirements and fight to ensure that these requirements are met.

In 2002, Cedars-Sinai Medical Center shelved a $34 million computerized prescriber order entry (CPOE) system after only a few months of use, in large part because rank-and-file physicians were not adequately represented on the team that developed and implemented it. The end users, who were accustomed to jotting notes on paper rather than typing them into a computer, were not fully informed about the changes the system would make on their practice. They lacked a sense of ownership of the system, and they found it slow and cumbersome. To its credit, Cedars-Sinai took this failure as an opportunity to evaluate the CPOE system and workflow procedures in all areas and hopes to try a computerized system again in the future.

As you plan your system for collecting and disseminating information, be sure that representatives from each discipline who understand end users' needs serve on the development team. This helps avoid scenarios like that at Cedars-Sinai Medical Center, which shelved an expensive computerized prescriber order entry system.

Using Universal Standards

Using universally understood electronic language that serves as "interpreters" between disparate electronic systems is important for disseminating information effectively. Much of the work done by organizations such as Health Level 7 (HL7) and the American National Standards Institute (ANSI) focuses on developing and endorsing such standards. (For more information on HL7, see Chapter 1, page 15.)

Internet browsers such as Internet Explorer and Netscape Navigator run on virtually all computing systems and can display data in the appropriate format for each. Extensible Markup Language (XML) is a programming code designed to allow data transmission and interpretation between different applications and organizations, thus improving information flow. Health care professionals, organizations, and institutions need to develop and publish data in a format—such as XML—that is understood by the browser or some other application and that reformats the data to suit the user's environment. Because no universal standard has been established, governmental regulation may be necessary in the future if health care is unable to reach a consensus on this issue.

Having Proper Infrastructure

The physical infrastructure must be set up so end users can receive, document, and display information. Because clinicians are constantly on the go, health care is moving toward a mobile delivery approach involving portable computing devices and wireless networking. This trend, which allows health care providers real-time access to information anywhere, involves adopting such equipment as:

Because clinicians are constantly on the go, health care is moving toward a mobile delivery approach involving portable computing devices and wireless networking.

- Handheld portable computing devices, such as PDAs, which provide personal information management as well as data capture and display capabilities.
- Smart phones, which are a combination PDA and cellular phone.
- Internet-enabled smart phones that connect to the Web and e-mail.
- Notebook computers and subnotebook computers (miniature notebook computers that are larger than a PDA but smaller than the traditional notebook computer).
- Tablet PCs (notebook computers with LCD screens that the user writes on with a stylus using digital ink).

For portable devices to be as functional as possible they must be part of a wireless, high-speed network infrastructure. This way, users have broadband access to the Internet and the institution's information system where they can access patient records, treatment protocols, and institutional policies.

Wireless fidelity (Wi-Fi), a current "hot" health care technology, provides inexpensive, user-friendly network access at high speeds for authorized users. Other wireless network options include high-speed cellular (EDGE and EV-DO), WiMAX, and Bluetooth (see Table 3-1). Although Wi-Fi is the most widespread wireless technology today, many others are competing with it and may receive broad support in the future. Ultimately, the specific type of wireless is less important than what it should provide—real-time access to information.

TABLE 3-1

Wireless Connectivity Options

Connection Types	Description	Example Applications
Wi-Fi (wireless fidelity)	Commonplace wireless broadband	E-mail and Internet at home and work
Bluetooth	Personal radio frequency	Wireless connections between computers, printers, PDAs, and other devices
802.15 (Wireless Personal Area Network or WPAN)	The wireless standard that is the basis for Bluetooth, but provides higher transfer rates	Broadband for personal devices such as PDAs and home entertainment
EV-DO (Evolution-Data Only)	Broadband for mobile phones; uses code-division multiple access (CDMA), a digital cellular technology involving spread-spectrum techniques	E-mail, Internet, clinical uses
EDGE (Enhanced Data Rates for Global Evolution)	Broadband for mobile phones using global system for mobile communications (GSM), a leading digital cellular system that allows several simultaneous calls on the same radio frequency	E-mail, Internet, clinical uses
WiMAX	High bandwidth over long distances (3-30 miles)	Wireless broadband over the "last mile," providing broadband wireless access in places that cable or digital subscriber lines (DSL) don't reach without disruptive or expensive installation
UWB (ultra wideband, also known as digital pulse wireless)	Digitally transmits ultra-low power radio signals with very short electrical pulses; sends voice and data over short distances at high speeds	Huge voice and data transfers between electronics equipment and appliances using low power, allowing multimedia networking between computers, high-definition televisions, PDAs, DVD players, etc.

When evaluating wireless networking, key considerations are speed, security, reliability, and accessibility. Although the first two are largely well in hand, accessibility is limited because developing and maintaining Wi-Fi access points on a national scale is expensive. And reliability can be an issue, depending on the location of the person accessing the wireless network. Despite these obstacles, cell phone companies, Wi-Fi companies, and other wireless industries are moving forward with national approaches to high-speed wireless access.

Fortunately for clinicians and administrators, health care institutions are beginning to see the benefits of wireless access and are implementing institutional wireless networks. Approved users can access the data or information they need from almost anywhere within the institution, while security measures ensure that patient confidentiality is maintained.

Increasing Efficiency in Managing Information

One clear way to remove inefficiencies and reduce errors in patient care and documentation is to switch to electronic health records. Records in electronic form can be used by many people at once, are accessible from many places, and contain system controls that recognize when a questionable data point has been entered. Electronic records should serve as the hub for all meaningful activity regarding patients, covering all clinical and administrative disciplines.

Enhance efficiency by using electronic records, removing information silos, and making information portable, so clinicians can access it when and where they need it.

Another way to enhance efficiency is to let data and information flow freely across discipline boundaries. We refer to this as removing "silos" in health care. Like the tall cylindrical structures that hold animal feed on farms, health care silos store information in separate locations with little to no communication between them. When silos are removed, laboratory data and pharmacy data, for example, can be freely exchanged as soon as they become available. This way, if the lab finds an elevated potassium level in a patient, it prompts the pharmacy system that action should be taken to adjust the patient's medication doses.

Clinicians also should be given information—such as laboratory results, a primary literature article, or a patient's medication history—when and where they need it in the format they desire. This means making it portable, if that's what clinicians want.

The Problem of Information Silos in Health Care

Storing information in separate locations with little to no communication between them—known as information silos—causes problems for many reasons:

- When practitioners cannot access the information they need, they must rely on human memory or conjecture-based decision making.
- Waste, errors, and variations in the delivery of care occur that could easily be avoided.
- Very little analysis or reporting of system-level performance takes place.
- Patients are asked the same questions at each encounter within the system— a poor use of time for both patients and personnel.
- When information is not integrated but instead exists in silos, personnel are more likely to tolerate paper-based references and documentation.
- Minimal data are collected, and when they are collected, the approach is unstructured.

Data-Processing Systems

Much information in the clinical and business sides of health care comes in the form of databases-bodies of related facts organized to produce information. Data-processing systems are a foundational technology, operating behind the scenes to support daily tasks.

The four primary data-processing systems are transaction-processing systems, management information systems, decision support systems, and artificial intelligence and expert systems. Characteristics of the four types of data-processing systems are compared in Figure 3-1.

FIGURE 3-1

Important characteristics of the four primary data-processing systems.

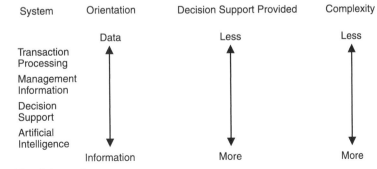

System	Orientation	Decision Support Provided	Complexity
Transaction Processing	Data	Less	Less
Management Information	↕	↕	↕
Decision Support			
Artificial Intelligence	Information	More	More

Source: Adopted from Reference 2.

ACTIVITY 3-1

Obtaining Critical Units of Data

Clinicians are best able to care for their patients when they can acquire necessary data and analyze them to produce useful information.

1. Within your organization and profession, determine and list fundamental units of clinical information that practitioners need. Use the examples below to help you think this through.

Critical pieces of data to a pharmacist counseling a patient with asthma might include:

- Medication history
- Details about the patient's adherence to therapy
- Measures such as the forced expiratory volume
- Presence and absence of medication side effects
- Events that precipitate an asthma attack
- Day-to-day quality of life

A nurse caring for a patient hospitalized for shortness of breath might want to know:

- Past medical history
- Family history
- Current medications
- Frequency and duration of symptoms
- Precipitating events
- Previous treatment measures

A pulmonologist examining a patient recently diagnosed with emphysema might want to know:

- Environmental conditions the patient has been exposed to
- Smoking history, if any
- When symptoms first appeared
- Severity of current symptoms
- The impact of symptoms on the patient's activities of daily living

2. From your list, select a single piece of data or information that is critical to you as a health care clinician. Identify where this information originates. Does the patient possess it? Is it part of the institution's formulary? Is it a clinical guideline promulgated by a professional society? Does another clinician have this information?
3. Diagram the flow of this piece of information from its origin to its ultimate use by you. Most likely this information is "handled" by someone or something else at several nodes along the way. Identify potential barriers at each node that could keep the information from reaching you in the manner you want.
4. Suggest potential solutions to overcome the barriers noted in number 3.

Transaction-Processing Systems

Transaction-processing systems (TPS) are the lowest-level data-processing systems. They process transactions that are part of an organization's normal business activities and produce a variety of documents and reports. Examples of TPS include order entry, inventory control, payroll, accounts payable and receivable, and general ledger systems.[2] By collecting, storing, processing, and sharing basic business data, TPS serve as the foundation for other data-processing systems.

The two primary approaches to TPS are batch and online processing. In batch processing, transactions are accumulated over a specified period and then, at a predetermined time, the group of transactions is processed together. The online processing approach performs real-time or near real-time processing of transactions as they occur.

The choice of which approach to use is based on available computing power, output expected from the processing (such as an inventory report), and how urgently the output is needed. A significant advantage of online processing is that databases reflecting the organization's business status are always up-to-date. Transactions such as payroll are run in a batch approach, however, because of the intervals at which they occur—bimonthly, monthly, etc.[2]

> *Transaction-processing systems process normal business activities such as inventory and payroll and produce documents and reports.*

Management Information Systems

Management information systems (MIS) handle ongoing data collection and analysis to provide managers with information that helps them plan, direct, and control activities. These systems use the data gathered by a TPS—organizing, summarizing, and displaying it—as well as data from external sources, such as suppliers, to produce information that managers and administrators use for ongoing decision making.[1] The MIS also produces reports that help managers oversee daily business operations and plan for the future.[2]

Management information systems often contain several subsystems organized by functional units within the organization. For example, an enterprise-wide MIS may be made of independent management information systems from payroll, human resources, manufacturing, shipping and receiving, and other categories. Regardless of the number of subsystems, an MIS needs to efficiently and appropriately share data across subsystems so users get the information they need on a timely basis.[2]

Decision Support Systems

Decision support systems (DSS), the next level of data-processing systems, help users solve unstructured problems and make decisions. A key distinction of decision support systems is that they give users access to large amounts of data and decision-making models.[1]

Among characteristics DSS have that increase their value to users is their ability to handle large amounts of data from different sources. A single DSS allows you to search multiple, independent databases simultaneously to solve a problem and lets you drill down to specific points of interest.

DSS are also flexible about the ways data and information are presented. While DSS users interact with the system through a computer screen, they can usually obtain printed reports, as well.[2,3]

Artificial Intelligence and Expert Systems

"Intelligent systems" is the general term used to describe the last class of data-processing systems, which is composed of artificial intelligence (AI) and expert systems (ES). Expert systems are actually a type of artificial intelligence that can repetitively and accurately solve problems using human expertise, stored knowledge, and inferences. The general goal of AI is to mimic the human brain's ability for intelligent behavior.[3]

Box 3-4 identifies key characteristics of intelligent systems. These functions are routinely performed by the human brain every day. Unlike depictions in science-fiction films, intelligent systems are not

---

BOX 3-4

Key Abilities of Intelligent Systems

1. Learn and apply knowledge gained from experience.
2. Handle complex situations.
3. Solve problems when important information is missing.
4. Determine what is important in making a decision.
5. React quickly and correctly to new situations.
6. Understand and interpret visual images.
7. Process and manipulate symbols.
8. Be creative and imaginative when problem solving.
9. Use heuristics (rules of thumb and decision-making shortcuts) in decision making.

Source: Reference 3.

---

designed to completely replace humans and cannot truly "think" as people do. Instead, intelligent systems can supplement or replicate human decision making for specific, well-defined problems.[2]

A primary advantage of AI/ES is that they offer nonexperts access to expertise in the form of computer systems. Artificial intelligence and expert systems go beyond TPS and MIS—which are information focused—to give you a knowledge base plus intelligence-like capabilities to solve a problem. You can also query the system for the rationale behind a suggested solution. AI/ES can be divided into several major branches, including robotics, vision systems, natural language processing, learning systems, and neural networks. These branches are related, with advances in one often influencing others.[2]

One obstacle to AI's adoption is people's reluctance to rely on it fully to solve critical problems—such as those that can directly affect someone's health.[1-3] Most likely, when users have several successful experiences with AI in critical situations their reluctance will decrease. For example, global positioning systems (GPS) are increasingly being incorporated into today's automobiles, but consumers were skeptical about them at first. "How can this box on my dash tell me where to go better than my traditional map?" Over the years, success with this technology has led to GPS becoming a high-priced accessory. Similarly, we can expect that repeated success with AI in the clinical realm will increase its acceptance.

Intelligent systems supplement or replicate human decision-making functions for specific well-defined problems.

Transaction-Processing Systems in Health Care

Clinicians may not think of their activities as part of a transaction, but they are. For example, a physician office visit involves record keeping, billing, and payments—transactions that can be processed in batch, online, or by hybrid methods involving both batch and online approaches. Transaction data can provide the physician or office manager with valuable information about the practice, such as number of patient visits per time period and at what reimbursement levels.

In community pharmacies, tens of thousands of transactions take place every day—with patients, wholesalers, third-party payers, and vendors—as pharmacists provide prescription and over-the-counter medications. These transactions can be processed using batch and online methods.

Transaction processing with third-party payers is extremely important to pharmacies. Each transaction transmitted to a third party has an associated processing fee that the pharmacy must pay as the "cost of doing business." Obviously, transmission methods that can decrease the cost per prescription are highly desired, such as batch mode, transmitting by Internet (rarely used for everyday prescription transactions), or using application service providers (third-party entities that allow companies to outsource their information technology needs) as the sole gateway for all pharmacy transactions.

Transaction-processing systems can add value to traditional health care services. For example, community pharmacies, which manage large amounts of medications they buy from wholesalers and sell to patients, have developed better methods for controlling their inventories. Thanks to extranet connections, which use Internet technology to securely and directly link pharmacies to wholesalers, pharmacies have real-time information about the availability of everything in the wholesaler's warehouse. This lets pharmacists give patients an accurate estimate of when, or if, a medication will be available and to order a medication at the moment the need becomes apparent.

From a business perspective, transactions between the pharmacy and patients provide the income necessary to "pay the bills." Maintaining transaction data is important for analyzing the pharmacy's business components, but it is also key to the clinical side of the pharmacy. Pharmacists use records that house a patient's complete history of dispensed medications to ensure appropriate medication therapy. Without these transaction data, pharmacists could not perform their role as medication therapy managers, as defined in the Medicare Modernization Act of 2003.

ACTIVITY 3-2

Transaction-Processing Systems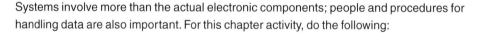

Systems involve more than the actual electronic components; people and procedures for handling data are also important. For this chapter activity, do the following:

1. Identify the most basic transaction occurring within your health care discipline. This transaction represents the lowest layer of data processing.
2. Identify the transaction-processing system(s) that collects and manages these data. List the people, procedures, data sources, and end users that make up this system.
3. Identify the transaction-processing system's output(s) that are used by clinicians and administrators, such as billing history, inventory requisitions, receipts, or similar information.

Management Information Systems in Health Care

Management information systems are one of the most visible types of data-processing systems in health care. Practically everyone involved in health care interacts with an MIS at some level. For example:

- Clinicians rely on MIS for important data and information they use in routine patient care, such as results of laboratory tests.
- Health system administrators rely on MIS to gain information about business aspects of the institution, such as general ledger information.
- Third-party payers use MIS to display and manage information about the people they insure, such as annual cost per life covered.

Patients are beginning to use MIS to manage components of their health care information by creating online health records through their local health care facility, pharmacy, or private company.

Because they're the gateway to virtually all data and information, MIS are vital to today's health care institutions. As the U.S. health system moves closer toward a completely electronic health record, the role of MIS will increase. Paper will be taken out of the equation to improve efficiency, patient safety, and ultimately, patient outcomes.

At many facilities, you can now access an MIS to input orders, review results of laboratory tests and radiology procedures, access information on staffing, and review institutional policies. In the future, additional clinical activities, such as communicating with colleagues, will be tied to an MIS instead of a paper chart or form. To interface with the MIS you will increasingly use personalized Web browsers, which, after you sign on using your password, display only the icons and options you've preselected so the browser is tailored directly to your needs.

If you work in a health system environment you've probably been exposed to what is generally called the "hospital information system"—often composed of individual departments' information systems. In the future, you should expect greater flow of data and information between the MIS of different departments due to integration—the removing of barriers between disparate departmental MIS and linking them to create a hospital-wide MIS.

As the U.S. health system moves closer toward a completely electronic health record, the role of MIS will increase. Paper will be taken out of the equation to improve efficiency, patient safety, and ultimately, patient outcomes.

ACTIVITY 3-3

Management Information Systems ✓

For this exercise you will need access to a clinical management information system.

1. Create a list of the important information you need to perform your daily clinical or administrative activities. For example, all clinicians need to know patient diagnoses. Physicians need to know current and previous medical history, current interventions, etc. Nurses need to know current medication regimens, daily schedules for treatments and radiology procedures, etc. Pharmacists need to know current and past medication history, medication allergies, therapeutic laboratory values, etc.

2. Identify which of these information items are found in the information system that you directly use on a routine basis, and which are in systems found in other departments.

3. Determine the optimal method of getting this information. For example, if you rely on an external information system for important information, what would be the best method for you to acquire this information? Is this method the one that is currently in place?

4. Using your customary procedures (username, password, biometrics, etc.) access the MIS you routinely use and answer the questions below.

   ■ How can the interface—that is, the means provided for you to interact with the MIS—be improved so it is more efficient for you to use? Is the interface cluttered with unnecessary information, links, or icons? Alternatively, are important links absent? Has your past experience with the interface uncovered design flaws that hinder your ability to use it efficiently?
   ■ Can you get access to all the information you listed in Step 1 above?
   ■ How much effort is required to access this information in terms of key strokes, mouse clicks, and/or touches of the screen?
   ■ How long does it take to access this information?
   ■ Is information external to your MIS readily available? In other words, can you get information from other silos quickly?
   ■ How much lag time exists between the appearance of information in an external MIS and its appearance in your MIS? (For example, how long does it take a laboratory value to appear in your MIS after it appears in the lab's MIS?)
   ■ Is the information presented in a way that best suits your needs? If not, how would you improve it?

5. If you see ways to improve the MIS, share your observations with colleagues, the information systems department, or your information system vendor.

Decision Support Systems in Health Care

If you're involved in direct patient care, DSS serve as valuable tools. Clinicians are increasingly expected to pull data and information from resources to make the best choice for a patient's care—and there is simply too much information available to keep up unassisted.[4] DSS bridge the gap between what clinicians know or remember and what they need to know to provide optimal care.

Computerized prescriber order entry (CPOE), described in Chapter 2 as a combination of hardware and software for capturing and transmitting medical orders, is potentially one of the most valuable decision support systems available today. To increase patient safety, CPOE systems give alerts and reminders as orders are created by prescribers. These alerts are triggered when the decision support component of the CPOE system "sees" a potential problem, such as ordering a medication for a patient who is allergic to that medication class. Or an order for a monthly lab test completed the previous day may trigger an alert that the lab result is already available. More sophisticated DSS approaches can be used to help prescribers select formulary medications or use the preferred schedule for a medication.[5] DSS can be developed to be institution-specific, allowing facilities or practitioners to tailor alerts to their individual needs.

DSS can also provide algorithms or decision trees for treating specific conditions. These help prescribers select therapeutic options based on patient-specific considerations, pulling data from multiple resources to show the optimal path for a patient's care. Even more advanced DSS can show potential outcomes of the selected therapies based on currently available evidence, but work in this field of DSS is still in its infancy.

While CPOE with a DSS component is relatively new, pharmacy has had widespread experience with DSS for many years. Management information systems used for maintaining patient profiles in pharmacies provide decision-support alerts—most often for drug interactions and allergies—when a new prescription is entered into a patient's profile. Alerts normally tell pharmacists the potential severity of the problem and the likelihood of the problem occurring.

When using CPOE or any DSS, it is extremely important that clinicians do not become complacent and simply "click through" the alert. You should always seriously consider these alerts in regard to the patient's care. When DSS are used in

When using decision support systems, carefully consider all alerts that come up: avoid becoming complacent and simply "clicking through" them.

health care, the clinician ultimately has the final say. DSS fill a supportive role, supplementing human memory and giving quick access to data to help ensure that treatment leads to the best results possible.

Artificial Intelligence in Health Care

Expert Systems

Expert systems rely on stored knowledge, inferences, and human expertise to solve problems.

Expert systems (ES)—which rely on stored knowledge, inferences, and human expertise to solve problems—are commonly used in pharmacies to manage inventory. For example, a pharmacist entering a medication order into the MIS may get a prompt from the ES saying that the desired medication is out of stock. The ES may ask if the pharmacist wants to check local pharmacies' stock for the medication. The ES uses stored routines and data about various pharmacies' inventories to solve the out-of-stock medication problem. It is not replacing the pharmacist but simply helping to solve a well-defined problem with available data.

Interactive Voice Response Systems

Interactive voice response (IVR) systems are used to route callers through menus based on the caller's response to questions. IVR systems use heuristics (rules-of-thumb that define

---

ACTIVITY 3-4

Becoming a DSS Champion

As DSS becomes more widely used in health care, this exercise may help you be receptive to it and advocate DSS features that best meet the needs of users in your institution.

1. Make a list of potential reasons why clinicians might react negatively to decision support systems.
2. Put yourself in the role of the clinician who is hesitant to embrace the DSS as a routine part of your daily practice. Identify what technological features would be required for you to be willing to use a DSS regularly.
3. Record your thoughts about what technological features would bring clinicians on board as champions of a DSS in your institution.

---

acceptable solutions) and built-in guidelines to solve the problem of getting callers to the right destination. (Verizon is one company that uses an IVR system with voice recognition to sort calls for customer service and refer callers to the appropriate department.) Because IVR systems help solve well-defined problems, they can also be considered ESs. IVR systems may not always be popular among callers, but they play a valuable role in handling routine functions so humans are free to perform more complex tasks.

Robotics

The exciting field of artificial intelligence known as robotics has to do with performing precise or tedious tasks.[2] Pharmacies use robots extensively to fill prescriptions quickly and accurately. Using information that humans enter in the pharmacy MIS, robots select the appropriate medication—including strength, dosage form, and count—and place it in the bottle. The pharmacist then doublechecks the bottle before distributing it to the patient. By filling prescriptions, robots give pharmacists more time to confer with patients and use their pharmaceutical knowledge in performing medication therapy management services.

At NewYork-Presbyterian Hospital, surgeons are testing a robot "scrub technician" that follows voice commands to identify surgical instruments, hand them to the surgeon, retrieve them, and put them back in place. The robot (known as the Penelope Surgical Instrument Server), which interacts with physicians and nurses only and has no direct patient contact, was first used in surgery in June 2005 in a procedure to remove a benign tumor from a patient's forearm. Among technologies incorporated into Penelope are continuous speech recognition software (see below), digital cameras, and advanced image-processing software. Penelope also includes software to predict what instrument the surgeon may need next and provide a detailed count of instruments that were used.[6]

Natural Language Processing

Natural language processing, commonly known as speech recognition, comes in three types: command, discrete, and continuous. Command recognition systems recognize individual words. Discrete recognition systems recognize dictated speech with pauses between words. Continuous speech recognition, the most advanced system, recognizes natural speech.[2]

In the field of robotics, devices are programmed to perform precise or tedious tasks in an effort to increase speed and accuracy.

Continuous speech recognition, the most advanced system form of natural language processing, recognizes regular speech.

Continuous speech recognition was used in "writing" much of this text. Using a $160 software program and a $20 headset microphone, we dictated up to 160 words per minute with 99% accuracy. Medical versions of the software we used allow users to speak medical terminology, such as medication names, which it then types on the screen. You can train the software to type phrases and paragraphs when a single word is spoken, greatly increasing efficiency when documenting routine tasks. You need minimal training to get started (about 5 minutes), and the intelligence in the software learns more about your speech each time the software is used.

You can pair continuous speech recognition with a portable recording device to document daily tasks. For example, you might make comments into a personal digital assistant or digital recorder and at the end of the day download the recording into your desktop computer, where a program that interprets your speech changes it to typewritten text. Currently, physicians are the leaders in this technology because their practice has such heavy dictation requirements. Soon handheld computing devices will be able to perform speech recognition.

ACTIVITY 3-5

Speech Recognition Software

1. Identify speech recognition software you can buy to help you in your professional and personal activities. To start your search, go to Google.com and search for "speech recognition." Adding the word "compare" to the search may provide additional useful hits.
2. Evaluate features. The best software allows you to dictate directly into any Windows-based program, learns your speech patterns with each use, and allows multiple user profiles on a single computer.
3. Compare prices. You can probably find a worthwhile program for around $160. Although this is not a small amount of money, it can be worth every dollar if you regularly spend as little as 30 minutes a day composing on the computer or responding to e-mail.

References

1. Carr HC, Snyder CA. *The Management of Telecommunications: Business Solutions to Business Problems.* Boston, MA: Irwin McGraw-Hill; 1997:1-29.

2. Stair RM, Reynolds GW. *Principles of Information Systems: A Managerial Approach.* 5th ed. Boston, MA: International Thomson Publishing; 2001.

3. Turban E, Rainer RK, Potter R. *Introduction to Information Technology.* 2nd ed. Hoboken, NJ: John Wiley and Sons, Inc; 2003.

4. Davidoff F, Haynes B, Sackett D, et al. Evidence based medicine. *BMJ.* 1995;310:1085-6.

5. Teich JM, Merchia PR, Schmiz JL, et al. Effects of computerized physician order entry on prescribing practices. *Arch Intern Med.* 2000;160:2741-7.

6. For the first time in medical history newly developed robot assists doctors and nurses in operating room [press release]. Office of Public Affairs New York-Presbyterian Hospital/Columbia University Medical Center; June 16, 2005. Available at: www.news.cornell.edu/stories/June05/med_robot.html. Accessed June 20, 2005.

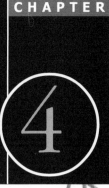

Information Systems in Health Care

Bill G. Felkey

Chapter Objectives

After completing this chapter, you should be able to:

- Explain the value of information technology in health care.
- Give examples of performance-enhancing technology in your workplace.
- Define the systems approach to health care technology.
- Name common components of health care information systems.
- Describe the attributes of a good computerized order entry system.
- Explain why information systems for outcomes measurement are useful.
- List key elements of an effective documentation system.
- Discuss benefits of automation in pharmacy.

Whⁿat do we mean by "information systems in health care," and how do these systems fit into the overall framework of informatics? Health care information systems include hardware, software, networks, and components that support clinical activities and functions important to your practice, such as scheduling and reimbursement. These systems are just one piece of health care informatics—which is essentially an information science. Health care informatics applies computer science and information technologies to advance health-related disciplines and specialties.

Practitioners who specialize in informatics usually provide a support role for their health care discipline, working to connect those providing patient care with evidence-based information. Ideally, this connection occurs in real-time so practitioners have the information they need right at the moment when they are making

FIGURE 4-1

An integrated hospital information system.

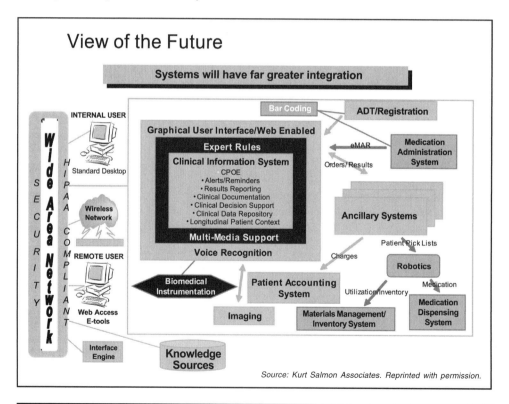

Source: Kurt Salmon Associates. Reprinted with permission.

decisions. Informatics specialists may also be responsible for collecting the data generated by each health care visit, test, and transaction and turning it into something useful—information that helps providers better render care in the future.

Unlike clinicians, who use only their own department's information system, informatics specialists usually understand all information systems used by a health system and have a larger view of the organization's information flow.

Figure 4-1 on page 78 shows the many components of a hospital information system and how, in the future, they will be fully integrated for better efficiency and quality of care. The diagram also illustrates the flow of information as practitioners care for patients.

Information technology helps overcome limits of human memory, reduces the use of opinion-based reasoning, and enables people to base decisions firmly on scientific evidence.

Automation and Performance-Enhancing Technology

It's hard to imagine any scenario in health care's future that does not involve technology. Automation in many forms is likely to increase, regardless of practice setting. One key purpose of technology is to take over repetitive, tedious tasks and free people for work that involves judgment, abstract thinking, and other high-level cognitive processes.[1] Another purpose is to enhance human work. With over 6000 articles published every week in the biomedical literature, it is impossible for anyone to "keep up."[2] Evidence-based medicine experts estimate that even in the narrowest specialty, you would need to read approximately 17 articles a day to maintain your professional competency at the highest level.[3] Information technology helps overcome limits of human memory, reduces the use of opinion-based reasoning, and enables people to base decisions firmly on scientific evidence.[4]

The use of bar codes in hospitals, nursing homes, and pharmacies is one example of performance-enhancing technology. By scanning codes throughout the medication order and dispensing process, right up to the point where medication is administered to the patient, busy practitioners can ensure that the right person gets the right drug at the right time, in the correct form, route, and strength. Use of bar codes in health care is proving to significantly reduce accidents and errors.[5]

A great example of performance-enhancing technology occurs at what is called the "point of administration" when nurses

The systems approach to technology in health care considers not only hardware and software but also the people who use it, the environment in which they practice, and the complex interactions involved—interactions that focus on the welfare of patients.

perform a medication pass in the hospital setting. Using a wireless, handheld device, a nurse enters a patient's room with a medication cart. She scans a bar code on her identification badge that verifies she is authorized to administer medication in the facility. She scans a bar code on the wristband that was put on the patient when he was admitted. She then scans each dose of medication that her electronic medication administration record (eMAR) tells her the patient is supposed to get at this time. If each drug, strength, and route is appropriate, she administers the medication. If any aspect of the drug is inappropriate or if the medication has been discontinued, she is warned by the pharmacy system immediately. Everything she does is documented automatically without the need to fill out paper forms or type on a computer keyboard.

The Systems Approach

Using appropriate technology, such as the medication scanning described above, can increase the efficiency and effectiveness of physicians, nurses, and pharmacists—especially when that technology is integrated into a larger system. Our discussion of information systems in health care emphasizes the word "system"—going beyond individual parts to look at the role each part plays in the larger whole so teams can work effectively. The systems approach to technology in health care considers not only hardware and software but also the people who use it, the environment in which they practice, and the complex interactions involved—interactions that focus on the welfare of patients.

Medicine, pharmacy, and nursing are subsystems of a larger, comprehensive health care system that increasingly relies on multidisciplinary teams to provide care. In addition to sharing a common vision for patient care, the disciplines must be able to share information quickly and effectively. Thus all work areas should be interconnected and contain multiple interfaces that allow information systems and devices to "talk" or exchange information with each other. Because of the variety of hardware and software applications that may be used, these interfaces must be built to allow the systems to "speak the same language." Single interfaces are called point-to-point interfaces. In a complex system, when many interfaces are required, it can be cost-effective to use an interface engine—usually an additional computer that serves as a translator for all the hardware and software to which it is connected. For example, in a community-based outpatient clinic, the following functional areas would be desirable:

- Patient intake.
- Processing of insurance.
- Fulfillment of interventions, goods, and services.
- Quality assurance that assists in process improvement.
- Counseling and disease management services.
- Delivery of additional health care services beyond addressing the patient's chief complaint.
- Knowledge management of health-related problems to assure appropriate documentation and follow-up care.
- External connectivity to other providers, payers, and regulatory agencies.

Customer relationship management (CRM) software is increasingly being used in health care to capture information about patient preferences and anticipate appropriate elective services a patient may be interested in.

Each functional area uses specific technologies. The intake area might include electronic prescribing, interactive voice response systems, a fax server (computer-based fax machine), and predictive fulfillment applications that identify appropriate intervals for reexamining the patient, refilling medications, and conducting preventive health screening. Just as in the business world, customer relationship management (CRM) software is increasingly being used in health care to capture information about patient preferences and anticipate appropriate elective services a patient may be interested in. So in a dental practice, for example, patients who regularly schedule dental cleaning visits may be offered whitening services during their next appointment reminder.

Overall, key goals of integrating the components of a health care operation into the larger system should be:

- Taking work out of the system that would normally be performed by costly personnel.
- Reducing errors.
- Providing value-added services such as home care that could prevent expensive rehospitalization.
- Making decision support more efficient.
- Eliminating waste, errors, and unnecessary variation in practice.
- Allowing greater access to "just-in-time" electronic references that provide the latest information.
- Creating a more productive workflow for care providers.
- Automating the monitoring of errors and adverse reactions.

BOX 4-1

Acquiring New Components for Your System

Acquiring new components to add to an already complex information system can be challenging. As information becomes more integrated, any new hardware or software can cause a ripple effect throughout the whole system. Many information technology (IT) administrators keep a data dictionary just to track what each field of information is and what potential purpose the information can serve in the system.

For example, imagine identifying, selecting, and implementing a computerized prescriber order entry (CPOE) system for inpatient use in a large hospital. At the highest level, a selection committee will need to consider how the order entry process and software capabilities address the organization's needs, including implementation, operations, potential uses in the future, long-term vendor support, and finances.

Choosing and incorporating hardware and software components requires the following:

- Great attention to detail by the selection committee so they clearly visualize and understand how the new component will be integrated into the existing system.
- Considering training requirements and support issues (such as a help desk) for initial implementation, new hires, and ongoing updates to the equipment and software.
- Examining how the new information system affects other operations in the organization and establishing procedures for operation when unscheduled downtime occurs.
- Investigating the clinical impact of the system to determine the return on investment by looking at tangible savings, such as selecting less expensive drugs or saving labor.
- Gathering key performance indicators, such as clinical performance or compliance with accreditation standards, so the organization can continually improve.
- Assessing on an ongoing basis the technology's performance and impact on factors such as patient waiting time or accuracy of reimbursement coding.

Common Components of Health Care Information Systems

Many technologies need to be implemented in nearly every practice to make health care a truly digital industry. Failing to incorporate these components will compromise patient safety as well as provider efficiency and effectiveness. Every one of these components is necessary, but there are advantages to following a certain sequence for adoption.

Computerized Prescriber Order Entry (CPOE)

Computerized prescriber order entry (CPOE), also called electronic order entry, is an important component in the health care information system because it eliminates illegible handwriting, reduces medical errors, and improves patient care.[6] Electronic prescription entry is gaining momentum in response to today's concerns about patient safety. Estimates show that 20% of hospitals are actively planning or implementing CPOE systems. Less than 5% of prescriptions for ambulatory patients are currently processed using CPOE.[7]

Some people argue that electronic medical records need to be more widely adopted before CPOE can be implemented because they provide more complete information that results in better prescribing and ordering behaviors. Unfortunately, electronic medical records are more expensive to establish.

In 2004, for the first time, institutions placed a higher priority on creating electronic medical records than on purchasing and installing CPOE systems, according to an annual survey by the Healthcare Information and Management Society. Despite this shift in attitude, CPOE is coming along first because it's easier to install and is perceived to have a more quick and visual impact on patient safety.

Unfortunately, implementing CPOE without the presence of electronic medical records can result in "data holes"—missing data about allergic reactions or laboratory tests, for example— which could cause a medication to be ordered at an inappropriate strength or lead to a fatal adverse reaction.

People in organizations that adopt an electronic order entry system must undergo a huge change in behavior. Up to two years of committee work may be necessary to determine all the clinical decisions and guidelines that need to be associated with the process. The kinds of questions that must be answered include:

- If prescribers order a drug that has a significant drug interaction or disease contraindication with preexisting therapy, will they be allowed to override the warning offered by the system?
- If an override is implemented, will anybody else in the health system be notified of the override?
- Under what circumstances will prescribers be forced to try less expensive therapeutic equivalents before ordering extremely expensive options?

Organizations that adopt CPOE must undergo a huge change in behavior and lengthy committee work to determine which clinical decisions and guidelines must be associated with the CPOE process.

Physicians can be convinced to adopt CPOE if it is speedier or at least takes them no longer than manual systems for ordering prescriptions.

Individual hospitals are usually reluctant to accept clinical guidelines offered by national academies and organizations without modifying them. They are also concerned about "alert fatigue," in which prescribers are so inundated with computer alerts that they become less efficient. And there is the pharmacy verification issue: what sorts of medications can be administered to patients through the CPOE process without being electronically verified first by the pharmacy? In some institutions, patients cannot be given a Tylenol without pharmacist verification, but in others, narcotics are given without verification.

Physicians can be convinced to adopt CPOE if it is speedier or at least takes them no longer than manual systems for ordering prescriptions. Unfortunately, in many health systems CPOE is taking physicians longer. The personnel saving time are those who used to be charged with untangling order entry problems, such as clerks, nurses, or pharmacists. CPOE has been poorly received by physicians because it shifts responsibilities such as resolving formulary problems back onto them.[8] Institutions with strong pharmacy and therapeutics committees may use algorithms to automatically address therapeutic substitution issues, but some physicians feel that this automatic process undercuts their prescribing prerogatives. As described in Chapter 3, Cedars-Sinai Medical Center is an example of an institution that terminated a CPOE program because of physician resistance, poor planning, unsound implementation practices, and other frustrations.

Box 4-2 describes the attributes of a good CPOE system. Other key recommendations:

- Be sure a policy is set at the institution level on how—and if—overrides are permitted when a prescriber is warned about a drug interaction or other complications that could result when new therapy is added to an existing regimen. Instituting such a policy may be difficult because so many overrides depend on the prescriber's clinical judgment and the information he or she has at the time.
- Convene advisory panels to examine the implications of a CPOE implementation. Every clinical department should be represented as well as business units and even consumer advocacy groups. This approach helps people affected by the change accept the new procedures more readily.

■ Engage prescribers in the process and use early adopter "champions"—people who embrace rather than shun technology—to give encouragement to their peers. Plan on high levels of handholding at the beginning of implementation and at specific intervals throughout the first two years of adoption.

BOX 4-2

Best Attributes of Computerized Physician Order Entry (CPOE)

■ Signing into and out of the system is simple. Approaches may include a combination of password, biometrics (fingerprint scan), or proximity devices such as a radio frequency identification (RFID) button worn on a name badge.

■ Users can get easy access to information that helps them make decisions about patient care. Access is available from any location where patient care is rendered, including the pharmacy and physician's office. Prescribers should also have access from their homes or mobile devices via the Internet.

■ The system allows mobility. Prescribers can use both mobile and stationary devices, such as personal digital assistants and wireless computer workstations, respectively. Placement of these devices, ideally, should be wherever care is administered and convenient to the workflow of each practice location.

■ Navigation is from a main screen with direct links to screens designed for reviewing patient data, ordering, and searching information compendia. Moving forward and back to the main screen is clear and easy.

■ Patient data to support the ordering process are readily available electronically, including allergies, height, weight, current medications, laboratory values, radiology results, and a listing of the patient's medical problems.

■ Each screen presents the maximum amount of relevant information possible. In other words, content is more important than aesthetic design.

■ System response is fast and there is virtually no downtime.

Source: Reference 9.

Internet Usage in Health Systems

Patients are increasingly using the Internet to obtain medical information. A recent Harris poll estimated that 98 million Americans have retrieved health-related information online, an increase of 44 million since 1998.[10] The quality of information on the Internet is, however, highly suspect. In 2002, Eysenbach et al. conducted empirical content research on Internet health information directed toward patients and found significant problems,

BOX 4-3

CPOE Works Well at Brigham and Women's Hospital

One of the most mature implementations of CPOE is at the Brigham and Women's Hospital in Boston, Massachusetts. Operational for more than 10 years, the system was built specifically for the hospital through an internal process. A version of the software has been exported for commercial sale. David Bates, MD, chief of the Division of General Medicine, reports that clinicians who were trained at the hospital find it difficult to move to health systems where the technology has not been implemented.

The hospital's system creates an opportunity for a multidisciplinary approach to patient care by using information technology to connect prescribers with nurses and pharmacists on the care team. Having clinical decision support that is fully integrated into the system has generated a significant return on investment for the hospital.

including incomplete coverage of information, difficulty finding large numbers of high-quality sites with information that is not commercially targeted to sell a product, and lack of accuracy in the information presented.[11]

These days, nearly every organization in the United States is connected to the Internet, including hospitals, pharmacies, and medical clinics. Now that electronic adjudication of medical and prescription claims has gone mainstream, it's easier for organizations to justify acquiring high-speed or broadband Internet access. Claims-processing transaction fees levied by software vendors and claims-processing companies have decreased significantly, helping providers achieve an easy return on investment for broadband connectivity to the Internet.[12]

Levels of Web Site Quality

Nearly every health care system has a publicly viewable Web site directed at patients, but many of them are more like "placeholder" sites, used mainly for marketing and promotion. They may allow patients to review an online directory of providers or assist in recruiting employees, but typically they underuse the power of the Internet to connect with patients.

Web sites that make more advanced use of the Internet provide consumer health information and do a professional job of highlighting the brand name of the health institution sponsoring the site.

When the Internet is used on an even higher level, it gives patients access to health assessment tools and even a way to schedule appointments. And taking the Internet to the top level, patients can view their medical records and get engaged in self-care management.

For an example of a Web site that makes maximum use of its potential, look at Baptist Healthcare in Pensacola, Florida (www.ebaptisthealthcare.org). Baptist Healthcare is a winner of both the American Hospital Association's Most Wired Award and the Baldrige National Quality Award, given by the President of the United States to businesses, educational institutions, and health care organizations judged to be outstanding in leadership, strategic planning, knowledge management, and other key areas.

Web sites can be useful for highlighting the quality of health care services provided by a given institution. The satisfaction level of patients, the number and quality of procedures performed, medication error rates, and whether any litigation is currently in progress are all areas that may someday be posted for public access. A consumer market in health care is beginning to emerge where patients will shop by price and quality as they do in any other market.

When health care organizations use the Internet well, patients get access to health assessment tools, a way to schedule appointments, the ability to view their medical records, and self-care management opportunities.

Application Service Providers

In health care, Internet use at the point of care is lagging behind its use in front- and back-office operations. A major movement is under way toward application service providers (ASPs), which offer subscription-based access via the Internet to externally remote servers that allow the software that is normally stored locally on a computer to be accessed globally from any Internet browser. The many advantages ASPs offer include instantaneous upgrading of all software applications in use and redundant external storage of data if a natural disaster were to strike an installed user's location. Tremendous savings can be achieved by eliminating installation, media shipment, and paper documentation for systems.

ASPs are likely to be the information technology architecture that most physicians, pharmacists, and nurses use in the future because they offer the best opportunity to aggregate data generated by a workforce into a central data warehouse. These data can then be accessed in real-time by an entire organization through a simple browser interface. This technology is increasingly being adopted despite widespread concerns about the difficulty of protecting and securing critical information that is stored externally.

Patients and Providers Communicating by E-Mail

Many patients want to be able to communicate with their health care providers by e-mail. When Grover et al. examined patients' wishes for better access to health services, they discovered the following: "Patients were especially interested in getting e-mail reminders. They wanted online booking of appointments in real time...and wished to receive updates about new advances in treatment. Some wanted this information to be pushed to them according to a preference menu they would fill out. Thus, if a patient wanted information concerning women's health and cholesterol management, only news regarding those issues would be sent to them via e-mail. Patients were also interested in virtual visits for simple and chronic medical problems and for following chronic conditions through virtual means. We concluded that computer-using patients desire Internet services to augment their medical care."[13]

BOX 4-4

AMA Guidelines for E-Mail to Patients

Guidelines released by the American Medical Association for e-mail communication between physicians and patients (www.ama-assn.org/ama/pub/category/2386.html) stress that "new communication technologies must never replace the crucial interpersonal contacts that are the very basis of the patient-physician relationship," but should instead enhance communication. Among the AMA's recommendations:

■ Establish a turnaround time for messages and be cautious when using e-mail for urgent matters.

■ Make sure patients are informed about privacy issues and know who besides the physician processes messages during usual business hours, vacations, and absences.

■ Include a standard message block in all e-mails with contact information, security reminders, and emergency contact procedures.

■ Tell patients to put the category of transaction in the subject line so prescriptions, appointments, medical advice, and billing questions can be sorted.

■ Ask patients to put their name and patient identification number in the body of the message and to keep messages concise.

■ Avoid anger, sarcasm, criticism, and libelous references in messages.

■ If correspondence is too lengthy or prolonged, ask patients to call or make an appointment. If patients repeatedly fail to adhere to the guidelines, consider terminating the e-mail relationship.

Source: Reference 14.

A study in the journal *Pediatrics* found that despite some physicians' concerns that parents of their patients would e-mail them about billing, appointments, and other matters better handled by nurses and office staff, most e-mails asked legitimate medical questions about such things as symptoms and possible adverse reactions to foods or medications. The study, which examined 81 e-mail exchanges between two Massachusetts pediatricians with a primarily college-educated client base, found that 65% of the parents would be more likely to choose a pediatrician in the future based on his or her use of e-mail, and 80% think all pediatricians should use e-mail to communicate with parents.[15]

Patients are interested in e-mail reminders, online appointment booking, and updates about new advances in treatment.

Wireless Information Appliances

Thanks to the use of portable technology, something called "mobile care" is emerging, allowing practitioners to be connected whenever they wish to information, the Internet, and other members of the care team. The infrastructure that allows this portability is wireless networks (described in detail in Chapter 3), including cellular, wireless local area networks, Bluetooth technology, and infrared transmittal. These information technologies may weigh only a few ounces and fit comfortably into a shirt pocket, lab coat, or purse. The wireless infrastructure offers ever greater speed and connectivity and increasing coverage of U.S. communities.

Using Information Systems for Outcomes Measurement

An effective health care information system should provide feedback on how well interventions are working to achieve desired patient care outcomes.

Outcomes are divided into four categories: therapeutic, financial, quality of life, and patient satisfaction with the health care system. Outcome measures can be used in many ways[16]:

- To monitor the effects of interventions in both clinical practice and formal clinical trials.
- To assess changes within populations to see if the changes came about spontaneously or are the result of public health measures. Health systems can then measure the effectiveness of their overall impact of care.
- To monitor the course of an individual patient's illness as part of a management plan.

■ To identify changes brought about in larger groups because of interventions such as immunization or because patients migrated to other health care providers within a community or to another geographic area.

Software that prompts patients and the health care system to seek or provide preventive services at appropriate intervals can incorporate evidence-based resources at the point of care to assist in appraising patients' medical conditions. The software can suggest high-quality, empirically derived approaches for addressing problems and specify an appropriate evaluation period for ascertaining therapeutic outcomes. The scheduling system can include details for follow-up, monitoring intervals, and procedures to be done at follow-up visits. Table 4-1 describes ways to incorporate evidence-based materials and approaches into patient visits.

Therapeutic Outcomes

To determine therapeutic outcomes you must measure objective clinical results, such as blood pressure, blood glucose, liver enzymes, or some other health status indicator after patients in a clinical setting have been evaluated and treated. In many instances,

TABLE 4-1

Using Evidence-Based Approaches with Individual Patients

Approach	Explanation
Start with the Old	Do your normal clinical workup; appraise and interpret data before formulating the primary question to be pursued. Go through the other tools below and then decide your intervention, evaluation methods, and follow-up/monitoring scheduling.
Search and Match	Find guidelines, protocols, and other literature that match the needs of your patient and the setting in which you are practicing.
Estimate Outcomes	Use clinical judgment or decision analysis methods to see how your patient may respond relative to patients who were in a randomized, controlled trial.
Verify Resources	Check whether you have access to experts and other resources that may be useful.
Be Patient-Oriented	Listen to your patients and their families regarding the emotional, spiritual, and other nonbiological aspects of illness and be willing to share and ask, "What else?" until solutions match patients' values.

Source: Reference 11.

patients themselves determine whether a therapeutic outcome has been achieved; for example, whether their pain has been reduced.

Technology is available to help measure therapeutic outcomes and enter the measurements directly into a medical record or patient-specific Web page. For example, if a patient is diagnosed with hypertension, a key intervention is to prescribe medication to achieve a blood pressure reading of <140/90 mm Hg (the target set by the Seventh Report of the Joint National Committee on Prevention, Detection, Evaluation, and Treatment of High Blood Pressure). You can use blood pressure cuffs that digitally transmit the patient's results into a data field, which triggers the clinical decision support system to provide feedback and suggest further actions.

Technology is available to help measure therapeutic outcomes and enter the measurements directly into a medical record or patient-specific Web page.

Financial Outcomes

Financial outcomes have to do with the cost of bringing about desired results. In the example above of a patient with hypertension, the most cost-effective financial outcome would probably result from patient lifestyle changes, such as increased exercise levels and a healthier diet. If the patient needs medication, an inexpensive thiazide diuretic that achieves the therapeutic objective would be more favorable than a more costly calcium channel blocker or angiotensin II receptor blocker. Care management algorithms, practice guidelines, and decision support software, which include prompts at key points in the decision-making process, can help practitioners choose interventions that work well and keep down health care costs.

Quality of Life

Quality of life is a measure of the effects of health care on people's basic activities of daily living (bathing, dressing, and so on) as well as their physical and emotional performance at work, at home, and during recreation. Sometimes therapeutic and financial objectives can be met at the expense of quality of life. For example, a man in his 30s can get good blood pressure control via a beta blocker, but when he enters his 40s the same medication might cause fatigue and even impotence. Some health care systems administer quality of life scales to patients to assess how they are faring. Periodically, these instruments can be offered to patients remotely via e-mail or through Web pages so that the data can be incorporated into the medical record. When quality of life assessment results indicate significant problems in an individual patient, the system can signal care managers to consider different interventions.

Patient Satisfaction

Because managed care organizations are increasingly interested in measuring the quality of health services, they are placing more emphasis on assessing patient satisfaction. Health care organizations such as Kaiser Permanente and employers who pay for health care, such as General Motors, are giving patients a "report card" called the Health Plan Employer Data and Information Set (HEDIS) to assess the services rendered by their health care providers. Patients use Likert scales to respond to statements about the health services they have experienced, rating on a numeric scale such things as how long it takes to get an appointment with a primary care physician and how they are treated during their appointments. Depending on who is administering the survey instrument, it may be provided by regular mail, by electronic means, or in the waiting room while the patient is onsite. After the data are tabulated, some companies use them to demand a return of reimbursements when patient satisfaction does not meet a predetermined standard.

Documenting Interventions

There is a saying in health care, "If it wasn't documented, it wasn't done." Unfortunately, documenting care is time-consuming. When technology is properly put in place for documentation, it prevents extra work and saves time. The ideal system allows documentation to take place as a natural byproduct of patient care. Currently, most documentation is done after hours and is very costly because it involves the use of transcription services.

The best automated documentation system is stylus-based: the clinician or staff person simply touches the computer screen, choosing appropriate options from a pick list to populate a data field. For example, trauma to the lower left quadrant of the abdomen can be documented by one or two touches of the stylus on a computer screen. If a selection item is not available on the pick list, you can use speech recognition to place the nonstandard description into the record. This approach can be done in real-time—so there is no time lag in making the information available—at an approximate rate of 160 words per minute with over 99% accuracy. The combination of a stylus-based documentation system with speech recognition is proving to be one of the most efficient documentation methods available.

One medical record company uses the slogan, "When my last patient leaves, so do I." When documentation is truly a byproduct of providing patient care, it is exciting to see health care practitioners wonder how they ever did without such a system.

The best automated documentation systems combine a stylus-based touch screen and speech recognition technology.

Coding

Coding systems are important tools for documenting medical and drug-related problems and monitoring the effectiveness of interventions. Codes should be suitable not only for scientific studies but also for general use in health care settings and easy to use in a daily routine. It's best for coding systems to be structured as a decision tree so computer-aided versions can be developed. The coding system should consist of three parts[17]:

1. The classification of medical and pharmacy problems.
2. The intervention taken to solve the problem.
3. The degree to which the problem was solved.

Coding applications are currently being integrated into electronic medical records in such a way that appropriate procedural codes are generated at every patient encounter. Most practitioners tend to undercode their procedures because they fear audits that could result in accusations of overbilling. The rules for appropriate coding can be placed in an algorithm that creates defensible billing levels capable of surviving any audit. These software programs can optimize billing codes to achieve higher degrees of intensity, allowing additional revenues to be accrued to a practice. For example, if the coding application in a medical record suggests the evaluation and management code of CPT 99204 (new outpatient, comprehensive history and exam, moderate-complexity medical decision, moderate- to high-severity problem), the same software might suggest that, after a quick evaluation of previous data recorded at earlier visits, the intensity of this visit should be moved to a level reimbursed at 99205.

Intervention and Documentation Programs

We are at a point in time when the question should be asked, "When I am caring for patients, what should my supporting technology be doing?" It is not a question of whether applications exist to support every process—from appraising the patient

We are at a point in time when the question should be asked, "When I am caring for patients, what should my supporting technology be doing?"

through selecting and evaluating interventions and concluding with follow-up care and monitoring. All these applications exist, but they need to be integrated into the workflow of individual practitioners. This is the new frontier—an area under development that is poised for expansion.

Here's an example of the way it works. If a health care provider caring for a patient wants to learn an alternative dosing strategy for a medication, he or she can go online to access a review article, handbook, or textbook. The intervention and documentation program automatically grabs the name of the medication (and any patient information active in the medication field when the query is made) and places it directly into the decision support reference, populating all the appropriate fields. A pick list of alternative therapies that can be used for the same indication appears and equivalent dosing levels are automatically calculated. Voilà!

Thousands of practitioners routinely use applications for pain conversion medication selection in just this way. They input the drug and dose with which the patient is medicated and quickly receive information to help them select a replacement medication, along with equivalent dosing.

The idea behind this type of interactive software is to eliminate the typing of as much free text as possible. The software anticipates the most likely sequence of steps in the documentation process and automatically moves into the appropriate documentation form all the data necessary to complete the documentation process under most circumstances. Practitioners are prompted for any missing data that are necessary to the process.

Some health care software packages manage the entire practice management process and integrate clinical "to do's" into a provider's calendar. For example, if a provider is appraising a pediatric patient diagnosed with asthma, the software will give prompts for questions to ask. Then, if a problem is identified, the software prompts the provider toward evidence-based interventions. After the intervention is initiated, the software requires that the intervention be evaluated at appropriate intervals. When the evaluation is done, the software schedules the patient for monitoring and follow-up. All these functions are integrated into the software's time management features so that providers must respond or be "nagged" until they take the clinically appropriate action.

BOX 4-5

Essential Elements of Documentation

To be effective, documentation systems should offer the following:

- Unique patient identification. Identifies each patient when recording or accessing information—both within and across organizations.
- Accuracy. Promotes accuracy throughout each process: capturing information, generating reports, and transferring information among systems.
- Completeness. Identifies the minimum set of information required to completely describe the incident, observation, or intent and provides a way to ensure that recorded information meets legal, regulatory, institutional, policy, or other requirements for specific reports.
- Timeliness. Facilitates health care documentation during or immediately after each event so that information is recorded when memory is accurate and is immediately available for subsequent care.
- Interoperability across documentation systems. Provides the highest level of interoperability possible and enables authorized practitioners to capture, share, and report information from any system, whether paper or electronic.
- Retrievability. Is in accordance with worldwide consensus on how information should be structured. Requires use of standardized titles, formats, templates, macros, terminology, abbreviations, and coding and enables authorized data searches, indexing, and data mining.
- Authentication and accountability. Uniquely identifies each person, device, and system that creates or generates information, and requires the following:
  —All information is attributable to its source (person or device).
  —Unsigned documents are readily recognizable as such.
  —Providers or attending preceptors must review the documents before authentication.
- Auditability. Allows users to examine basic information elements, such as data fields. Audits access and disclosure of protected health information and alerts users to errors, inappropriate changes, and potential security breaches. Promotes use of performance metrics—key indicators for evaluating clinical performance—as part of audit capacity.
- Confidentiality and security. Adheres to applicable legislation, regulations, guidelines, and policies throughout the documentation process and alerts users to potential breaches of confidentiality and security.

Source: Reference 18.

Automation in Pharmacy Practice

Automated systems—in which machines used to perform work are controlled by a computer—can outperform humans in tasks that require tedious repetition, tiresome movement, intense concentration, immense memory retention, and meticulous record keeping. Automation presents opportunities to reduce errors, increase the volume of work performed, and manage costs in complex health care systems.

As health care tries to grow its capacity to deal with the aging baby boomers, it is experiencing acute shortages of personnel in a wide variety of health care disciplines and specialties. Certain kinds of work are being delegated to automation to help current personnel be more efficient and to allow them to focus more completely on direct patient care, especially where critical shortages exist.

When personnel are freed to provide direct patient care, customer satisfaction and service levels are enhanced. In some instances, new market opportunities emerge when automated systems are fully utilized. For example, one automated system used for dispensing may have the capability of supplying the needs of outpatient pharmacies and clinics in more than five hospitals. Ready-to-use products can be mass-produced and distributed within a system so they are available immediately when needed.

A Look at Automation: Applications in Pharmacy*

Although automation can be employed throughout the entire health care system, we're providing an in-depth look at just one area to give you a sense of automation's benefits. Automated systems fill about 125,000 of the 3 billion prescriptions dispensed annually in the United States to people in the community.[19] The first automated system—which simply counted tablets—was introduced in the 1970s. Roughly one in five independent community pharmacies uses automated dispensing now; in chain pharmacy, 80% of the members of the National Association of Chain Drug Stores have purchased automation for at least one of their pharmacies.[20] Figure 4-2 shows a popular automated prescription dispensing system, the ScriptPro 200.

*Note: This section was written by Kenneth N. Barker, PhD, professor and director of the Center for Pharmacy Operations and Design in the Harrison School of Pharmacy, Auburn University.

FIGURE 4-2

The ScriptPro SP 200 delivers filled, labeled vials at a rate of 100 prescriptions per hour. Bar code controls ensure accuracy. For more information: www.scriptpro.com.

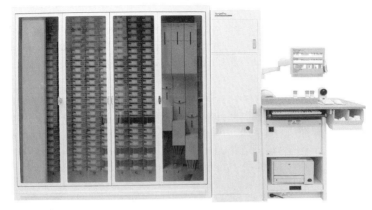

Source: Courtesy of ScriptPro.

Automation supports centralized unit-dose dispensing in 9.4% of hospitals, decentralized drug storage and distribution in 49.2%, production of intravenous medication in 27.5%, and transportation systems such as pneumatic tubes in 29.4%. Automation is more common in larger hospitals and those affiliated with a medical school.[20]

No universal standards exist for automated pharmacy systems, but most state boards of pharmacy have—or are in the process of writing—regulations for use of automated systems. Other groups, too, have taken action, such as the Joint Commission on Accreditation of Healthcare Organizations, which in 1998 published accreditation requirements and standards for automated medication distribution systems.[21] That same year a coalition of pharmacy associations, state boards of pharmacy, and automation industry representatives released the White Paper on Automation in Pharmacy to address quality, safety, manpower, and professional issues.[22]

In pharmacy practice, automation can be used to enhance the following tasks:

- Storage
- Packaging
- Compounding
- Dispensing
- Medication distribution

Systems may be centralized, pharmacy-based devices, or decentralized devices in locations outside the pharmacy, such as nursing units or long-term care facilities. There are two types of pharmacy-based automated pharmacy systems:

1. Systems that repackage medications from bulk.
2. Robotic systems that "overwrap" unit-dose medications in another package that the robot can recognize or manipulate.

Decentralized automated pharmacy systems can be interfaced to a central pharmacy computer to maintain control over drug storage and distribution. Some devices dispense multiple-dose packages, while others dispense unit doses. Some systems package the doses, while others dispense only prepackaged medications.

BOX 4-6

Benefits of Using Automated Pharmacy Systems

- Saves time that pharmacists, technicians, and nurses can devote to other tasks.
- Increases productivity.
- Improves accuracy and reduces medication errors.
- Improves documentation of patient care activities.
- Increases authorized access to both medications and information by requiring user authentication through authorized accounts and passwords for all personnel.
- Enhances security.
- Relieves on-the-job stress, thus reducing pharmacist turnover.

General Steps in the Process

Prescription processing begins when someone enters an order into the pharmacy management computer system. The order is sent to another computer that operates the automated pharmacy system robot, which then initiates these steps: printing barcoded labels and receipts, selecting the prescription bottle, labeling the container, filling, and capping. Before the bottle is capped, the system displays a video image of the drug inside the bottle for the pharmacist to check after he or she scans the bar code linked to that bottle. Other tasks the technology contributes to include pricing the prescription, adjusting the inventory, documenting the transaction, and billing the third-party payer.

Mail Service Pharmacy

Mail service pharmacies use "assembly line" automated drug distribution systems to dispense prescriptions, which are checked by a pharmacist and mailed with patient information directly to the patient. Mail service pharmacy has taken advantage of the economies of scale offered by automation, and is attractive for serving some patients with chronic diseases who are taking maintenance medication and need to have prescriptions delivered to their homes.

In large, fully automated mail service pharmacies, the patient medication database is integrated with automated drug distribution systems to dispense thousands of prescriptions per day. In the Veterans Affairs (VA) system, consolidated mail outpatient pharmacies (CMOPs) across the country use automation to fill 8000 to 10,000 prescriptions in a 10-hour day, freeing pharmacists to spend more time on direct patient care.[23]

Here's how the system works[24]:

- Medication orders are entered into patient databases at the local VA medical center and are electronically transmitted to the CMOP.
- A CMOP technician scans the bar code of a tote bin that will hold all items to be dispensed to an individual patient.
- A computer screen indicates which items are needed to fulfill a complete order for the patient. Each item is verified for accuracy against the original order as the tote proceeds.
- The technician places the tote on a conveyor belt, where prepackaged items in racks overhead are automatically dispensed onto part of the belt the computer has designated for the order.
- The machine sends the items through a chute into the appropriate tote.
- The tote travels to the final dispensing area, where the automated bottle filler scans it to determine which oral solids (tablets, capsules) are to be dispensed.
- The machine prints a label containing both patient and medication information and applies it to the plastic vial for each medication.
- The machine fills and caps each vial (see Figure 4-3).
- Before releasing the vial, the computer verifies the tablet count, cap integrity, and label placement.
- When the order is complete, a pharmacist checks the items and sends the tote to technicians who prepare the medications for mailing.

FIGURE 4-3

Automated filling and capping of vial.

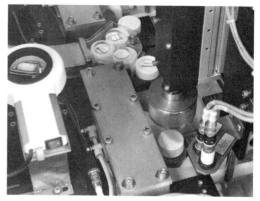

Source: Courtesy of AutoMed Technologies, Inc.

Pharmacy Automation in Institutions

Hospitals and long-term care pharmacies use a variety of centralized automated pharmacy systems, integrated with the pharmacy information system, to repackage and label solid oral medications. These systems count, package, and label medication (including patient, date, and time) in unit-dose, multidose, or patient "med packs"—in which all medications for a particular administration time are packaged together. Steps in these systems include the following:

- Technicians manually load bulk medications into individual, medication-specific canisters calibrated according to the size and shape of the specific drug product. Each canister will fit only into its assigned location (see Figure 4-4).
- Some systems incorporate bar-code labeling on the canister, which can be scanned against the bulk medication supply to ensure accuracy.
- With information downloaded from the pharmacy information system, the automated system packages medication in unit-dose packets, labels each packet with the required information, and dispenses medications in the order in which they appear on the fill list.
- To fill patient medication cassettes in unit-dose medication carts, which hold all doses for administration to an individual patient, integrated robotic systems receive orders from the pharmacy's medication dispensing system. They process orders

efficiently and accurately and read bar-coded, overwrapped, unit-dose packages to organize them for patient administration. These systems also can return unused medications to stock and handle injectables, suppositories, and liquid unit-dose containers in addition to oral solids.

Comprehensive, electronically sophisticated automated pharmacy systems count, package, and label patient-specific medications in unit-of-use envelopes and sort the envelopes by patient in the order in which they are to be administered. These systems can be used centrally in the pharmacy or in decentralized patient care areas. Decentralized systems in nursing units feature dispensing cabinets similar to automated teller machines (ATMs) in banks, which offer secure, computer-controlled access to medications and supplies.

If the decentralized system is linked with the pharmacy computer system, the nurse can request a medication dose as soon as a prescriber inputs an order and the pharmacy verifies it. There are also mobile dispensing cabinets that can be moved from bedside to bedside. Computer terminals can be mounted on these cabinets, from which personnel can enter and review medication orders (see Figure 4-5). An important optional feature allows the dose being administered at the patient's bedside to be checked by bar code.

FIGURE 4-4	**FIGURE 4-5**
A canister fitted snugly in its position.	An ATM-like dispensing cabinet and mobile bedside unit with a computer terminal.

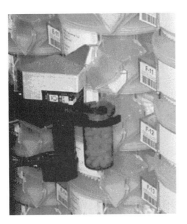

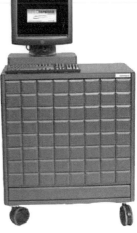

BOX 4-7

Integrated Drug Distribution on the Horizon

Today, automated systems are being planned to meet the needs of an entire community by providing seamless distribution of medications to primary care clinics, hospitals, long-term care facilities, and private homes. This concept, known as integrated drug distribution, allows large health care systems to refill drug distribution machines at sites where care is delivered, so patients receive the medications they need on time.

In the central fill concept, another type of integrated drug distribution, a group of pharmacies operates one high-volume dispensing facility where prescriptions are filled and then delivered to the patient's local pharmacy. Telepharmacy, which provides medications from a distance by remotely controlled dispensing technology, has been shown by the Veterans Healthcare System and others to be a workable way of providing pharmacy services to sites where demand is too small to justify employing a pharmacist.

Source: References 25 and 26.

Automation and Patient Medication Safety

In 1999, the death rate associated with medication errors in hospitals was estimated to be about 7000 per year.[27] In 2002, when researchers studied the relative frequency of medication errors in 36 hospitals and skilled nursing facilities in Georgia and Colorado, they found errors in almost one of every five doses. The percentage of these errors rated "potentially harmful" was 7%, or more than 40 per day in a typical 300-patient facility.[28]

In 2003, a study of 50 community pharmacies in six major cities found that 1.7% of prescriptions filled contained one or more errors—a rate of about four per day in a pharmacy filling 250 prescriptions daily. The percentage rated "potentially harmful" was 7%. Given that 3 billion prescriptions are filled annually in the United States, these findings suggest that 51.5 million contain one or more errors, of which 3.3 million are potentially dangerous.[29]

Evidence suggests that automation could prevent many of these errors. In a prospective, controlled clinical trial conducted in 1969, the error rate declined from 13% to 1.9% when a system was introduced where dispensing envelopes were attached by a fastener to the patient profile. The envelopes, containing unit doses, were labeled with the complete physician's order and

BOX 4-8

Bar Codes

Bar codes are a great way for machines to identify all kind of products—including medications—throughout the manufacturing, wholesaling, and dispensing process. In community pharmacy practice, the benefits of bar coding appear so evident and achievable that three major organizations, the American Pharmacists Association, the National Association of Chain Drug Stores, and the National Community Pharmacists Association joined in recommending the use of bar code verification in all pharmacy practices by 2006.

In hospital pharmacy practice, bar coding drug products at the unit-dose level is attractive in theory, but the complexity involved has thwarted years of attempts to achieve this goal. Among problems to overcome are the small size of unit-dose packaging, the pharmaceutical industry's unwillingness to offer larger packages, barriers to a standardized approach, and hospitals' reluctance to pay the extra cost when they can save money through in-house packaging.

Source: References 30 and 31.

delivered to the patients' bedside for administration.[32] In 1975, a similar system reduced the error rate from 7.35% to 1.61%,[33] and in 1984 at a medical-surgical nursing unit, a bedside unit-dose dispensing machine system controlled by a pharmacy computer reduced the error rate from 15.9% to 10.6%.[34]

More recently (1995), two studies found that using automated Pyxis devices reduced errors from 16.3% to 5.4%[35] and 16.9% down to 10.4%.[36] Studies underway at Auburn University have demonstrated that using the ScriptPro automated system reduced the rate of dispensing errors from 2.8% to 2.1% in an independent pharmacy and from 0.3% to zero in a chain pharmacy.[37]

Health Care Informatics Technology on the Horizon

Health care is continually moving toward becoming a truly digital industry where systems are paperless and integration is at high levels. Technologies that can improve efficiency and patient care quality are readily available. Industry observers think we have reached a "tipping point" with regard to the readiness of health care personnel and patients to embrace new systems.

BOX 4-9

Error-Reduction Features in Automated Pharmacy Systems

Research shows that the following features in automated pharmacy systems are useful for reducing errors:

- **Comprehensive controls.** Decision-support software, bar codes, and wireless connectivity to confirm order status are used right from when orders are entered to the point where medications are dispensed or administered, and are integrated with the pharmacy or facility information system.
- **Electronic identification.** All components, including the drug, patient, and person dispensing, are identified by electronic means, such as bar coding.
- **Limited access.** Access to medications is limited through the use of lockable security cabinets and software-controlled access to operate the technology. Controlled substances are accessible only when a patient needs them, and only by authorized personnel.
- **Automatic documentation.** When medications are dispensed and administered, the system captures and stores this information automatically.
- **Immediate access to drug use information.** Leaflets and references to support provider decision making are provided where medication is dispensed. Access is immediate, in both electronic and print formats.
- **Labeling.** A labeling machine prints labels or medications and supplies, which are then affixed to products.
- **Secure controls.** When someone overrides a function in the system, it immediately emits a visible or audible signal. The system also documents the override electronically.

Source: Reference 38.

New technologies such as radio frequency identification (RFID) are moving rapidly into health care settings. These small chips that send out a signal to scanners are quickly helping authenticate and locate patients, providers, and equipment in organizations. Biometric scanners are replacing digital signatures by reading fingerprints or retinas rather than using the slower approaches of user ID and password authentication. Patients are receiving increasing access to their own medical records and some organizations are issuing affinity cards that identify patients as they enter a building and even give them the ability to transfer medical records access to medical specialists or emergency departments they may visit in other parts of the country.

Chapter 16 provides more detail on the future of health care technology. An important factor is for organizations to promote a culture where change is embraced and is seen as a constant, expected part of doing business. They need to resist the temptation to wait for "perfect" systems to be developed before taking action and adopting technology.

> Organizations must promote a culture in which change is embraced and seen as a constant, expected part of doing business.

ACTIVITY 4-1

Familiarize Yourself with Software, Systems, Planning, and Training

1. Create a listing of all major hardware and software systems that support patient care delivery in your practice. Determine which are interfaced and/or fully integrated. Add to this list all vendors that have interfaced new products to your existing systems.
2. Use the advanced search feature of the Google search engine, with the "file format desired" set to PowerPoint. Search for the phrase "health care information systems" and create a PowerPoint presentation that describes the opportunities offered by information technology within your practice setting.
3. Construct a diagram of the computer system network in your organization using the example provided in Figure 4-1. Try to map out information flow, personnel involved, and major departments in your organization
4. Identify a progressive health care organization geographically close to your location. Perform a site visit with a counterpart in that organization to see how other health care practices manage information systems.
5. Create an information systems business plan for a new service offered in your practice. If you are unfamiliar with how to create a business plan, go to www.google.com and type in the search text "how to write a business plan" to locate samples and assistance in business planning.
6. Evaluate how training was used to support the implementation of your last hardware or software installation in your practice. Determine what should be done differently for both short-term and long-term support if a new hardware or software system were to be installed in the near future.
7. Determine the composition of the ideal Information Technology Advisory Committee for your organization. To be a workable committee, it should have a representative from every functional unit. You should begin with a needs assessment and identify barriers as well as perceived opportunities for enhancing operations.

References

1. Felkey BG, Barker KN. The power of information in an integrated health care system. *Am J Health Syst Pharm.* March 1995;52(5):537-40.

2. Arndt KA. Information excess in medicine. Overview, relevance to dermatology, and strategies for coping. *Arch Dermatol.* 1992;128:1249-56.

3. Davidoff F, Haynes B, Sackett D, et al. Evidence based medicine. *BMJ.* 1995;310:1085-6.

4. Felkey BG. The role of the home of medical and from medical informatics in future healthcare systems. *Int Pharm J.* 1995;9:108.

5. Knowlton CH, Penna RP. *Pharmaceutical Care.* 2nd ed. Bethesda, MD: American Society of Health-System Pharmacists; 2003.

6. Felkey BG, Buring SM. Using the Internet for research. *J Am Pharm Assoc.* 2000;40:546.

7. Brown E. EMRs for small physician groups. Forrester Research Report. December 2003; 21. Available at: www.forrester.com/ER/Research/Report/ Summary/0,1338,16518,00.html. Accessed December 21, 2004.

8. Felkey BG. Building the clinical workstation: software for the health-system pharmacist. *Am J Health Syst Pharm.* 1997;54:1505.

9. Davidoff F. In the teeth of the evidence: the curious case of evidence-based medicine. *Mt Sinai J Med.* 1999;66:75.

10. Taylor H. Explosive growth of "cyberchondriacs" continues. Available at: www.harrisinteractive.com/harris_poll/index.asp?PID=104%20. Accessed March 25, 2003.

11. Eysenbach G, Powell J, Kuss O, et al. Empirical studies assessing the quality of health information for consumers on the World Wide Web: a systematic review. *JAMA.* 2002;287(20):2691.

12. Felkey BG, Fox BI. Using the Internet to enhance pharmacy-based patient care services. *J Am Pharm Assoc.* 2001;41:529.

13. Grover F, Grover F Jr, Wu HD, et al. Computer-using patients want Internet services from family physicians. *J Fam Pract.* 2002;51(6):570.

14. American Medical Association. Guidelines for Physician-Patient Electronic Communications. Available at: www.ama-assn.org/ama/pub/category/2386.html. Accessed July 7, 2005.

15. Anand SG, Feldman MJ, Geller DS, et al. A content analysis of e-mail communication between primary care providers and parents. *Pediatrics.* 2005;115(5):1283-8.

16. Felkey BG, Fox BI. *Pharmacotherapy Self Assessment Program.* 4th ed. Kansas City, MO: American College of Clinical Pharmacy; 2001:117-143

17. Field MJ, Grigsby J. Telemedicine and remote patient monitoring. *JAMA.* 2002;288(4):423.

18. Silverman M. Choosing the right outcomes. *Allergy.* 1999;54(49):35.

19. Levy S. *Drug Topics.* May 21, 2001:46-8.

20. Automation in pharmacy initiative: white paper on automation in pharmacy. Proceedings from the Sesquicentennial Stepping Stone Summit One. *J Am Pharm Assoc.* 2003;43:140-7.

21. *Technological Solutions to Standard Compliance: Automated Dispensing* [audiotape]. Oakbrook Terrace, IL: Joint Commission on Accreditation of Healthcare Organizations; 2000.

22. Schacht HM, Dorup J. Wireless access to a pharmaceutical database. *J Med Internet Res.* 2001;3(1):4.

23. Gostin LO. National health information privacy: regulations under the Health Insurance Portability and Accountability Act. *JAMA.* 2001;285(23):3015.

24. Schaefer M. Discussing basic principles for a coding system of drug related problems: the case of PI-Doc. *Pharm World Sci.* 2002;24(4):120.

25. Data from Tessier C. The continuity of care record. *Healthc Inform.* 2003;20:87.

26. Landis NT. Patient care fills out VA pharmacists' schedule, as automation lifts the dispensing load. *Am J Health Syst Pharm.* 1995;52:584,587-8.

27. Johnson CL, Carlson RA, Tucker CL, et al. Using BCMA software to improve patient safety in Veterans Administration medical centers. Proceedings of Bar Code Administration Conference; April 25, 2003:12-4.

28. Knapp DA. Professionally determined need for pharmacy services in 2020: report of a conference sponsored by the Pharmacy Manpower Project, Inc. March 25, 2003:1-22. Available at: http:/ courses.washington.edu/pharm560/ CRPC/4634_needsconferencefinalreport.pdf. Accessed December 21, 2004.

29. Kohn LT, Corrigan JM, Donaldson MS. *To Err Is Human.* Washington, DC: National Academy Press; 1999.

30. Rupp MT. *America's Pharm.* January 2002:11-3.

31. Ringold DB, Santell JP, Schneider PJ. ASHP national survey of pharmacy practice in acute care settings: dispensing and administration. *Am J Health Syst Pharm.* 2000;57:1759-75.

32. Barker KN, Flynn EA, Pepper GA, et al. Observation method of detecting medication errors. *Arch Intern Med.* 2002;162:1897-903.

33. Flynn EA, Barker KN, Carnahan BJ. National observation study on dispensing accuracy in 50 pharmacies. *J Am Pharm Assoc.* 2002;43:191-200.

34. Barker KN. The effects of a medication error system on medication errors and cost. *Am J Hosp Pharm.* 1969;26:324-33.

35. Means BJ, Derewicz HJ, Lamy PP. Medication errors in a multidose and a computer-based unit dose dispensing system. *Am J Hosp Pharm.* 1975;32:186-91.

36. Barker KN, Pearson RE, Hepler CD, et al. Effect of an automated bedside dispensing machine on medication errors. *Am J Hosp Pharm.* 1984;41:1352-8.

37. Borel JM, Rascati KL. Effect of an automated, unit-based dispensing system on medication errors. *Am J Health Syst Pharm.* 1995;52:1875-9.

38. American Society of Health-System Pharmacists. Report of the Joint Commission on Accreditation in Healthcare Organizations. *Am J Health Syst Pharm.* 1998;55:1403-7.

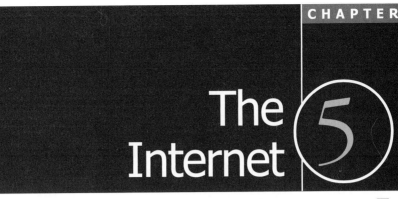

The Internet 5

Bill G. Felkey

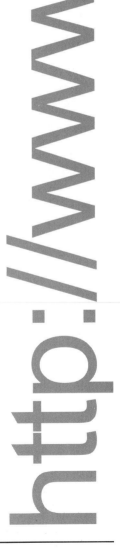

Chapter Objectives

After completing this chapter, you should be able to:

■ Describe how the Internet was formed and how it evolved to its present-day configuration.

■ Describe functions you can use your browser for.

■ Describe functions you can use a search engine for.

■ Discuss the four main types of Web sites.

■ Describe the advantages of a Netcentric, patient-focused approach.

■ Explain the purpose of the Internet2 consortium.

We used to think of the Internet as a network in which every computer in the world is communicating with every other computer. Today, we define the Internet as every computer, cell phone, personal digital assistant, and pager in the world talking to every other computer, cell phone, personal digital assistant, and pager in the world.[1] In 2005, 935 million users in over 200 countries were actively using the Internet. Projections have the number of Internet users at 1.35 billion in 2007.

However, most people don't realize that the development of what today is commonly called the Internet began with Sputnik. In 1958—after the USSR launched the first satellite into space—the United States formed the Advanced Research Projects Agency (ARPA). The mission of ARPA was to regain a U.S. global technological lead in all things military.

By the 1960s, many researchers believed that the typical U.S. configuration of large, centrally formed communications networks was vulnerable to nuclear attacks. As a result, ARPA underwrote several projects aimed at developing a decentralized communication network. The network eventually called ARPANET represents the earliest known infrastructure of what would eventually be renamed the Internet.

In the 1970s, major U.S. and international research universities were connected by computer through the ARPANET, and similar commercial networks began emerging. The first e-mail was sent and the first reported use of emoticons began—those little sideways faces such as :) (smiling) and ;) (winking).

During the 1980s, ARPANET was halted by the accidental introduction of a virus. Although communication was interrupted for a brief time, the network was restored and safeguards were installed to prevent future attacks. Domain name servers (DNS) were introduced, and more than 1000 host computers were on ARPANET—a number that by the end of the 1980s grew to more than 100,000 computers in over 10 countries. Conferences and academic studies relating to the communication protocols promulgated on ARPANET occurred regularly.

In the beginning of the 1990s, ARPANET officially closed and Internet telephone dial-up access started being offered. Although the word "Internet" was used in the late 1980s, it wasn't taken up by the media and public until the early 1990s. In 1991, the term "World Wide Web" was coined and a congressional act, called the U.S. High-Performance Computing Act (sponsored by Sen. Al Gore), established the National Research and Education Network. Faster access, the Internet Society (formed to oversee standards used on the network), and over a million host computers were in place by 1992. By 1994, you could order pizza online in some U.S. cities, and by the end of the 1990s, the Internet was exploding globally, with hundreds of millions of connected computers.

Infrastructure of the Internet

Nobody owns the Internet. It is a vast entity that spans the globe and even jumps off the planet through orbiting satellites. Every device and computer that connects to the Internet is a part of a small network. Internet service providers (ISPs) host small networks to give us access to the overall Internet. Small networks connect to larger networks; the very largest networks on the Internet are described as backbones.

Routers, another important part of the Internet's infrastructure, send data traffic through computers and networks to the destination that the sender intends. Every device on the Internet has a distinct Internet Protocol (IP) number, also called a machine address, which you can think of as being synonymous with a telephone number. An example of a typical IP would be 131.207.38.128.

Because these IP numbers would be difficult to remember, a system of domain names was created to provide unique identifiers for each Internet site. An example of a domain name is IBM.com. The domain name is part of a Web site's uniform resource locator (URL) or "address." IBM's URL is http://www.IBM.com.

Initially, some users feared that the infrastructure of the Internet would collapse from a lack of capacity. Fortunately, large fiber-optic backbones provide the capability for managing data in large volumes for the foreseeable future. Huge Internet servers make global communication instantaneous, and even high-demand telecommunication traffic, such as transmittal of digital movies, can be accomplished for millions of users.

Communication Protocols

Because there are so many different computer systems and devices in the world, many different communication protocols have been developed—a concept akin to languages in human speech. One communication protocol that came out of the Internet's formation was Transmission Control Protocol/Internet

Some users feared that the infrastructure of the Internet would collapse from a lack of capacity. Fortunately, large fiber-optic backbones provide the capability for managing data in large volumes for the foreseeable future.

Protocol (TCP/IP), which today is the universal "language" of the Internet. This means that huge mainframe computers and tiny cellular telephone devices are all built to communicate via TCP/IP.

TCP/IP supports many functions of the Internet, including:

- File Transfer Protocol (FTP), which allows Internet users to share documents and applications.
- TELNET, which allows remote access to computers via the Internet.
- Electronic mail messaging, which generally runs on TCP/IP protocol.
- USENET News, which creates communities of Internet users with common interests who subscribe to posted news and discussion issues.
- Hypertext Markup Language (HTML), which displays content in a specific format used in creating Web pages and other information that is viewable in a browser.

> Today's Internet browsers combine graphical capability, sound, and video in a fairly intuitive, single application.

Browsers

A browser is a software application used to display Web pages. The most popular browsers today are Microsoft Internet Explorer and Netscape Navigator. Other good ones are available as well, such as Mozilla Firefox and Avant. Today's Internet browsers combine graphical capability, sound, and video in a fairly intuitive, single application. Instead of typing out syntax-specific instructions and commands, you can click with a pointing device to transfer or copy files and perform many other useful functions.

Intranets

Organizations that use the Internet need to add extra layers of security to protect their privacy and confidentiality. For this reason, intranets—which use the backbone of the Internet for data transmission—provide closed-access security through user identification, passwords, and machine-specific restrictions. Intranets typically operate through the Internet but are secured by organizations. This security, called a firewall, combines both hardware and software to keep out unwanted intruders.

Extranets

Extranets provide organizations with another type of connectivity and, like intranets, are not open to public viewing. In essence, an extranet is an intranet that is partially acces-

ACTIVITY 5-1

Becoming Familiar with Browser Functions

Carry out the tasks below to make sure you know how to do key functions in your Web browser.

- Go to a specific Web address.
- Identify and open a hyperlink—a word or phrase that is underlined to allow you to link (move) to another location on the Internet.
- Go backward and forward in this sequence by using the Back and Forward buttons of your browser.
- Add a Bookmark or Favorite by clicking on the browser button labeled as one of these two words.
- Organize Bookmarks or Favorites by using the Help function of your browser to explain how to do this function.
- Turn off images on Web pages for faster viewing using these steps:
  1. On the Tools menu, click Internet Options.
  2. Click the Advanced tab.
  3. Under Multimedia, clear one or more of these check boxes: Show Pictures, Play Animations, Play Videos, or Play Sounds.
- Save images from a Web site to your PC by right-clicking on an image and saving it in your My Pictures folder.
- Interrupt a page download using the Stop feature—the button depicting a big red "x" on a piece of paper in your browser tool bar.
- Find a particular word on a Web page by holding the Ctrl key and the "f" key at the same time to produce a search box.
- Open multiple windows in your browser by clicking on the "File" pulldown menu, then clicking New and then Window. Resize the two windows so you can see them both without overlap, which is useful for comparing two Web pages.

sible to authorized outsiders, such as business partners and suppliers. A drug wholesaler may need to connect to a health system via an extranet to maintain a "just-in-time" inventory. As the health system uses goods for patient care, messages are sent to the supplier to indicate that the health system needs replenishment of product inventory. Patient identities and other protected details should never appear among this information.

Internet Connection Options

An important aspect of the Internet is how you connect to it. Options today range from old-fashioned dial-up, the cheapest and slowest method, to broadband and wireless. Table 5-1 lists the various options available today.

Creating a Web Presence

Have you ever been embarrassed by having to tell someone who asked for your business card that you don't have one? In today's world, not having a Web presence indicates that your business or practice is not really a going concern. When potential patients move into your community, it's possible that they will select health care providers based entirely on their Web presence. For example, a mother might enter "pediatrician" and "Detroit Michigan" into a search engine on the Internet and choose her children's physician from that list. Most consumers will not search beyond the first 20 "hits" that a search engine locates. This reality has brought about a type of business called "Internet optimization services" that use keywords and other strategies to procure a high ranking in the results of popular search engines, thus driving more traffic to the Web site.

Publish Stage

Nearly every professional Web presence starts with a place-holder Web site. This is known as the publish stage. (Very simple place-holder sites are often referred to as a Web page. "Web site" and "Web page" tend to be used interchangeably, but the latter actually refers to one document in a Web site, which is an entire collection of Web pages for a specific organization). These place-holder Web sites have static text and photographs that acquaint you with the name, logo, address, telephone number, and mission of the organization. This level of Web site seems to suffice for some groups because it creates a presence, no matter how small. Many people believe that Web sites are a better return on investment than Yellow Page ads in the telephone book.

Interact Stage

The next stage of Web development attempts to engage constituencies through interaction. Adding useful information and ways to connect with an organization 24/7 is both a service to users and a promotional tool for the organization. Interactive features may be things that take work out of the practice, such as having patients fill

TABLE 5-1

Characteristics of Internet Connection Options

Type	Speed Down/Up (approx)	Time to Download 10 MB file (minutes)	Price (per month)	Pro	Con	Urban	Suburb	Rural	Home	Power User	Office
Cable	200 KBps–30 MBps/128 KBps–3 MBps	1.4	$30–$55	Blazing downloads; comparatively quick installation	Limited upload speed; bandwidth sharing can degrade performance	Good	Good	Poor	Good	Good	Satisfactory
DSL	144 KBps–8 MBps/128 KBps–8 MBps	1.8	$29–$500	Variable-bandwidth services can be tailored to your needs and budget	Higher bandwidth costs more; sometimes difficult installation	Good	Good	Poor	Good	Good	Good
Fixed wireless	500 KBps/150 KBps	2.7	$60	Nice if you can get it	Not yet widely available	Poor	Poor	Poor	Satisfactory	Good	Good
Satellite	400 KBps–500 KBps/28.8 KBps–256 KBps	3.4	$30–$80	New bidirectional services bring DSL-like speeds to rural users	Inexpensive one-way service requires dial-up modem for upstream communication	Good	Good	Good	Satisfactory	Poor	Poor
ISDN	128 KBps/128 KBps	10.7	$70–$150	Provides two analog lines or a 128-kbps Internet connection	Not fast enough for the price	Good	Good	Satisfactory	Satisfactory	Poor	Satisfactory
Analog Dial-up	56 KBps/33.6 KBps	28.4	$8.95–$24.95	Cheapest Internet connection	Provides a fraction of broadband speed	Excellent	Excellent	Excellent	Satisfactory	Poor	Poor

Source: Reference 3.

out online forms before office visits or providing interactive health assessments that engage patients with information on key lifestyle changes. Health care professionals might benefit from interactive surveys that match a person's continuing education needs with available programming. Anything that begins to customize the Web experience while avoiding the "one-size-fits-all" approach to disseminating information is an improvement over static information.

Transact Stage

Today, Web pages can perform transactions that significantly reduce the need for personnel involvement. For example, the ability to book flights and make hotel reservations online without human assistance has had a major effect on the travel industry. Initially, airlines gave consumers incentives to book flights online—incentives that were removed as people became comfortable with the transactional process. Now travelers seeking the lowest fares often have no choice but to book online.

Web sites that are at the transact stage integrate Internet resources into daily operations. A good example in health care would be having patients use an online scheduling application—which also decreases the use of personnel—or displaying pictures of newborn infants on a hospital site, which is becoming a popular way for family members who live far away to view their new relatives.

Anything that allows patients to do business with a health care organization without the need for human intervention can have a positive effect on the overall cost of rendering care. In every planning session, organizations should ask, "How can we use the Internet to do (or support) this process in our organization?"

> Anything that allows patients to do business with a health care organization without the need for human intervention can have a positive effect on the overall cost of rendering care. In every planning session, organizations should ask, "How can we use the Internet to do (or support) this process in our organization?"

Integrate Stage

The ability to integrate online transactions with management systems enhances customer support. For example, a hospital can be more efficient by allowing ambulatory surgery patients to register online and transferring the data directly into scheduling systems. Consumers, when surveyed, fully expect that health care will offer these levels of connectivity, like the banking and finance industries do. They want to have the option of using the Internet to interact with their own medical records and with health care professionals.

Transform Stage

Many organizations now want to integrate the Internet into all aspects of their service offerings. They realize that not all customers use the computer but they understand that the Internet provides an opportunity to enhance service levels and lower the costs of transactions.

It has been found that patients and physicians are both willing to substitute face-to-face office visits with online visits when appropriate. This type of interaction has been well received by California citizens, managed care organizations, and physicians involved with the USCF Stanford Health Care System.

Pharmacists, too, can offer a full level of patient care services using telecommunication channels. For example, through its Web site and e-mail, Walgreens accepts prescription refill requests, answers patients' drug-related questions, and displays potential interactions between over-the-counter medicines and prescription medicines. Nurses are using videoconference equipment placed in the home to provide care to high-risk patients and to determine when patients need face-to-face care. Organizations are moving toward a single, Web-based, electronic medical record for each patient that covers both inpatient and ambulatory care.

TABLE 5-2

Stages of Maturity of Health Care Web Sites

Stage	Description
Publish	Build Web awareness and a presence with customers and employers by publishing static information.
Interact	Engage the community by providing relevant information; enable the community to interact with the site and the organization.
Transact	Deploy robust self-service capabilities and online transactions.
Integrate	Integrate automated transactions in an effort to automate the entire array of business functions.
Transform	Transform the enterprise by seamlessly integrating all processes through end-to-end, Web-based interactions with customers and business partners.

Source: First Consulting Group and Cisco Systems. Adapted with permission from HEALTHvision.

ACTIVITY 5-2

Establishing a Web Presence

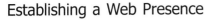

1. Investigate the availability of a desirable Internet domain name that you want to purchase.
2. Investigate the cost of a commercial Web hosting service to house a Web site you would like to create.
3. Determine the cost of an optimization service to increase the likelihood that your Web site will be highly placed in Internet search results.

To do this, they use a framework known as enterprise information technology architecture,[2] which pulls various functions and processes together in one place.Table 5-2 on page 117 defines the stages of maturity of health care Web sites.

Fundamentals for Establishing a Web Site

Establishing a Web site is initially a business decision. Organizations with limited resources need to decide whether a Web presence is consistent with the business image of the practice and is an appropriate way to spend money when compared with other potential expenditure areas. Because the Web presence may be the public's first (and only) impression of your organization, we recommend that you take care to ensure that your Web site transmits the kind of image you want. Developing a Web site is an excellent opportunity for an organization to revisit or even update its mission and goals.

Establishing a Web site is initially a business decision. Organizations with limited resources need to decide whether a Web presence is consistent with the business image of the practice and is an appropriate way to spend money when compared with other potential expenditure areas.

Domain Names

Establishing a Web presence for either personal or professional purposes starts with acquiring a domain name. Traditionally, domain names or Uniform Resource Locators (URLs) have three parts. The first is "www," which stands for World Wide Web. This is followed by brief wording that usually represents the organization name (e.g., Auburn, IBM, WalMart, etc.). The third part of the URL typically tells you what kind of organization owns the Web site, such as university (edu), government (gov), or business (com). A fourth designation can sometimes be found that informs you about the organization's country of origin, such as uk for the United Kingdom or ca for Canada.

Domain names can be acquired through Web sites such as www.register.com for approximately $35 per year and are usually maintained for a 2-year period. They must be reregistered or they will be made available to others who wish to take over that name.

Most U.S. Web sites do not carry a country designator associated with their domain names. Many businesses in foreign countries are registering U.S.-looking domain names that make the sites appear to be physically located in the United States. For example, one health care practitioner in New Zealand is selling wines from his vineyards through a .com Web page, which at a glance looks like it could be in the United States because it does not have a country designator. Only a few companies, such as Underwriters Laboratories, include the .us country code in their addresses.

Interestingly, many associations were a little slow when domain name registration became available, so their URLs are not always what you would expect. For example, www.ama.org was snapped by the American Marketing Association before the American Medical Association tried to acquire it, so you have to access the latter group at www.ama-assn.org.

Web Site Hosting

When an Internet user enters a Web site address (URL) into a browser, a computer called a domain name server (DNS) looks at the URL and connects the user to the designated computer on the Internet that "hosts" the Web site. Some Web sites are small enough and receive low enough traffic that users on a continuous connection to the Internet (such as a cable modem, local area network [LAN], or digital subscriber line [DSL]) register their domain names to their own computers. Each computer on the Internet has a specific number that can be permanently or temporarily assigned when the computer accesses the Internet.

High-traffic Web sites require large-capacity, high-speed servers. These servers offer high-bandwidth connectivity and redundant backup so that users gain easy access to Web sites.

Web hosting services also offer complementary features and tools. For example, one computer hosting company we are familiar with charges subscribers $7.95 per month for 500 MB of Web page content storage. For this price, the hosting company also will create and manage up to 300 separate e-mail accounts and provide unlimited transfer of data (uploading data to the server and downloading data from the server), multimedia capabilities, content subscriptions for news and issues, registration on popular search engines, and a shopping cart capability for e-commerce transactions performed on the site.

When shopping for a Web host, locate the subscription service with the best features first. Then, determine if the business will be around in the years to come. You can start your selection process with a Web search, but you should do a good deal of comparison shopping for the features offered and check to see that the hosting company is financially viable before making a final selection.

Web Page Authoring

When creating a Web site, your first decision is whether to buy it or build it. Constructing a Web site can be highly rewarding but

> When shopping for a Web host, check its financial viability, and compare the features it offers with those of other hosting services.

Preregistering patients for office visits, registering meeting attendees, purchasing transactions, and thousands of other uses are waiting for what we call "aha moments" when we realize that the Internet is a solution looking for problems.

time-consuming. As the Internet has grown in popularity, productivity tools such as word processors, spreadsheets, databases, and presentation programs have been developed that easily create "Internet ready" documents. For example, Microsoft Word has a Web page wizard that will help you create a complete Web site. However, it doesn't contain all the bells and whistles that programs like Microsoft FrontPage, Dreamweaver, and others offer.

If you hire Web masters to create your Web site, count on spending at least $500 to $1000 for a reasonably complex startup site. Change orders and updates are usually billed at an hourly rate of $75 to $110.

Netcentric, Patient-Focused Thinking

Everyone, from health system corporate leadership to entry-level office staff, should be trained to think about what things the organization can present on the Internet. Remember, a great deal of work can be delegated to Web transactions. Preregistering patients for office visits, registering meeting attendees, purchasing transactions, and thousands of other uses are waiting for what we call "aha moments" when we realize that the Internet is a solution looking for problems.

FIGURE 5-1

The structure of a netcentric, patient-focused strategy.

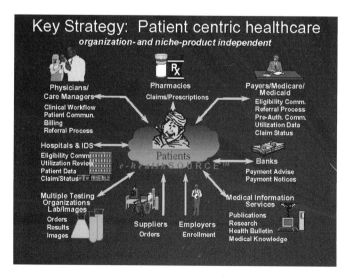

Source: Reprinted with permission from HEALTHvision.

A netcentric approach assumes that all aspects of patient care delivery and business processes will be conducted on the Internet in the near future. As seen in Figure 5-1 on page 120, many innovative health systems using a Web-based approach can be highly patient-focused. The patient-focused strategy to enhancing an organization's operations begins with a question: "Of all of the things we could do to improve our organization, what would benefit the

BOX 5-1

Internet Health Care Web Site Profiles

Here's a detailed overview of two useful Web sites that also happen to be among the most popular sites with patients.

eDiets.com

With over 1.3 million subscribing members and 13 million opt-in registrants, eDiets was rated by ClickZ Network, which monitors traffic on the Internet, as the most active Web site in the health care market in 2003. It's easy to see why—the majority of Americans say that weight management is their highest disease management concern. In addition, membership costs as little as $5 per week. The site uses a personalized assessment to analyze user preferences and offers a variety of plans and menus. Besides receiving customized diet recommendations and newsletters, members can share in a community forum with other eDieters.

The Web site's stated mission is, "building a global online diet, fitness, and motivation destination to provide consumers with solutions that help them realize life's full potential." The company was formed in 1996 and is staffed by licensed dietitians and psychologists.

WebMD.com

WebMD, a highly visited health destination for both professionals and patients, has more than 5000 employees and 12 million registered users. Registration is required for users, but many services are free. Initially, WebMD Corporation sought to serve as a link for all clinical and business processes in health care, helping to streamline administrative and clinical processes. The company has had to push back its timetable for achieving this lofty goal, but the site remains popular for health information.

Medscape is a WebMD service that gives health professionals access to continuing education, specialized resources, conference coverage, patient information, and expert advice. With a membership of more than 575,000 physicians and 1.6 million allied health care professionals worldwide, Medscape reaches more health care providers than any other online professional destination.

Source: References 4, 5, and 6.

patients we serve to the greatest extent?" With all the excitement of using technology, we should never lose sight of the fact that its purpose is to relieve human suffering and increase the quality of life of patients.

When you make patients the central focus in a health care system, several obvious Internet applications become apparent. For example, providers of care—such as physicians, nurses, pharmacists, dietitians, physical therapists, disease managers, and all other types of care managers—can use the Internet to perform health risk assessment surveys, create patient action plans, transmit medical knowledge through self-education modules, and form virtual communities of people dealing with a similar disease. Patient communication can be expanded to include online billing and virtual encounters, in which telecommunication connects the provider and patient. Primary care referrals, personalized health calendars, home monitoring of therapeutic outcomes, feedback from patients on such outcomes as quality of life and satisfaction with the health system, and even practice site evaluation are all possible online thanks to Internet connectivity.

At the acute care level, health care systems can be connected with payers and third parties to verify patient eligibility and provider credentialing, perform institutional utilization review to look at formulary compliance, and determine reimbursement status of insurance claims. The Internet can also facilitate direct connections with financial institutions, employers, and equipment suppliers.

Using Search Engines

Of the popular search engines available today, Google receives the highest ratings for validity and reliability in health care searches.

Dictionary.com defines search engine as, "A Web site whose primary function is gathering and reporting information available on the Internet or a portion of the Internet."[7] For some reason, people tend to confuse browsers, which are used to display Web pages, with Web-based search engines. Some of the confusion may stem from the fact that recent browsers contain a button labeled "Search." When users click on this button, however, it launches a search engine on the Internet that is associated with that particular browser.

Of the popular search engines available today, Google receives the highest ratings for validity and reliability in health care searches. This is probably because Google uses a keyword search format whereas other search engines arrange the Internet in a topical hierarchy. Google indexes every important word on more than four billion Web pages. When you search a word or phrase, Google uses mathematical formulas to rank order the pages it finds, and it displays them on your browser in order of greatest likelihood of containing the information you requested.

The Google search engine has a Directory tab that displays categories of information including Arts, Business, Computers, Games, and Health. Clicking on the word Health in the main directory links you to a display of topics ranging from Addictions to Women's Health. Most health topics contain thousands of Web sites that are organized under subtopics. Under the Nursing hyperlink, for example, there are 1816 available nursing sites, with subtopics including Care Plans, Education, Employment, and References.

Regardless of how you search the Internet, it's helpful to become familiar with the "tips on searching" supplied by each search engine. Basic tips describe how to select keywords to quickly narrow your search results. You can also learn how to connect

BOX 5-2

Tips for Searching Google

- Put quotation marks around a phrase to ensure that the search engine seeks only that exact phrase when searching Web pages—for example, "smoking cessation."
- To retrieve pages that include either word A or word B, use an uppercase OR between terms. To search for hospitals in either Dallas or Houston, for example, type: hospital Dallas OR Houston.
- Use the plus sign (+) in front of a word to be sure it is included in the search along with the primary term you are searching, such as salsa +dance to avoid getting sites that have to do with Mexican food.
- Use the minus sign (–) in front of a word to exclude terms. This is helpful when the word you're searching for has more than one meaning, such as "bass," which can refer to fishing or music. Typing bass –fish would avoid turning up fish-related entries.
- Use the tilde (~) in front of a word to search for synonyms. For example, typing in ~food ~facts would yield food facts as well as information on nutrition and cooking.
- If you know which Web site you want to search but aren't sure where the information is located in that site, you can use Google to search only that domain. Type in the term you are seeking followed by the word "site" and a colon, and then put in the domain name. For example, to find faculty information at Harvard University's Web site enter: faculty site:www.Harvard.edu.
- Keep in mind that in Google, putting * after the stem word does not produce better results, like it does in some search engines. For example, searching for book* will not return Web pages that contain books, booking, bookie, or bookstore.

two words in the search engine's logic. In Google, using quotation marks around a phrase forces the search engine to look for that exact phrase when searching Web pages. For example, searching for smoking cessation (without enclosing the phrase in quotation marks) could result in Web pages about smoking car engines and cessation of taxation being displayed. Searching for "smoking cessation" will force the two words—smoking and cessation—to appear in exactly that sequence for the Web page to be considered for display.

Search engines each differ slightly in the logic they employ to display Web pages that respond to your queries. Some search engines sell page ranking placement to the highest bidder. As a result, searching for the phrase "laboratory software" could display a company Web page in the top five only if that company paid for its placement. Because many Web searchers only look at the top 10 to 20 Web sites displayed by a search engine, optimizing the placement of search results can be financially important to a commercial Web site.[8]

ACTIVITY 5-3

Practicing Searching Skills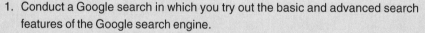

1. Conduct a Google search in which you try out the basic and advanced search features of the Google search engine.
2. Search for an example of information from a health care Web site located in Italy that appears to be country specific. For example a drug may be labeled for a use in Italy that is not be legally approved in the United States. You may have to use the translator services of Google (translate just one paragraph) if the site is written in Italian.
3. Search for a health care–oriented Web site created in a language other than English by using the advanced search function of Google, and identify a free translation service for this Web content in Google that attempts to translate the whole Web site.

Global Web Sites

One interesting problem the Internet presents to health care regulators is the global display of information. For example, a product by a multinational pharmaceutical company might be approved to be used for an indication in Italy that would be considered off-label in the United States. This situation raises the question of whether the Food and Drug Administration should attempt to block access to this information for U.S. citizens or require that the pharmaceutical company limit its display of information. One way that some Web developers are dealing with this problem is to require that users indicate their country of origin before they can obtain information.

Unfortunately, fraudulent vendors can operate Web sites focusing on health care from countries that do not regulate advertising or use good manufacturing procedures. These same countries may exclude extradition of criminals from their borders. Consumers who buy health care goods and services, as well as professionals seeking information for decision support in their practices, must be vigilant about the source, quality, and relevance of the information they acquire over the Internet.

> Online reference sources have several advantages over books and CD-ROMs, including frequent updates and accessibility anytime from anywhere in the world.

Advantages of Online Content Resources

Practitioners used to rely on books for information to help them in their medical decision making—with some publishers sending out monthly or quarterly inserts to keep the material as current as possible. When electronic resources became available, the first CD-ROMs merely placed on the computer screen the same information contained in the book version and sent out quarterly updates. Now, because so many health care providers have no time to read full monographs when they are making a decision, many electronic publishers provide "punchier" nuggets of information that practitioners can locate quickly on the computer screen. These electronic publications are called off-line products because they are usually stored locally on a hard drive or CD-ROM. Networked versions are also available to place on mainframes or local networks so that multiple users have access to the resource.

Placing information online has several distinct advantages over off-line products:

- The publisher can update the information instantly whenever necessary. For example, if a major product is recalled or is found to be associated with a significant therapeutic problem, the next time a user of the resource logs in to the site, he or she receives only the most current information. Users can even sign up for alerts and messages from the publisher to receive immediate notification about significant events.
- Practitioners can access the information resource from any location where an Internet connection exists. If authorized, a practitioner can access information anytime from home, office, library, or Internet café anywhere in the world.

Health Care Portals

A portal is a Web site that serves as an entry point to other Web sites. Portals have also been described as "one-stop shopping" sites on the Internet. Very often a portal contains a search engine. Yahoo, considered a general portal on the Internet, allows users access to Internet resources on shopping, travel, education, communication, entertainment, and just about anything esle.

Professional associations typically try to become portal sites for their members. Other sites try to connect health practitioners with complementary services but are owned by commercial companies, such as nurse.com and virtualnurse.com. Physician.com has services for physicians but is also connected with a service for creating virtual office visits with patients. Pharmacist.com, owned by and connected to the American Pharmacists Association, contains news and other information geared to the interests of pharmacists.

The Internet2 Consortium

Today, over 200 universities are forming a high-speed, broadband network called Internet2 that facilitates education, research, and other applications requiring unusually high transmission of data. As part of this process, academic research centers, industry, and government leaders are taking on revolutionary initiatives that include tremendously powerful connection speeds to maximize data transfer in all digital modes. Everything from powerful data-processing analysis to large videoconferencing sessions for scientific collaboration will allow information exchange that far exceeds the capability of the current Internet bandwidth used by most nonmember universities. Because the Internet2 is a not-for-profit organization, its development will proceed similarly to the original Internet.

The Internet2 is not a replacement strategy for the original Internet. Rather, the new consortium is using the expanded network capabilities to test revolutionary applications that would consume an inordinate amount of resources on the standard Internet. New computer workstations and applications will have capabilities offered by the Internet2 network to process data at speeds many times faster than available now. Member institutions will purchase workstations that allow full usage of the increased bandwidth available through Internet2. Additional initiatives, such as the Next Generation Internet (NGI), have similar goals. The masterminds behind these efforts are trying to harmonize them for interoperability, so that all equipment will function on either platform.[9]

Greater Connectivity, More Options

With all the available options for connectivity, health care is only beginning to tap the Internet's capabilities. Any person charged with system planning in a health care organization needs to maximize the Internet's power to achieve quality, safety, and efficiency goals.

At one time, experts predicted that an implosion would occur as system demands outstripped available Internet infrastructure. Now, however, we realize that our excess capacity for speed and access will stretch far into the future.

All of us must continue to move toward greater connectivity and speed. This will improve care for our patients and help our organizations operate at peak efficiencies.

ACTIVITY 5-4

Becoming Familiar with Basic E-mail Functions

Carry out the tasks below to make sure you know how to do key functions in your e-mail program. If you need assistance, use the Help feature of your e-mail package.

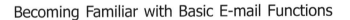

- Read new mail that has been sent to you.
- Reply to a message you have received (without rekeying the sender's address).
- Reply to a message without including the original message.
- Delete a message once you have read it.
- Keep a message you have read, so you can read it again later.
- File your mail in folders.
- Send the same message to two people.
- Send a message to someone and a courtesy copy (cc) of it to someone else.
- Keep copies of messages you have sent.
- Add your own remarks to a message you received and forward it to someone else.
- Use an address book to enter the personal information of the people with whom you frequently communicate.
- Check back through old mail in stored locations.
- Print an e-mail message.

Becoming Familiar with Advanced E-mail Functions ✓

Carry out the tasks below to practice advanced functions in your e-mail program. If you need assistance, use the Help feature of your e-mail package.

1. Search in Help to see how to set up a distribution list so you can e-mail groups of people by entering a single group address in the To: portion of your e-mail.
2. Send someone a message prepared in a word processing program.
3. Send someone a document file as an attachment.
4. View a document file that someone has e-mailed to you.
5. Set up your e-mail to automatically add your personal Signature to e-mails by searching Signature in your Help feature.
6. Turn your signature off or set up a feature so you are prompted before adding a signature to your message.
7. Sort your mail (by date, sender, subject, etc).
8. Filter incoming mail to eliminate spam by looking at the word "filter" or the phrase "spam filter" in the Help feature of your e-mail application. If you are a part of a large organization, you may want to call your information technology support for help with this activity.
9. Join a state, national, or global discussion list by searching a topic that interests you. For example, you could try using "diabetes discussion forum" in Google.
10. Back up your e-mail onto a floppy disk or CD. You can use the Help feature here, or try clicking on the File pulldown menu and then Save As. You can usually choose MS Word or generic text as the desired file format.

ACTIVITY 5-6

Internet Research ✓

1. Locate on the National Library of Medicine's site the most recent research on professional use of the Internet for health care–related purposes.

2. Locate the most recent research on patient use of the Internet for health care–related purposes using search terms such as health care Internet statistics. Groups such as Forrester Consulting publish these data to help organizations plan their priorities.

3. Identify what the intranet in your work or school setting is being used for. If an intranet is not in place, identify potential areas of need for this technology.

4. Determine what extranet connections are in place in your health care setting or school. What type of information is being transmitted over each of these connections? If an extranet is not in place, what are potential areas of need for this technology in your organization?

5. Determine what security measures are in place on your workstation and your organization's networks.

6. Identify universities, industries, and governmental organizations that are participating in the Internet2 initiative in your local geographic area. Determine what type of activities these organizations perform in the Internet2 initiative.

References

1. Zakon RH. Hobbe's Internet Timeline. Available at: http://www.zakon.org/robert/internet/timeline/. Accessed July 26, 2004.

2. Armour FJ, Kaiser SH. *Enterprise Information Technology Architecture: A Practical Approach.* Hoboken, NJ: John Wiley & Sons Inc; 2005.

3. Broadband Comparison Chart. YZ Technology. Available at: www.yztech.com/Broadband.html Accessed July 27, 2004.

4. Users shrink, sites expand, healthcare trends and statistics. Available at: http://www.clickz.com/stats markets/healthcare/article.php/3298631. Accessed July 27, 2004.

5. Company Overview, eDiets, Inc. Available at: www.ediets.com/company/index.cfm. Accessed July 27, 2004.

6. Company Overview, WebMd, Inc. Available at: www.webmd.com/corporate/index.html. Accessed July 27, 2004.

7. Online Dictionary, Lexico Publishing Group, LLC. Available at: http://dictionary.reference.com /search?q=search%20engine. Accessed July 27, 2004.

8. Basics of Search. Google search engine. Available at: www.google.com/help/basics.html. Accessed July 27, 2004.

9. About Internet2. Internet2 Consortium Web site. Available at: www.internet2.edu/. Accessed July 27, 2004.

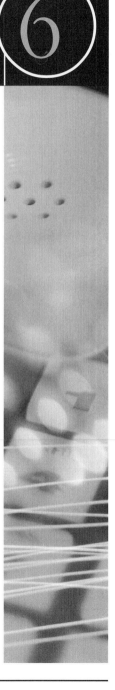

CHAPTER

Telecommunication in Health Care ⑥

Brent I. Fox

Chapter Objectives

After completing this chapter, you should be able to:

- Understand the basics of telecommunication.
- Define the various types of telecommunication media.
- Identify everyday examples of telecommunication.
- Discuss ways that telecommunication is used in health care.
- Describe various communication protocols.
- Understand the clinician's role in implementing a telecommunication system.

Telecommunication is part of our everyday personal and professional lives. Like many other technologies, telecommunication systems have become so common that we don't even give them a second thought. As of November 2003, 94.7% of U.S. homes had telephone service. Unlike early data communication technologies—the landline telegraph, radio telegraph, and teletypewriter[1]—today's telephones can transmit both data and voice anywhere in the world, making it truly intregral to today's society.

But what about other telecommunication technologies? How do they transfer information? What factors should you consider when evaluating a new telecommunication system? And how can you potentially use these systems to communicate with providers and care for patients?

Telecommunication System Components

A communication medium is anything that carries a message between the sender and the receiver.

Communication and telecommunication are closely related activities that we perform daily almost automatically. Even newborn babies are able to partially communicate, but unfortunately, their parents can't always understand them.

Basic communications can be thought of as transmitting a message (or signal) from a sender through a medium to a receiver. In the example above, the newborn baby is the sender and its parents are the receivers. A communication medium is anything that carries a message between the sender and the receiver. In most cases of face-to-face human communication, air is the communication medium. Figure 6-1 depicts the basic components of a communication system.

Successful communication means that several independent processes must occur at all three points represented in Figure 6-1. In human communication, the sender must be able to translate

FIGURE 6-1

The three components of a communication system.

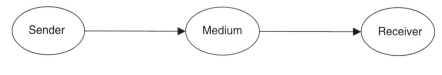

Source: Adapted from Reference 1.

internal thoughts into audible sounds. Then, the sender's message must be successfully transmitted to the receiver, and the receiver must be able to accept and interpret the message. The receiver and sender must speak the same language and share common meanings of words in the message.

Telecommunication systems have essentially the same core components as human communication. But whereas a face-to-face human communication system uses people and air vibration to transfer an audible message, today's telecommunication systems use many types of media to transfer a message, generally between two or more electronic devices. The telephone, the most obvious example of a telecommunication system today, translates the sender's audible voice into a signal that is transferred to the receiver's telephone, which then translates the signal back into an audible message the receiver can understand. Many types of media, such as copper wire or fiber-optic cable, can serve as the transmission medium in a telecommunication system.

The "tele" component of telecommunication, which comes from Greek and means "far off," indicates that communication is occurring over a distance. Before the widespread use of electronic devices, telecommunication involved smoke signals, signal flares, and other nonelectronic devices, whereas today it refers to transmitting sound, images, text, or other types of data over distance using some type of electronic or light system. Here are a few examples of the ways telecommunications have decreased limitations of time and distance in our everyday lives.

- Reports from war zones are transmitted directly into our living rooms.
- We are able to get real-time updates of the Dow Jones stock market reports.
- Health care providers can function virtually in war zones where it is too dangerous for them to be physically located.
- A top surgeon can operate virtually on a wounded soldier through a surgical technician or remotely controlled robotics.
- Our e-mail inboxes and personal digital assistants automatically receive updated drug information, procedure information, and health-related news as it becomes available.
- Distance education allows students and professionals across the country to "attend" classes taught by the field's experts.

Before the widespread use of electronic devices, telecommunication involved smoke signals, signal flares, and other nonelectronic devices, whereas today it refers to transmitting sound, images, text, or other types of data over distance using some type of electronic or light system.

An example of encoders in health care today are picture-archiving and communication systems (PACS), which store, retrieve, distribute, and display digital medical images such as radiology films.

In all these examples, some type of message is electronically transferred over distance between a sender and a receiver. Messages can either be sent in real-time or by the "store and forward" method.

Telecommunication Terminology

The primary terms in telecommunication systems—sender, medium, and receiver—can be exchanged with source, channel, and destination, respectively. Basic telecommunication components are also usually accompanied by several other elements—encoders, decoders, transmitters, receivers, and noise.

Encoders

Encoders translate the message from its original form into a form suitable for transmission. In the human communication example, encoding occurs when the human brain translates thoughts into audible sounds. In telecommunication, electronic devices translate data or information into a form that can be electronically transferred to the final destination.

Among encoders actively at work in today's health care environment are picture-archiving and communication systems (PACS), which are increasingly being adopted to store, retrieve, distribute, and display digital medical images. For example, PACS allow clinicians to remotely access radiology films via computer.[2] In this process, encoders translate the radiology films into an electronic version that can be transferred to the ultimate user.

Decoders

Telecommunication messages contain more than the information sent by the source. The encoding process adds additional information to the message to assist the transfer process. Decoders work on the other end of the system, where the message is received.

The process of decoding involves taking the entire electronic message sent by the source and pulling out of it the information useful to the receiver. Decoders must be able to "speak" the same language as the encoder and reconstruct the information back into its original format. Using our PACS example, the clinician's computer decoding component must reconstruct the radiology film into the exact image that was originally sent.

Transmitters and Receivers

Transmitters and receivers work between the encoding and decoding components of a telecommunication system. As the name implies, a transmitter takes the encoded message and sends it through the communication medium to the receiver. In this case, the receiver is not the ultimate end user of the message. The receiver is the actual physical component within the telecommunication system that accepts the message before the decoding process.

Because the word "receiver" can be used in many ways, we will use "destination" here to describe the end user of the information. In the PACS example, the destination is the clinician using the radiology information to provide care to a patient.

High signal-to-noise ratios are preferred in a telecommunication system because they indicate that the signal strength is much higher than the accompanying noise.

Noise

Noise in a telecommunication system is any unwanted signal that interferes with the desired signal.[1] Noise takes many forms and can be introduced at any point in a telecommunication system. Therefore, high signal-to-noise ratios are preferred in a telecommunication system because they indicate that the signal strength is much higher than the accompanying noise. Figure 6-2 depicts the components of a typical telecommunication system and the points where noise may interfere with the signal.

FIGURE 6-2

A complete telecommunication system.

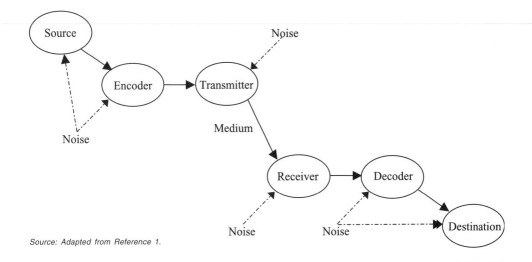

Source: Adapted from Reference 1.

Synchronous and Asynchronous Communication

Other common terms in telecommunication, synchronous and asynchronous, are often discussed in the context of data communications—the special form of telecommunication that collects, prepares, and sends data.

Synchronous communication allows the destination to receive the message when it is sent. Everyday examples of synchronous communication include face-to-face, telephone, and chat room conversations. Synchronous is also used to refer to situations where communication flows freely between source and destination at the same time. In asynchronous communication, the destination receives a message at a point in time after it has been sent.[3] E-mail is a common example of asynchronous communication.

The Telephone's Significance

Today's telephone is a descendent of the original electrical device for communicating over distance—the telegraph. Invented in 1837, the telegraph was followed by the radiotelegraph and the teletypewriter. Each device improved on the data communication capabilities of the original telegraph.[1]

Although the telephone, patented in 1876, is a spinoff of the telegraph, it is an analog device while the telegraph, radiotelegraph, and teletypewriter were all digital. Analog devices record sound as waves; digital devices use a series of numbers to record sound. This key difference allowed people to use the telephone without help from a telegraph operator, except to make connections.[1] The fact that people can use the telephone independently along with its ability, unlike the telegraph, to allow voice communication, spurred its widespread use.

The global adoption of the telephone, including today's wireless forms, allows connectivity just about anywhere in the world for both people and machines, voice and data. The popular digital subscriber lines (DSL) that provide high-speed Internet access to homes and businesses use existing telephone lines for connectivity, and much of the information transmitted in health care systems is sent over telephone lines. In fact, many community pharmacies still rely predominantly on telephone lines to submit reimbursement claims to third-party payers, and for health care providers the telephone is a key tool for professional communication due to its simplicity, availability, reliability, and affordability. In effect, Alexander Graham Bell's telephone laid the groundwork for much of today's telecommunications.

The popular digital subscriber lines (DSL) that provide high-speed Internet access to homes and businesses use existing telephone lines for connectivity, and much of the information transmitted in health care systems is sent over telephone lines.

Telecommunication Media

A telecommunication medium is essentially anything that carries an electronic signal between a source and destination. Telecommunication media are made of various materials, including light waves in the air. The material making up the medium plays a key role in how the medium acts as a data carrier.

Two common characteristics used to compare telecommunication media are transmission capacity and speed. In health care, there is a growing push to move toward computerized prescriber order entry (CPOE) and a completely electronic health record (EHR). As we inch closer to these goals, telecommunication media will have to be identified, evaluated, and implemented that have both the capacity to carry huge amounts of data and the speed to deliver it.

Telecommunication media are also evaluated in terms of their cost, security, ease of installation, susceptibility to noise, and signal attenuation (weakening) characteristics. Ideally, a telecommunication medium would provide unlimited communication capacity, travel at the fastest speed possible on a secure channel that is immune to noise and signal attenuation, and be easy to install and maintain—all at a really good price. Of course, health care doesn't operate in a perfect environment, so you have to make the best of available resources.

Health care clinicians usually do not have the final say in selecting a telecommunication system, but they may participate in multidisciplinary committees that evaluate systems from the clinical end-user perspective. If you find yourself in this role, you must try to match your needs, your colleagues' needs, and the needs of the organization with the capabilities of various telecommunication system options. You may also need to select a telecommunication system for your home or clinical practice setting. Among aspects to consider are:

- The goals of the overall telecommunication system.
- The type and volume of data to be transferred.
- The telecommunication system's scalability; that is, the ability to modify its size.
- The physical, financial, and human resources available to the owner of the system.
- The implementation time frame.

Keep these considerations in mind as you read the following section that describes common telecommunication media.

> Two common characteristics used to compare telecommunication media are transmission capacity and speed.

Twisted-Pair Wire

Whether you realize it or not, you encounter twisted-pair wire every day, a telecommunication medium that consists of two insulated wires—usually made of copper—twisted around each other. The twist decreases interference, or noise, in the signal transmitted on the cable. Because the pairs are insulated, a twisted-pair wire can be composed of one or many pairs. The most common use of twisted-pair wire is in telephone lines. Figure 6-3 shows a twisted-pair wire.

FIGURE 6-3

Twisted-pair wire.

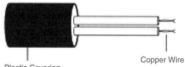

Copper Wire

Plastic Covering

Reprinted with permission (not copyrighted).
www.ictp.trieste.it~radionet/1998_school/networking_presentation/MEDIA.html

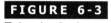

Twisted-pair wire can be unshielded (UTP) or shielded (STP) with an extra layer of insulation to reduce interference. STP is classified in five categories (CAT 1 to CAT 5) according to the number of twists and other features.

The two types of twisted-pair wire are shielded and unshielded. As the name implies, shielded twisted-pair wire (STP) is surrounded by an additional protective layer of insulation, while unshielded twisted-pair (UTP) does not contain this protective layer. The extra layer of insulation in STP reduces interference entering or leaving the cable and greatly affects the capabilities and uses of twisted-pair wire. Shielded twisted-pair wire is classified in five categories (CAT 1 to CAT 5) according to the number of twists and other features.[1]

Both types of twisted-pair wire are used in telecommunication systems, often in local area networks (LAN). The additional insulation layer in STP wire enables it to be used in higher-speed networks than UTP. In general, twisted-pair wire of both types is less expensive than alternative telecommunication media and has a lower installation cost, so it has historically been used in computer and telephone networks. Also, it is easier to work with than higher-capacity telecommunication media. Twisted-pair wire does suffer from two primary limitations, however: it has considerably less capability to transmit data (i.e., bandwidth) than other telecommunication media, and it is susceptible to electrical interference that can substantially affect the signal transmitted.[1,3,4]

Coaxial Cable

Coaxial cable, used to deliver cable television to homes and businesses, has greater data transfer speeds than twisted-pair wire. Coaxial cable wires are not twisted around each other and instead are made up of a main wire surrounded by another wire that is either braided or a solid sheath. The main wire contains the signal and the surrounding wire is the ground. A layer of insulation is placed between the two wires and an outer layer of insulation protects the entire cable. Figure 6-4 shows the components of a coaxial cable.[1]

FIGURE 6-4

A coaxial cable and its components.

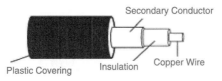

Reprinted with permission (not copyrighted).
www.ictp.trieste.it~radionet/1998_school/networking_presentation/MEDIA.html

The physical structure of coaxial cable provides a transmission medium that is less susceptible to interference than twisted-pair wire, but it is more expensive and is easily tapped, making it relatively insecure. Amplifiers are used to boost signals carried on coaxial cable because the signals are subject to much greater attenuation than those sent on twisted-pair wire.[1]

Microwave

Microwave transmission does not use a physical transmission medium but instead occurs through the air (or space) between stations. This type of transmission is known as "line-of-sight" because there must be an unobstructed path between transmission points for data to be sent successfully. Sending and receiving stations are arranged in a line, with one station transmitting the message, the next receiving it and then transmitting it down the line to subsequent stations. Figure 6-5, which depicts the wireless spectrum of electromagnetic waves, includes the range for microwave telecommunications, which have shorter wavelengths than radio waves but longer than infrared, ultraviolet, and x-rays. Figure 6-6 shows the relationship between waves in the electromagnetic spectrum.

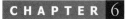

FIGURE 6-5

The wireless spectrum.

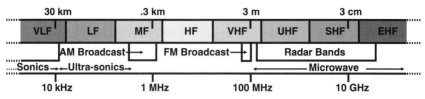

Reprinted with permission (not copyrighted).
www.ictp.trieste.it~radionet/1998_school/networking_presentation/MEDIA.html

FIGURE 6-6

The size of waves in the electromagnetic spectrum.

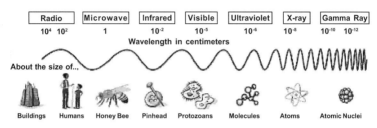

Source: http://imagers.gsfc.nasa.gov/ems/waves3.html

FIGURE 6-7

A microwave tower in Montgomery, AL.

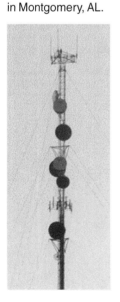

A key benefit of microwave transmission—that it does not rely on a physical cable to carry the message—is also a limitation. Messages sent by microwave channels lack many of the security features in messages sent by physical media. Also, microwave devices are costly, and the line-of-sight nature of microwave transmission limits its range.

Typically, microwave stations are placed 30 to 70 miles apart to ensure that the stations can "see" each other. Figure 6-7 shows a typical microwave tower. However, effective, high-speed data transfer can take place between buildings in a city by placing microwave transmission stations at both the sending and receiving ends. It takes considerably less time to set up a microwave transmission channel than to lay cable over the same distance.

Satellite

Satellites are a special type of microwave transmission station in space, approximately 22,300 miles above the Earth's surface. Communication satellites are so expensive that governments and huge corporations are the only entities that can afford them.

An advantage is that three geosynchronous satellites—orbiting the Earth in the same direction and at the same speed as the Earth's rotation—can completely cover the Earth's surface, allowing communication across oceans and over desolate terrain. Beyond their prohibitive cost, satellites suffer from a transmission delay of approximately 1/4 second, often making voice communications difficult.[1]

Because satellite and microwave transmission both rely on line-of-sight communication channels, they are subject to interference from the weather. Rain and snow can significantly affect satellite and microwave signals—as you know if you've watched satellite television during bad weather.[1,4] Like microwave transmission, messages sent via satellite are relatively insecure compared to other transmission media. However, satellite transmission can employ encryption as a security measure, altering data to make it unreadable unless you have the proper tools to translate it.[1,4]

Cellular

From 1998 to 2003, residential use of landline phones for long distance calls decreased from an average of 97 to 52 minutes a month. Over the same time period, wireless phone use for long distance calls increased from an average of 4 to 34 minutes a month. These data indicate that many people no longer use landline phones. In fact, recent reports indicate that nearly 15% of the U.S. population now uses wireless (i.e., cellular) telephones exclusively. This percentage is expected to double by 2008.[5]

Current cell phone service provides much more than just voice communications. Optional "data plans" let cell phone users transfer data at three to four times the speed of current dial-up modems. Digital cameras are now commonplace on cell phones, which are being combined with personal digital assistants (PDAs) into devices called "smart phones."

Like microwave and satellite transmission, cellular phone service uses the air as the transmission medium. Transmission speeds vary considerably depending on the service provider and the individual user's plan. Cellular transmission methods essentially break up geographical locations into cells, with each cell containing one or more transmission towers. As cell phone users move within a cell and between cells, their signal is transferred from one cell tower to another. Figure 6-8 shows a cellular telecommunication tower.

Today, the cost of cell phone service is decreasing, while hardware, service features, and functionality are increasing. The primary

FIGURE 6-8

A cellular telecommunication tower.

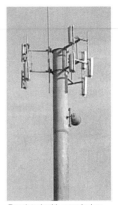

Reprinted with permission (not copyrighted). Steve Romaine. www.geckobeach.com

limitation is the inconsistency of the cellular phone service itself. Signal reliability is one of the primary features that service providers use to distinguish themselves from their competitors. Generally, reliable coverage within major cities is not a problem, but coverage begins to dissipate as cell phone users travel into rural areas.

Infrared

Infrared is another line-of-sight transmission method that uses air as the transmission medium. As with twisted-pair wire, many people use infrared daily, since it is the telecommunication medium of choice in television remote controls and other audio/video devices. If you have ever used your PDA to "beam" information to a printer, computer, or another PDA, you have used infrared transmission.

Unlike most of the transmission media discussed above, infrared actually uses light waves to transfer data. Infrared range is generally limited to less than a few yards, and transmission speeds usually run about 115 kilobytes per second, which is roughly twice the speed of dial-up modems. Use of infrared transmission technologies is generally localized to the room where the devices are located. Infrared is often used to connect computer peripherals, such as printers. Infrared is relatively inexpensive, easy to install, and easy to move, but infrared transmission is not secure.[1,4]

Fiber-Optic Cable

Fiber-optic cable is the fastest transmission medium today. Like infrared, it uses light waves to transfer data, but the transmission range for fiber-optic cable is exponentially larger than infrared. Also, infrared is transmitted through air, while fiber-optics use high-quality strands of glass or plastic to carry the signal as light waves. A fiber-optic cable consists of glass or plastic fibers, a thin coating called "cladding" around the fibers, and a protective "jacket." Figure 6-9 depicts a fiber-optic cable.

FIGURE 6-9

Fiber-optic cable.

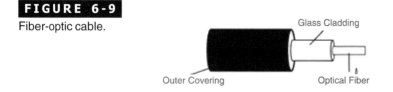

Glass Cladding

Outer Covering

Optical Fiber

Use of fiber-optic cables is limited by price, the equipment required to transmit data through the cable, and the fragility of the actual medium, which makes installation and maintenance difficult because the cable does not bend like coaxial or twisted-pair wire. Broken fiber-optic cables are hard to repair and their delicate nature makes it difficult to splice them with other communication media.[1]

Among key advantages of fiber-optic cable over other telecommunication media is that it can transmit data in digital format, the natural form for computer-generated data. Fiber-optic cable is not susceptible to electrical interference because it uses light waves, providing a clearer signal that can travel farther than other media. Fiber-optic cable's small physical size is a plus when there is limited room for additional cabling. Single strands of fiber-optic cable (about the thickness of a human hair) are often bundled together to form cables whose diameter is appropriate for the specific application. Finally, fiber-optic cable has high data-transfer speeds as well as the ability to carry large amounts of data.[1,3] Table 6-1 compares the speed of various telecommunication media and puts fiber-optic cable's superior transmission rate into perspective, where its slowest speed is 2.5 to 5 times faster than the fastest speeds for infrared, microwave, satellite, and coaxial cable.

Fiber-optic cable has security advantages because its signals are difficult to split and it is virtually impossible for someone to tap into a fiber-optic cable without being detected.[1,3]

Although fiber-optic cables are subject to attenuation, it occurs much less frequently than with other media. Signal attenuation occurs because the fiber absorbs some of the light passing through it. Amplifiers are often placed every 50 to 75 miles along a fiber to handle this problem. Recent advancements have helped increase the carrying capacity of fiber while also reducing the need for amplifiers.[4]

> Fiber-optic cable's advantages include high transfer speeds, good security, high-volume capacity, and the ability to transmit data in digital format.

TABLE 6-1

Telecommunication Media Speed Comparison

Twisted-pair Wire	300 bps (bits/second)–10 Mbps (million bits/second)
Infrared	115 Kbps (thousand bits/second)
Microwave	256 Kbps–100 Mbps
Satellite	256 Kbps–100 Mbps
Coaxial Cable	56 Kbps–200 Mbps
Fiber-optic Cable	500 Kbps–25 Tbps (trillion bits/second)

Source: Reference 4.

Geographical Networks

A variety of telecommunication media can be used in a single network. A local area network (LAN), for example, may include twisted-pair wire, coaxial cable, and infrared transmission.

As discussed in Chapter 2, the four types of geographical networks include local area networks (LANs), metropolitan area networks (MANs), wide area networks (WANs), and wireless local area networks (WLANs). Geographical coverage of a LAN is smaller than that of a MAN, which is smaller than that of WAN. Wireless local area networks are special LANs that are wirelessly connected.

The use of telecommunication media in networks cannot be divided into neat categories. While one type of medium may be more common in a particular geographic network, several media might be used in a single network.

For example, the vast majority of LANs are based on UTP wire, but many of the other media discussed above can also be found in LANs. Because of infrared's short transmission range, its use in networks is limited to LANs, often within a single room. Coaxial cable and UTP can be found in LANs, MANs, and WANs.

Microwave transmission is ideal for cities, where towers can be placed on the tops of buildings, and satellite transmission is ideal for WANs because of its geographic coverage. The speed, bandwidth, and security of fiber-optic cable make it an ideal choice for WANs, as well. However, fiber-optic is seldom run all the way to the end user; usually it is the backbone of large network channels.[4] Box 6-1 contains a listing of criteria that are important to consider when evaluating telecommunication media.

BOX 6-1

Telecommunication Media Evaluation Criteria

- Secure: free from danger or risk.
- Reliable: dependable.
- Affordable: within available financial means.
- Scalable: able to increase in size.
- Extensible: able to extend in capability.
- Economical: requires the minimum of time and resources for effectiveness.

ACTIVITY 6-1

Telecommunication Media Evaluation Matrix

Using the evaluation criteria in Box 6-1, create a matrix for evaluating each of the telecommunication media discussed above. For your evaluation categories, use the characteristics that would be most important to you in a new LAN that provides real-time access to patient, laboratory, and other clinical information.

For example, you are considering implementing a LAN that will employ a microwave telecommunication system. The matrix (i.e., table) would have the items in Box 6-1 listed in the horizontal axis at the top of the table. The vertical axis on the left side of the table would contain the desired functional capabilities (i.e., evaluation categories) of the system. Using a 1-5 ranking (1 lowest and 5 highest), score the microwave system on its ability to meet the functional capabilities (vertical axis) while providing the desired features of a telecommunication system (horizontal axis). Add up each column to create a score for each feature. Add up each row to create a score for each functional capability. Compare these scores with scores for the other telecommunication media.

Telecommunication Media in Health Care

Telecommunication channels that carry health care information must be reliable and provide consistent service regardless of the time, distance, or environmental conditions. Health care telecommunication channels must also transmit data accurately and avoid introducing extraneous or erroneous data into the message being sent. The sensitivity of health care information requires that telecommunication channels protect patient information from external dangers of any kind, such as manipulation or unauthorized access.

Telecommunication Standards

A common problem when transferring data across devices from different manufacturers is the ability for the data to retain its integrity, that is, its original form and presentation. This is because hardware manufacturers often develop their own proprietary standards for handling data flowing across their devices, which can limit the success of telecommunications regardless of the medium used. Proprietary standards may offer a technological advantage in instances where a single manufacturer's components are used, but in health care, a top priority is integrating software and hardware components from a variety of vendors.

"Open standards" are not specific to a single hardware manufacturer or device. Accessible by anyone, open standards enable data to flow across hardware and software from different manufacturers. One of the most visible open-source (i.e., nonproprietary) technologies is the Linux operating system.

Interoperability—the ultimate goal of communication standards—refers to the capability of two or more devices to freely transmit data regardless of the device manufacturers.

Open Systems Interconnection (OSI) Model

In Health Level 7, an organization that sets standards for exchanging clinical and administrative data in health care, the "7" is an important component of its name because it indicates a focus on layer 7—the application layer—of the Open Systems Interconnection (OSI) model, which defines a networking framework for implementing protocols in seven layers. Layer 7 provides application services for e-mail, file transfers, and other network software functions. Although the OSI model once received widespread support from vendors, poor definitions and widespread use of proprietary standards have made it more of a teaching model for other protocols.[1,2]

Despite certain limitations of the OSI model, it is the basis of several commonly used standards and it makes developing interoperable software and hardware from different manufacturers significantly easier. Figure 6-10 details the seven layers of the OSI model.

FIGURE 6-10

The OSI model depicting the flow of data from the sender on the left to the receiver on the right.

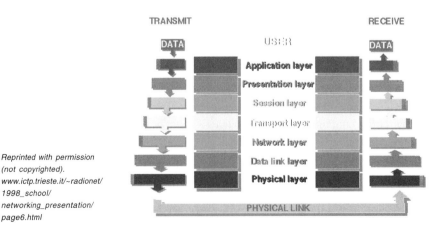

Reprinted with permission
(not copyrighted).
www.ictp.trieste.it/~radionet/
1998_school/
networking_presentation/
page6.html

Each layer of the OSI model—beginning with the physical layer at the bottom and continuing to the application layer at the top—defines how communicating networks will interact to achieve the specific functions of that layer. This technically complex set of activities is defined in Box 6-2.

BOX 6-2

Activities Carried Out at Each Layer of the OSI Model

Layer 7. Application: User-oriented; determines data to be transmitted, the format of the data, and transaction codes to identify the data on the receiving end.

Layer 6. Presentation: Formats and displays the data; performs data encryption and data compression.

Layer 5. Session: Organizes and maintains sessions, which are periods of interactive communication between user processes.

Layer 4. Transport: Ensures reliable service for message transmission between computer processes.

Layer 3. Network: Manages the routing of messages from end to end.

Layer 2. Data link: Establishes and controls the physical paths for message transmission; handles errors that occur in the physical layer.

Layer 1. Physical: A node-to-node protocol describing the characteristics of the telecommunication system.

Source: References 1 and 3.

Transmission Control Protocol/Internet Protocol

Transmission Control Protocol/Internet Protocol (TCP/IP)—also known as the "Internet Suite"—is the number one global communication protocol of the Internet. The U.S. government has selected the OSI model to replace TCP/IP, but until the full GOSIP (U.S. government implementation of OSI) protocol can be implemented, TCP/IP will remain the government's primary networking protocol. Furthermore, businesses and schools still rely on TCP/IP as their primary networking protocol.[1,3,6,7]

The OSI model and TCP/IP handle data in a similar way. As shown in Figure 6-11, the Internet Suite (TCP/IP) has four layers as compared with OSI's seven. The primary difference between these two approaches is that the Internet Suite focuses solely on establishing a connection between hosts and transferring the message. The Internet Suite does not concern itself with the contents of the message, making it more efficient and simple than the OSI model, which is often viewed as being too complex to be practical in implementation.

TCP/IP is a set of rules that establishes the method with which data are transmitted over the Internet between two computers. Eventually, the OSI model, favored by the U.S. government, will replace it.

FIGURE 6-11

The OSI model versus the Internet suite.

OSI	TCP/IP
Application	
Presentation	Application
Session	
Transport	Transport
Network	Internet
Data Link	
Physical	Host to Host

The telecommunication implementation cycle is a stepwise process for developing and implementing telecommunication systems.

Other Communication Protocols

Four additional protocols are:

- **Ethernet**, a protocol that allows multiple devices to share a single cable as well as all network resources attached to that cable. In LANs using the Ethernet protocol, bus topology (described in Chapter 2) is the standard topology.
- **Systems Network Architecture (SNA)**, an architecture model that was designed for IBM systems. Due to the popularity of IBM hardware, many other manufacturers have incorporated this protocol into their systems.
- **X.400**, a protocol published in 1984 for the exchange of e-mail, which was called Inter Personal Message at the time. Because X.400 is more complex that other e-mail protocols, its usage is limited.
- **X.500**, a protocol for electronic directories such as white pages

Box 6-3 gives examples of just how widespread the use of telecommunication is in health care.

Telecommunication Implementation Cycle

Similar to the systems development life cycle (SDLC), which is the process for developing information systems, the telecommunication implementation cycle is a stepwise process for developing and implementing telecommunication systems. Clini-

BOX 6-3

Scenario: Telecommunication at Work in Health Care Today

Here's an example of how telecommunication advances are affecting health care providers and the way they function. TF, a 53-year-old African-American male, makes an appointment to see his physician because of an expanding skin rash, flulike symptoms, and myalgia. At the same time that TF is on the telephone setting up his appointment, the physician is using the local hospital's intranet to download regional and national health plan formulary updates to his PDA before conducting his morning rounds. While on rounds, the physician uses the bedside touchscreen computer display to access the most recent laboratory values and radiology results for his patients and incorporates this information into his patients' care.

Earlier that same morning, the pharmacist who regularly rounds with the physician used her broadband Internet connection at home to download the most recent updates to her PDA-based drug information software. When she arrives at the hospital, the pharmacy director tells her about the department's new intervention documentation software, which has the feature of being both workstation- and PDA-based. The director beams the software to the pharmacist's PDA using infrared connectivity. The pharmacist then hurries out the door to round with the physician.

While she is on rounds, a patient's renal insufficiency prompts her to recommend a change in therapy, which the physician implements. The pharmacist documents the change in the new intervention-tracking software on her PDA. When she returns to the pharmacy, she wirelessly synchronizes her PDA with the department's information systems with a single tap of the PDA's stylus on the PDA screen, automatically transferring the documented intervention. Now the intervention is stored in the department's intervention database for further analysis.

The nurses are using a newly installed wireless voice communication system that is saving them 30 to 45 minutes per day. Like something straight out of Star Trek, nurses wear a communication badge on their shirts that they press when they need to communicate with personnel located throughout the hospital. They speak the name of the person or department they desire, and the badge connects them with that party. The receiving party presses the communication badge and accepts the connection. No longer do nurses have to leave a patient's room to speak with another health care provider.

After completing his morning rounds in the hospital, the physician grabs a quick lunch and heads to his office for his regular afternoon activity of seeing patients. TF is his first patient. The physician discusses TF's symptoms and performs a physical examination.

continued on page 150

BOX 6-3 *continued*

Following a differential diagnosis procedure using a decision algorithm in his PDA, the physician is convinced that TF has contracted Lyme disease. After further discussion with the patient, he discovers that TF spends many hours outside each day, which helps support his suspicion that TF was bitten by a tick carrying Lyme disease. Using his recently updated formulary list, the physician generates an electronic prescription for TF that he sends over the Internet to the pharmacy of TF's choosing before either person leaves the examination room.

The pharmacist at a local community pharmacy receives the electronic prescription from TF's physician directly into her pharmacy information system, which flashes a small alert in the top right corner of the computer display. She clicks on the alert, views the entire prescription, associates the prescription with TF's profile using a few keystrokes, and begins to fill the prescription. While processing the prescription, the new medication is checked against TF's current profile by the pharmacy information system for any allergies or potential drug-drug interactions. The pharmacist electronically transmits the prescription claim to TF's health insurer and receives electronic notification that the submission is approved for payment. The pharmacist prepares the prescription, which is waiting for TF when he arrives.

The pharmacist presents the medication to TF and discusses with him how to take it, side effects to watch for, and key aspects of Lyme disease. After ensuring that TF has no further questions or concerns, the pharmacist offers TF the opportunity to use the computer in the patient counseling area to access patient education materials on Lyme disease. TF politely declines and goes home. Once home, TF logs into the Internet and spends three hours researching Lyme disease on his own.
Source: Reference 8.

cians are often involved in developing these systems because, as the ultimate end user, they are often best able to identify necessary features. Clinicians taking part in this process must understand the goals of each step so they can provide the maximal contribution. Box 6-4 defines the five stages of the telecommunication implementation cycle.

The initial stages of the implementation cycle are very important. The later in the cycle an error is identified, the more expensive it is to be corrected—a problem that is compounded

ACTIVITY 6-2

Telecommunication Applications

Identify the 17 instances of telecommunication use in the scenario described in Box 6-3.

The Telecommunication Implementation Cycle

In these steps, the term "system" is used to designate the object or goal of the implementation cycle (such as, for example, a picture archival communication system).

Step 1: Problem Investigation. Define the problem to be solved or the opportunity to be seized, and define the project objective in terms of the organizational goals.
Step 2: Analysis and General Design. Identify the requirements, strategy, and architecture for the system.
Step 3: Detailed Design. Create a detailed functional design of the system or modifications to be made to an existing system.
Step 4: System Implementation. Gather and assemble the functional components and put them in place; train the users.
Step 5: System Maintenance and Review. Ensure continued functionality and modify the system as needed; evaluate the overall project.
Source: References 1 and 3.

by the fact that end users do not receive the final product until the system is almost complete.

The Cedars-Sinai Medical Center computerized order entry system (CPOE) mentioned in Chapter 3 gives a sense of what can go wrong during a telecommunications implementation. This highly respected institution was in the process of putting in a CPOE system when, approximately 8 weeks into the planned 14-week department-by-department rollout, the system was taken down due to physician resistance. The medical executive committee, composed of 40 physicians, was involved in developing and implementing the CPOE system, but physicians who were not on this committee believed that the committee did not represent their interests and felt that the system did not follow their normal workflow. They also felt that the CPOE system was slower than their previous methods and they refused to use it.

Also, Cedars-Sinai's administration realized that the CPOE system affected ancillary departments outside the physician community in ways they hadn't anticipated. For example, it did not allow orders to be attached to patients during the admission process, which caused patients to arrive in urgent care areas, such as the cath lab, before their admission orders arrived.[9] The system is expected to be reinstalled after a thorough review of the problems.

Cedars Sinai Medical Center ✓

In the Cedars Sinai example on page 151, strategic errors were made at several points in the telecommunication implementation cycle outlined in Box 6-4. Visit the Web addresses listed in references 9 and 10 to learn more about the Cedars Sinai experience. After reading these two short articles, use your knowledge of the telecommunication implementation cycle to develop a plan for reimplementing the computerized order entry system at Cedars Sinai.

The Clinician's Implementation Role

As a clinician, your role in telecommunications initiatives will be to provide your input and expectations for the system.

The best way to initiate a telecommunication implementation is to bring together the users to define the problem to be solved and the overall goals of the system. As a clinician, your role in telecommunications initiatives will be to provide your input and expectations for the system. The best way to do this is to follow a systematic approach.

1. Define the Problem. The clinician's first job in a telecommunication implementation is to concisely define the problem from the user's perspective. For example, perhaps the institution's pharmacists are unable to access patients' laboratory results through the pharmacy side of the hospital information system. When defining this problem, you should determine if all patients' results cannot be accessed, the problem only applies to patients in a specific unit, only a certain set of laboratory results cannot be accessed, only a subset of pharmacists have this problem, or some other combination of circumstances leads to the problem.

2. Limit the Problem. The second step is to determine the limits of the problem. In the example above, if the problem only occurs with patients in the medical/surgical unit, manpower and technical resources should be used to identify which unique properties of this unit distinguishes it from the others. In today's cash-strapped health care environment, any resource that can be redirected toward other problems is essentially money and time saved.

3. Analyze the Problem. Next, you must thoroughly analyze the problem. After determining that the problem is with a specific unit in the hospital, you can help recreate the exact situation that leads to the problem's occurrence. In fact, end users are best able to perform the analysis step because of their intimate familiarity with the system and the situations that lead to the problem. A thorough analysis phase with clear documentation helps develop the best possible solution.

4. Propose a Solution. The fourth step is to develop specifications for what is essentially a proposed solution to the problem and give them to the technical crew (or other appropriate personnel in your institution, depending on the problem) responsible for actually correcting the problem. Here, you serve as a resource to clarify any points of confusion and provide the user's perspective of the problem.

5. Test the Solution. In the fifth step, you test the solution—either in a prototypical environment or in a fully functional version. At this point, clinicians need to thoroughly evaluate the solution based on evaluation criteria previously established.

6. Provide Feedback. As a clinician, your final step is to give feedback to the system developer so the system put in place as the solution to the original problem can be continually modified and maintained, an ongoing process.

Increasing Your Use of Telecommunications

Most telecommunication applications discussed in the following sections require high-speed Internet connections. Table 6-2 compares the download capability of the most popular Internet connection types, including high-speed options, known as broadband connections.

TABLE 6-2

Download Speeds for Various Internet Connection Types

Type	Download Speed	Time to Download			
		5 KB e-mail	5 MB file	10 MB file	30 MB file
Dial-up	56 KBps	1 sec	15 min	28.4 min	80 min
Cable	200 KBps–30 MBps	< 1 sec	40 sec	1.4 min	4 min
DSL	144 KBps–8 MBps	< 1 sec	1 min	1.8 min	7 min
ISDN	128 KBps	< 1 sec	8 min	10.7 min	40 min
Satellite	400–500 KBps	< 1 sec	2 min	3.4 min	15 min

Source: References 12 and 13.

Broadband describes telecommunication media that can carry multiple data, voice, or video channels simultaneously. Broadband media include coaxial cable, fiber-optic cable, and satellite.

Technically, broadband describes telecommunication media that can carry multiple data, voice, or video channels simultaneously. Broadband media include coaxial cable, fiber-optic cable, and satellite. Broadband service includes cable modems, digital subscriber line (DSL) modems, and satellites, and is generally more expensive than dial-up connections. An estimated 55% of adult Internet users have broadband access at home or work.[11]

Cable modems are often rated as one of the fastest broadband options available. While this is generally true, cable modems are sometimes subject to significant decreases in speed because users in a common area share the network. Box 6-5 provides addresses of two Web sites you can visit to test your Internet connection, which will give you a reference point for the discussion that follows.

BOX 6-5

Test Your Internet Connection Speed

The sites below let you test the speed of your Internet connection for free simply by supplying quick, basic information about your connection type.

- Bandwidth Place: http://bandwidthplace.com/speedtest
- CNet.com: http://reviews.cnet.com/7004-7254_7-0.html?tag=cnetfd.dir

E-mail

One of the greatest benefits of e-mail is the ability to add an attachment. Where you previously used an overnight courier service to send an important file, e-mail attachments allow you to save time and money by appending files to an e-mail message. E-mail also allows you to wait until the last possible minute to complete the document before sending it.

E-mail is also very useful for mass communication. Distribution lists, listservs, and other group-oriented functionality give e-mail users the ability to communicate with literally thousands of people through a single action. In health care settings, various kinds of group lists are often used to give practitioners the most recent treatment updates or to let staff know about upcoming meetings.

Push Technology

You may already be using push technology without realizing it. Push technology is user-requested e-mails periodically sent out about content categories that the e-mail recipient has specified. If you have signed up to have information sent to you by e-mail on subjects you have designated, you are using push technology. Push technology is not "spam," which is unsolicited junk mail sent as e-mail messages.

Push technology can be a way of automatically keeping up with information with little to no effort on your part. If you have a topical area of interest, you can probably find a Web site devoted to the area that will let you sign up for push e-mails. Push technology also comes at a great price—it's free.

Many Web sites use push technology service as a way to obtain e-mail addresses for marketing purposes, so you should read the fine print when signing up for push e-mails.

Push technology allows information to be delivered automatically over the Internet to a preselected audience.

ACTIVITY 6-4

Push Technology

Perform the following push technology activities:

1. Identify five Internet Web sites that provide a push e-mail service. A good starting point is to visit your favorite news Internet site and explore it for the option to receive e-mail updates.
2. Register to receive push e-mail messages in three content categories that interest you, such as clinical trial information, new treatment options for a disease of interest, or international news. Then perform the steps that the e-mail service outlines to unsubscribe. How easy is the process? What problems do you see with it?
3. Resubscribe to at least one of the e-mail services you selected and after an adequate trial period, decide if you would like to keep it. Why or why not?

Instant Messaging

Instant messaging (IM) is closely related to e-mail, except that people who use it share a common display area where their typed messages appear as soon as they press the Enter key. You do not deal with the transfer delays that occur with regular e-mail messages when you are in an IM session.

Instant messaging is not just for kids and college students. Many IM software applications allow much more than simple text messages to be displayed. Users can send and receive files, share a whiteboard on which participants in the message session can draw pictures, and share the messaging session with multiple users. Other IM functionality includes voice and video shared over the same connection as the text-based message. Most IM software programs are free, making them economical and easy to use. Box 6-6 lists some of the available IM programs.

BOX 6-6

A Sampling of Free IM Software

- **AOL Instant Messenger:** www.aim.com. The most popular IM program today
- **ICQ Instant Messenger:** www.icq.com. One of the first IM programs available
- **MSN Messenger:** http://messenger.msn.com. The second most popular IM program.
- **Praize Instant Messenger:** www.praize.com/IM. An IM program for Christians
- **Windows Messenger:** Part of Microsoft Windows XP
- **Yahoo! Messenger:** messenger.yahoo.com. Includes games and personalized radio stations

---

Several IM programs have an embedded feature that allows users to share applications. In the sharing mode, person A grants person B control over his computer and/or specific software programs. Person B is then able to remotely control person A's computer via the shared connection, an ability used by hardware and software vendors to help troubleshoot their customers' problems. As frequent users of computer-based applications, health care professionals can expect to find themselves participating in these types of sessions.

File Transfer Protocol

File Transfer Protocol (FTP), closely related to TCP/IP, is the primary means of transferring files across the Internet and uses TCP/IP as its communication protocol.

Webmasters commonly use FTP to transfer Web sites from their local computer to the server where the Web site is stored. The popular online music swapping Web sites (that have become the targets of the Recording Industry Association of America) often use FTP to transfer files between users' computers. Transferring files through instant messaging applications also uses FTP. There are many FTP programs available for download directly from the Internet, including free versions. Figure 6-12 shows an example of FTP.

FIGURE 6-12

File Transfer Protocol is the underlying application allowing file downloading (and uploading) via the Internet.

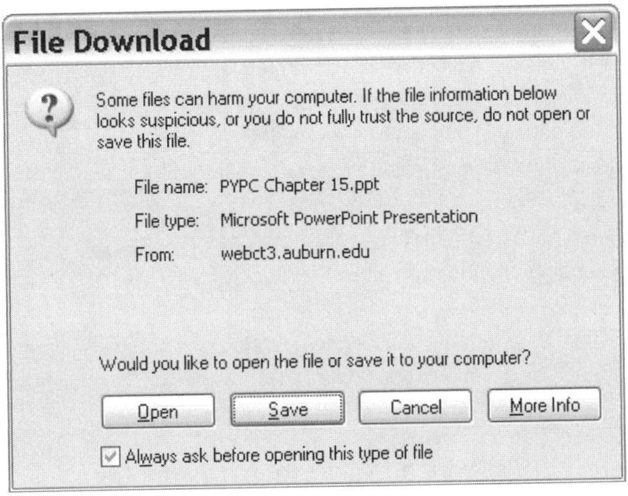

FTP is not used simply for "recreational" purposes. When you are trying to send very large attachments, File Transfer Protocol offers a significant advantage over customary e-mail because many e-mail inboxes have a preset maximum allowed attachment size—especially Web-based e-mail services. FTP allows users to directly transfer a file over the Internet that may be too large to send or receive as an e-mail attachment. Using the Internet address of the receiving computer, the sender is able to directly transfer the file.

The Health Insurance Portability and Accountability Act of 1996 (HIPAA) has received enormous attention because of the requirements it places on health care clinicians and health systems when transferring patient-identifiable information. Fortunately, developers of FTP software are aware of the implications and requirements of HIPAA, and have developed HIPAA-compliant software. Ipswitch, a Massachusetts-based company that develops network management, messaging, and file transfer software, has a useful White Paper on its Web site that discusses HIPAA and security, available at www.ipswitch.com/products/ws_ftp/industry/healthcare.asp.

File Transfer Protocol (FTP) ✓

1. Identify five free FTP programs located at www.tucows.com.
2. Pick one of these programs and complete the following with a colleague, friend, or family member:
   a. Download it and acquaint yourself with its user interface.
   b. Explore the program's compliance with the security requirements of the Health Insurance Portability and Accountability Act (HIPAA). This may involve visiting the software developer's Web site.
   c. Find the information that explains how to initiate a file transfer and share this information with your FTP partner.
   d. Select files of various types and sizes and send them.
   e. Evaluate how easy the program is to use.

Pick another of the five programs you identified in step one and repeat items a-e. Go through this process for each program until you find an FTP program you like, then uninstall the others.

Software and Document Distribution

i Application service providers are third-party entities that manage and distribute software-based services across a network from a central data center.

To share documents and software, users must be connected to a network with a central server that houses the specific applications and documents. Users initiate a request for an application or a document on their local machines. The server recognizes the request and "serves up" the requested file to the user.

This type of software and document distribution requires a high-speed network that can accommodate extremely large traffic volume. Today's health care environments are starting to implement the necessary telecommunication channels to handle such data flow, but connection speeds faster than 56 Kbps will be required as clinicians' demand for access increases.

Application service providers (ASP) are closely related to the type of network described in the first paragraph of this section. ASPs are entities external to a health care institution that provide software-based services to their customers. Using a centralized data center and high-speed connectivity, health care institutions can outsource much of their software and hardware technology needs to the ASP organization. In turn, all software maintenance and updating is handled by the service provider, freeing clinicians to perform clinical services. In some ASP models, all clinical data reside with the ASP, including patient data and practice support data that the clinician relies on to provide care. Using an ASP gives clinicians a software interface and high-speed connection at their clinical practice site that lets them access all software and data that reside at the ASP's location.

Some community pharmacy operations offer excellent examples of ASPs in action. The pharmacy uses a high-speed, full-time Internet connection to connect to the ASP vendor, which houses and maintains the pharmacy's patient database, clinical decision-support database, and third-party payer database. All dispensing transaction processes occur at the ASP site, which allows the pharmacist to focus on dispensing prescriptions and counseling patients instead of troubleshooting software or maintaining databases.

Videoconferencing

Videoconferencing allows multiple users in different locations to communicate over the Internet with voice, data, and video capabilities. All videoconferencing software has core components including text chat component, shared whiteboard, file transfer, application sharing, and audio/video.

Videoconferencing software applications and hardware components are differentiated based on their ease of use, sophistication, operating system platform compatibility, and price. For example, several of the free IM software applications have features beyond simple text chatting, but their level of sophistication can be limited. The decision quickly becomes whether a free application can meet your needs or if you should spend thousands of dollars to purchase a professional level suite. Box 6-7 lists some videoconferencing software and hardware sources.

BOX 6-7

Sample Audio and Videoconferencing Software/Hardware

Centra: www.centra.com
Click to Meet: www.radvision.com/EnterpriseSolutions/videoconferencingproducts/ClicktoMeet
Conferencing.net: www.conferencing.net
Connex International: www.connexintl.com
eStreamingMedia: www.estreamingmedia.com
Genesys Conferencing: www.genesys.com
Helpmeeting.com: www.helpmeeting.com
Netspoke: www.netspoke.com

This decision of whether to go with a free service or pay for professional videoconferencing equipment may not be difficult if the system is for the boardroom of a major health care institution, where the ability to have several microphones and video cameras positioned throughout the room is much more desirable than a single video camera and microphone shared by all. The average cost to set up a typical group videoconference room is $60,000.[3] On the other hand, you can set up a personal videoconference system at home or at an office for as little as $200. Using the Windows Messenger application that comes standard with Windows XP, a $100 Web camera, and a $50 headset microphone, you'll still have $50 left to pay for the first month's high-speed Internet service you'll need for videoconferencing.

ACTIVITY 6-6

Videoconferencing

Learn more about videoconferencing by performing the activities below. You will need a microphone and speakers connected to your computer, a high-speed Internet connection, and someone to share your videoconference.

1. Determine if your computer has preinstalled videoconference capabilities called NetMeeting using the Help feature. (Type "videoconference" in the search field. If this feature is already installed, skip step 2.)
2. Obtain free videoconference software:
   a. Users of Windows 95, 98, Me, or NT 4.0 should use Windows NetMeeting. (Go to Microsoft.com and type in "NetMeeting.")
   b. Windows 2000 users should click on Start – Programs – Accessories – Communications – NetMeeting.
   c. Windows XP users should click on Start – All Programs – Windows Messenger.
   d. Users of Mac OS X Panther should use iChat AV.
3. Establish and experiment with a text chat session.
4. Share the whiteboard and take turns drawing on it.
5. Transfer files between your computer and the computer of your videoconference colleague.
6. Experiment with the application-sharing capability of the program by sharing an Internet browser with your conferencing partner.
7. Experiment with the program's audio capabilities by speaking into your computer's microphone and listening as your conferencing partner does the same on his or her computer.
8. If Web cameras are available, experiment with the program's video capabilities by having a live videoconference your conferencing partner.

Distance Learning

Distance learning is not limited to college students anymore. All health care professionals are required to maintain competency within their disciplines, and the number of online learning options is increasing. Although national association meetings are great places to fulfill continuing education requirements because of the high-caliber experts brought in to speak, clinicians are not always able to take time away from their practices to attend. Recognizing this problem, event organizers have come up with accessible alternatives, such as placing the speaker's slides on the Internet along with an audio recording of the presentation to create a Web-based version. Clinicians can view the presentation with full function controls, take the posttest, and receive continuing education credit—all made possible through a high-speed Internet connection. Figure 6-13 shows an online distance education program offered by the American Society of Health-System Pharmacists. On the left of the screen, you can see the controls available to the user, such as "take notes" and "take CE test."

FIGURE 6-13

A distance education program. Note the various controls on the left that are available to the program viewer.

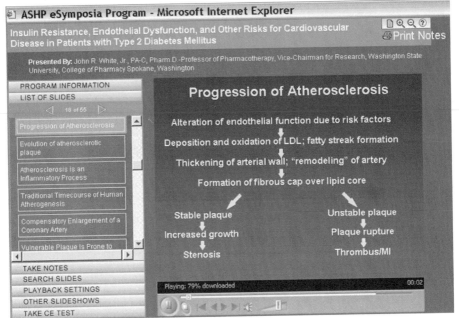

Reprinted with permission of the American Society of Health-System Pharmacists.

Clinicians are beginning to identify and explore potential telecommuting roles as the aging population places more demand on their time.

Telecommuting

Telecommuting (also known as telework) allows people to work away from the office, usually at home offices equipped with the essentials of traditional offices. High-speed Internet connections are the norm, connecting the telecommuter in real-time with resources back at the office. Telecommuters often split their time each week between working from a home office and going to work onsite, but some work from home exclusively. Research indicates that companies can save approximately $10,000 per year for each employee who telecommutes, in part through reduced office space and supply expenses.[3] By some estimates, workers achieve a 10% to 40% increase in productivity by telecommuting.[14] Telecommuting also helps reduce pollution and traffic, allows workers flexible schedules to meet demands of family life, and benefits people whose physical constraints prevent them from commuting or working onsite.[3]

Radiologists have been reading films remotely for years, but even so, telecommuting is new to the health care environment. Clinicians are beginning to identify and explore potential telecommuting roles as the aging population places more demand on their time. Telenursing allows nurses to monitor patients in their homes from anywhere, including the nurse's home. Automated dispensing technology allows pharmacists to remotely dispense medications in isolated areas that are too small to support traditional pharmacy services. This variant of telecommuting is one way that telecommunication technology facilitates patient care. The key feature of telecommuting is that it allows work from any location.

We are standing on the tip of the telecommuting iceberg. The changing demographics of the U.S. population will place considerable demands on the health care system. Patients will increasingly desire to remain at home to control their conditions, and telecommunication technology will connect these patients with their caregivers. Telecommunication technology will also help meet the demands placed on the health care system by geographical limitations that create barriers to adequate care and will help clinicians connect to patients, resources, and other health care providers to facilitate care regardless of time and place.

References

1. Carr HC, Snyder CA. *The Management of Telecommunications: Business Solutions to Business Problems.* Boston, MA: Irwin McGraw-Hill; 1997.

2. Baldwin FD. Traveling in PACS. Healthcare Informatics Online. Available at: www.healthcare-informatics.com/issues/2003/11_03/cover.htm. Accessed March 28, 2004.

3. Stair RM, Reynolds GW. *Principles of Information Systems: A Managerial Approach.* 5th ed. Boston, MA: International Thomson Publishing; 2001.

4. Turban E, Rainer RK, Potter RE. *Introduction to Information Technology.* 2nd ed. New York: John Wiley & Sons; 2003.

5. Greenspan R. Callers hanging up on wireline phones. ClickZ Stats. Available at: www.clickz.com/stats/big_picture/hardware/article.php/3319251. Accessed March 1, 2004.

6. Leiner BM, Cerf VG, Clark DD, et al. A brief history of the Internet. Internet Society. Available at: www.isoc.org/internet/history/brief.shtml. Accessed January 13, 2004.

7. CyberAtlas. Population explosion! Available at: http://cyberatlas.internet.com/big_picture/geographics/article/0,1323,5911_151151,00.html. Accessed January 13, 2004.

8. Vocera Communications. Vocera communications system helps improve staff communication. Available at: www.vocera.com/PDF/stvincents.pdf. Accessed April 17, 2004.

9. Chin T. Doctors pull plug on paperless system. *American Medical News.* Available at: www.ama-assn.org/amednews/2003/02/17/bil20217.htm. Accessed April 17, 2004.

10. Bass A. A big rollout bust. Cio.com. Available at: www.cio.com/archive/060103/tl_health.html. Accessed April 17, 2004.

11. TechWeb News. Surge in DSL pushed broadband in the home. DigitalConnect.com. Available at: www.digitalconnectmag.com/showArticle.jhtml?articleID=18902136&_. Accessed April 21, 2004.

12. Lonestar Broadband. How fast is fast? A broadband comparison of download speeds. Available at: www.lonestarbroadband.org/background/howfast.htm. Accessed April 21, 2004.

13. YZ Technology. Broadband comparison. Available at: www.yztech.com/Broadband.html. Accessed April 21, 2004.

14. European Telework Online. Telework (telecommuting): The benefits and some issues! Available at: www.eto.org.uk/faq/faq03.htm. Accessed April 21, 2004.

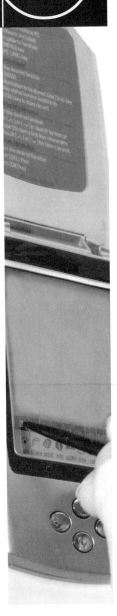

CHAPTER

Point of Care 7
Technology

Bill G. Felkey

Chapter Objectives

After completing this chapter, you should be able to:

- Describe briefly at least four technologies that focus on the point of care.
- Discuss key components to include in a computerized prescriber order entry (CPOE) system.
- List options for ensuring privacy on CPOE systems.
- Describe ways that personal digital assistants (PDAs) can be used in health care.
- Describe four potential levels of bar code point of care (BPOC) systems.
- Discuss issues to consider when implementing an electronic clinical data repository (CDR).
- Describe how the Veterans Health Administration has used technology to enhance the point of care.

P oint of care, one of the largest growth areas in health care, is also one of the most exciting. The "point of care"—the place where providers render care to patients—is taking on a whole new definition as technology becomes more mobile. Thanks to advances in computing technology, patients and providers benefit from powerful information systems and appliances in ways not imagined decades ago—such as delivering evidence-based medicine and monitoring therapeutic and financial outcomes at the point of care.

Wireless networks and mobile hardware are allowing broader access to patient information so that now, a growing number of clinicians can retrieve data almost anywhere in their health care setting. In other words, point of care technology is no longer in a few fixed spots, such as the physician's office or the bedside. Point of care includes "near patient" locations—nursing units, physician lounges, cafeterias, satellite pharmacies, and clinic or hospital hallways—where colleagues collaborate to prevent, identify, and resolve medical and drug-related problems.

In fact, the point of care is becoming less physical and more virtual as "mobile care" becomes more prevalent,[1] giving health care professionals access to information wherever they are. Mobile care, a relatively new term, relates to the ability to render care wherever providers find themselves.

Even more relevant may be the concept of "moment of care"—where the provider's clinical skills are supported by evidence-based information to reduce the level of uncertainty as decisions are made. Information technology and portable devices can support care not only by providing reference-based information, but also by supplying alerts and key details as soon as they become available. Knowing that a medication has been discontinued because of allergic reaction problems is of little value after you've already pushed the syringe.

Many clinicians have taken a grass-roots approach to point of care, acquiring their own personal technology. At the same time, institutions are launching organized initiatives to address the information needs of practitioners by rolling out a variety of point of care solutions. Providers generally like to be able to pick technology that meets their own set of personal criteria. For example, while one practitioner is willing to carry a tablet PC, another wants an appliance that fits in a shirt pocket.

Mobile care, a relatively new term, relates to the ability to render care wherever providers find themselves.

Some focus on clinical references while others stress connectivity. This chapter highlights major areas related to point of care technology.

BOX 7-1

Mobile Technology Devices

Here's an overview of devices that are making health care delivery at the point of care more widespread:

- **Personal digital assistants (PDAs):** These pocket-sized information appliances are now powerful enough to do almost all the information processing that health care professionals need. When combined with the cellular telephone they allow connectivity wherever you want it. The main drawback of the PDA is its small screen size, which limits the amount of viewable information displayed at a glance.
- **Notebook computers:** These portable computers only weigh between 2 and 8 pounds but can be as powerful as any desktop computer. Usually sized at approximately 8.5 by 11 inches and between 1 and 3 inches thick, they offer a full-sized keyboard and integrated pointing device as well as the processing power to provide continuous speech recognition. Although heavier than the PDA, they provide the power of a fixed workstation.
- **Tablet-based computers:** Similar to a notebook computer in size and weight, these portable computers offer a stylus-based method for data entry. Their handwriting recognition capabilities let you write with the stylus on the touch-sensitive screen; in many medical applications, the device offers pick lists of structured information that you normally enter during the medical visit.
- **Wirelessly connected computers on wheels (COWs):** These workstations can offer full-sized displays and extra-long battery life for mobile health care professionals. The computer is integrated into a movable stand that can accompany you as you move about a hospital or nursing wing. Since the units are on wheels, a large battery is part of the typical configuration.
- **Touch screens:** These permanently installed workstations at bedsides or in nursing units or exam rooms make information readily available. Some operations prefer these devices because they allow normal coaxial networks to connect terminals to a common database for data integration.
- **Wireless air panel:** Functioning much like a tablet PC, this device remotely accesses an office-based personal computer. Ideally the air panel has a large-screen display—15 to 21 inches—with long-life battery power, high-speed, secure wireless connectivity, bar code scanning, and the ability to port the information it generates onto a PDA screen for use outside the walls of the facility.

The Clinical Information System

The Clinical Information System is a complex combination of hardware and software operating on a network that moves data to where clinical departments and practitioners need it. The overall clinical information system serves as the infrastructure to the point of care system components.

At the point of care, tools must be efficient and effective, formatting information for quick retrieval—what is called a "granular" format.

Because many appliances used at the point of care are wireless, the ability to move and integrate data displays into many formats is necessary to support clinical decision making. This requires a sophisticated information technology (IT) staff who can anticipate the ways in which data are going to be used at the point of care and ensure that these data can be properly displayed on whatever device is used.

At the point of care, tools must be efficient and effective, formatting information for quick retrieval—what is called a "granular" format. When you are trying to decide how to dose a patient with renal impairment, having to read a complete drug information monograph would not be productive. Instead, point of care information allows you jump quickly to the critical nugget of information. This granular format reduces information overload and what is described as information "noise"—anything that does not help solve the clinical problem at hand.

BOX 7-2

Patients Central to Setting Priorities

Using a patient-focused strategy is the best way to set priorities when implementing new technology, given the many options available. This means that maximizing the quality of patient care ranks first in determining the sequence of implementation. For example, any technology that improves patient safety outcomes would be chosen over those that create better working environments for support departments. Technology for clinical departments that render direct patient care would also be high priority.

Electronic Medical Record

The centerpiece of all point of care information is the electronic medical record (EMR), which presents what has gone on before and what is known in the present—the repository of all interventions and evaluations that relate to the patient's future. Because EMRs are electronic, they are viewable by every person from every discipline and specialty who is applying knowledge for the benefit of any individual patient.

Built in to EMRs are clinical decision support systems that alert caregivers to possible complications arising from their actions, such as allergy warnings, duplicate therapy warnings, redundant laboratory orders, and medical clues to precipitating events. EMRs can be customized to capture the workflow preferences of each provider, so the family practitioner sees one presentation of the medical record, the ophthalmologist sees another.

One of the most important attributes of the best point of care EMRs is the synopsis view, which at a glance alerts any care provider to the availability of relevant information about a patient, such as impressions recorded by a radiologist or chart information posted by a nurse. The EMR can aggregate the data on a combined line chart and even display normal values for reference and color code the data.

The best point of care EMRs offer a synopsis view, alerting you at a glance to relevant information about a patient.

Computerized Prescriber Order Entry

Although computerized prescriber order entry (CPOE) should be an integrated part of the clinical information system, many organizations are developing it as a standalone application that does not mesh fully with the EMR. We believe it's critical for the EMR to be fully implemented before adopting CPOE so that all the technologies work together.

In integrated systems, for example, you are supplied the patient's body mass from the EMR when you dose a medication, allowing for precision. When systems are not integrated, the medical record might indicate that a patient has asthma but the order entry system will not have this information, and thus will not send an alert if an order is placed for a drug contraindicated in patients with asthma.

Documentation Systems

Another critical component of clinical information systems is the ability to document care provided by each member of the team. In fact, being able to document care efficiently plays a major role in whether users will accept the system. Right now, handwritten documentation or oral dictation that must be transcribed is the norm. Transcription costs health systems and group practices hundreds of thousands of dollars. Moving to a combination of speech recognition and stylus-based menus should greatly facilitate clinical workups and documentation of care.

Decision Support Systems

Thousands of clinical decisions are made every day that represent potential life-and-death consequences for patients. The software in decision support systems (DSS) figuratively "looks over the shoulder" of the person making the decision and flags potentially significant medical problems that could stem from a particular action. Some of these flags may suggest alternatives or concurrent actions to safeguard the patient. For example, if bed rest is ordered, the DSS would suggest the use of heparin. The DSS would also suggest how often laboratory studies should be scheduled to monitor potential toxicities of a drug and give warnings of allergies, duplicate therapy, and drug interactions.

Order Entry at the Point of Care Poised for Growth

As the medication use process in hospitals and health systems grows more complex, reliance on four technologies to help practitioners improve safety, efficiency, and overall patient care is becoming more important. One of these is CPOE, which digitally transmits legible medication orders into pharmacy management software without an extra data input step—a step rife with opportunity for error. Because CPOE systems contain DSS, they enhance the quality of care through evidence-based product selection. EMRs are also key, as are electronic medication administration records (eMARs) and bar code verification of medication in hospitals and at bedsides. Increasing internal and external pressure is causing at least 40% of U.S. hospitals to begin planning and installing order entry technologies, and the other technologies are at similar levels of adoption, according to the Health Information and Management Systems Society's 2005 survey.[2]

Before adopting order entry systems, many inpatient institutions are waiting for major health information system companies to add them to their product offerings. In ambulatory care, state-level Blue Cross/Blue Shield organizations are beginning to roll out CPOE systems for use by affiliated prescribers. In focus groups, prescribers mention that they like such immediate benefits as refill authorizations of chronic prescriptions that reduce the number of calls from pharmacies, but are less enthusiastic about moving to CPOE for generating new prescriptions. Incentives from the federal government and state legislation will continue to push adoption, as will performance incentives such as a differentiated reimbursement for those using order entry systems.

Although many health systems began moving to CPOE before implementing EMRs, this trend is reversing. As mentioned above, an order entry system that is not fully integrated into a medical record does not possess all the critical patient data that influence what kind of medication, strength, duration, and route of administration to prescribe. A recent study reported in the *Journal of the American Medical Association* found that a leading hospital CPOE system exacerbated 22 types of medication error risks, even though these systems are widely regarded as the technical solution to such errors.[3] Many of these errors, such as ignoring antibiotic renewal notices on paper charts, would not occur in integrated EMR systems. David Bates, MD, professor at Harvard Medical School and a champion of information technology to reduce medical mistakes, noted that the study focused on a relatively old CPOE system. His own studies through the federally funded Centers of Patient Safety and Research indicate that adopting appropriate technology should bring "a hundredfold reduction in the medication error rate in the inpatient setting."[4]

An order entry system that is not fully integrated into a medical record does not possess all the critical patient data that influence what kind of medication, strength, duration, and route of administration to prescribe.

Implementation Approaches

At least four types of implementations, listed below, are being used for CPOE. More research is needed to determine which works best in terms of ease of transition, error rates as personnel adapt, and so on.

1. Direct cutoff: the manual system is discontinued on a given day and the organization starts the CPOE method.
2. Parallel implementation: both manual and computerized ordering is done and the manual method is eventually eliminated.
3. Pilot type: selected nursing units are given the new system and new units are added as the system proves its merits.
4. Phased implementation: some types of electronic order entry are implemented initially and the full array of CPOE is reached over time.

Key Components

Key components to include in CPOE applications include:

1. DSS that provides active alerts and guidelines.
2. Integration with existing systems.

3. Ability to scan the existing medication regimen for potential drug-drug interactions, allergies, medications that affect the accuracy of laboratory results, and contraindications.
4. Knowledge rules, which take 18 to 24 months to establish. A knowledge rule is an "if-then" statement usually monitored by the DSS. For example, if the system detects that a potentially life-threatening and therefore highly significant drug interaction will occur when a new medication is ordered, a knowledge rule will require that a pharmacist verify the appropriateness of a prescriber's override.
5. "Smart prompts" from the order entry system suggesting other evidence-based actions that can be taken to optimize patient care practices. For example, if a particular beneficial medication is known to frequently cause stomach irritation, alternative medications or combination medications may be suggested for the prescriber.
6. Display of primary literature (short monograph reviews or access to full text articles) to help in decision making.

One note of caution about all the possible "help" CPOE software can offer: a well-documented problem called "alert fatigue" can occur when these systems interrupt the workflow too often. People who implement the CPOE systems may need to pick their battles carefully to avoid user frustration during the order entry process.

BOX 7-3

Options for Ensuring Privacy on CPOE Systems

■ Encryption, which converts plain text information into code to prevent unauthorized viewing of protected health information.
■ Incorporating information appliances that offer their own internal security, such as password protection or biometric fingerprinting, so only authorized users can access the unit.
■ Using "thin clients," which are low-cost computing devices that access applications and data from a secure central server over a network without storing them locally on a PDA or other point of care device. When using thin clients, you must protect against fraudulent use so unauthorized personnel cannot enter orders for substances of abuse.

Patient Safety at the Point of Care

In 1999, when the Institute of Medicine (IOM) published its landmark report *To Err Is Human,*[5] much attention became focused on patient safety—already a major topic of public concern thanks to some high-profile medical errors reported by the press. A study by the American Society of Health-System Pharmacists found that the major concern of hospitalized patients is experiencing a medication error.[6] Concern about patient safety is the chief drive for adopting such point of care technologies as bar codes and CPOE.

Research performed by the IOM has shown that information transfer problems are the root cause of many patient safety issues. Point of care technologies such as PDAs, which are growing in popularity among health care providers, should significantly reduce medication and medical errors when they are connected to bar code scanning and specialized wireless communication applications. In a study conducted in 2002, one in five American families (8.1 million households) reported experiencing a serious medication error during hospitalization.[7] The authors noted that most of these errors—which occurred during the ordering process and at the point of administration—could be eliminated by increased use of wireless PDAs and bar code scanning.

Point of care technologies such as PDAs, which are growing in popularity among health care providers, should significantly reduce medication and medical errors when they are connected to bar code scanning and specialized wireless communication applications.

BOX 7-4

Leadership Needed to Address Patient Safety

Health care leaders must take the forefront in guiding organizations through the attitudinal and behavioral changes needed to address patient safety. Today's environment tends toward "blame and shame," so that health care workers are reluctant to report errors for fear of retribution. To make real headway in reducing error rates and improving patient outcomes, a culture must be fostered that looks at errors as a symptom of a disease that can be cured (sometimes with the help of technology).

1. Continuous quality improvement (CQI) teams made up of each discipline and specialty should examine the errors occurring and address appropriate ways to identify, prevent, and resolve future errors.
2. Using a systems approach, each component of the health care system should be examined for ways it contributes to errors and ways it can prevent them.
3. Error detection methods should move toward direct observation and away from voluntary reporting.
4. When personnel make errors, nonpunitive risk-management approaches should be employed. Retraining rather than removal should be the first response to errors whenever possible.

Bar Code Point of Care (BPOC) Systems

Bar code technology at the point of care can be an effective tool for decreasing medication errors and enhancing patient safety, studies indicate. Bar code point of care (BPOC) systems for medication administration at various levels of sophistication have shown documented decreases in medication errors ranging from 65% to 74%.[8,9]

BPOC systems constitute the final safety net before patients receive their medications. In addition to using bar codes and scanning technology to electronically verify medication administration, BPOC systems collect critical charting information such as:

- Patient identity.
- Patient demographics.
- Status of orders.
- Specific characteristics and timing parameters for each scheduled administration of a medication.

Users can also enter into the system clinical observations such as pain scale ratings, adverse reactions, or atypical pulse. If the system provides accurate and complete medication administration records, hospitals can eliminate paper processes entirely, saving hours of nursing administrative work per shift.

Bridge Medical, a southern California-based provider of patient safety technology, has proposed a useful approach to addressing medication errors: levels of BPOC administration systems.[10] These levels are described below.

Level 1: 'Five-Rights' Checker Systems

These systems are very basic, simply verifying the "five rights" of medication administration:

- Right patient
- Right medication
- Right dose
- Right time
- Right route of administration

The pharmacy sends orders and schedules of drug administration times electronically to the BPOC system. When the nurse scans the patient's wristband and the medication's bar codes using a handheld scanner, the system automatically doublechecks via a wireless network to ensure that the appropriate patient is about to receive an appropriate medication and that no medications have been discontinued or dosages altered since the original medication order was placed. Level 1 systems provide a complete and accurate eMAR and full patient information at the point of care, in a real-time, single-source presentation.

Level 1 systems cannot intercept mistakes in the medication order, such as dosing a drug at a level 10 times too high because of a transcription error. Key features that Level 1 systems may include:

- Customizable work lists for nurses that establish the most efficient sequence for delivering medications within a unit.
- Alerts for missed doses.
- Online access to the hospital formulary.
- Storage of data collected by the bar code scanner in an electronic format for retrospective analysis.

Level 2: Integrated Online Medication Reference Systems with Enhanced Pharmacy Communication

More evolved systems go beyond checking the five rights to give providers more information about medications and facilitate electronic communication with the pharmacy. For example, a pharmacist can enter a customizable comment for any medication in the formulary, which clinicians can see when they order the medication. Prescribers also receive information from online reference libraries about the medications they order, such as:

- An image of the tablet or capsule.
- Usual dosages in which the medication is supplied on the formulary.
- Details of proper administration.
- Contraindications.
- Warnings.
- Adverse reactions.
- Pregnancy risk factors.

Level 2 systems may also allow patients to review educational pamphlets online or print them at the nursing station. The most sophisticated Level 2 systems integrate dose calculation tables. Although these systems do not alert providers to potential errors in medication orders, they do provide tools for the medication administration nurse to proactively research a medication order.

Level 3: Embedded Computer Logic and Alert Engine Systems

The third level of BPOC technology incorporates "rules engines" into the process of verifying the five rights—that is, intelligence based on "if-then" parameters from actual experience that not only identify potential problems but also suggest resolution options. Level 3 systems are able to compare the pharmacy order and the nurse's actions against preprogrammed standards. For example, suppose an order specifies "acetaminophen 500 mg orally every 4-6 hours for pain or fever" and the maximum dose is 4 grams of acetaminophen, or a total of 8 tablets, in a 24-hour period. At each administration, the software will refer to a rolling 24-hour count of doses given and signal the nurse when an additional dose would exceed the maximum 4 grams of acetaminophen.

The system will also alert nurses to the potential for confusion over look-alike/sound-alike medications and tell them the intended use of the medication they are about to administer. Having been made aware of the potential for an error, the nurse may opt to verify the order with the physician or pharmacist.

These advanced systems may also include:

- High-risk medication warnings: alerts to potential errors that could produce drastic consequences.
- Prompts telling the prescriber to record additional clinical information for certain medications.
- Reports of near-miss errors such as process errors that are caught upon inspection.
- Order reconciliation that reports the steps necessary to resolve problems.

The order reconciliation capability allows health care providers to use the system safeguards when they administer pending or standing (stat) orders that have not yet been verified by a pharmacist. In some facilities, these may account for up to 30% of all orders. Without the ability to enter a stat order into the system when patients receive unscheduled doses and to later link it with the pharmacy order, medications may be double-dosed when regularly scheduled drugs duplicate stat orders.

Level 3 systems are combined with online reference materials and tools to prevent errors proactively and give nurses access to key clinical knowledge during the medication administration process.

Level 4: Expanded Point of Care Safeguard: Blood Transfusion and Specimen Collection

This level is sophisticated enough to go beyond medication administration and address bedside errors. It also includes other critical point of care safety checks for blood transfusions and laboratory specimens.

The most common transfusion error is giving correctly labeled blood to the wrong patient. The blood transfusion software application allows hospitals to ensure that patients receive the specific units of blood that have been typed and crossmatched for them. Before a transfusion begins, the nurse scans the patient's bar coded identification bracelet and the transfusion identification number on the unit of blood. If there is a potential error, the software generates an audible alarm and visual warning.

The systems can be programmed to remind clinicians to perform any checks the hospital requires, such as documenting vital signs before, during, and after a transfusion and recording reactions. All documentation generated during this process is entered into the patient's electronic chart.

Level 4 systems can also verify that laboratory specimens are correctly identified, solidifying the link between patient and specimen. Mislabeled laboratory specimens can lead to inappropriate results, misguided therapy, and unnecessary additional collection of specimens.

The Level 4 system lets clinicians add tests not ordered via the laboratory information system and generate labels bearing all pertinent information, thus eliminating the hazard of difficult-to-read handwritten labels. Clinicians can view collection instructions and correctly calculate the amount of blood needed for all tests ordered to prevent having to redraw the sample again if blood is collected inappropriately. These features are of tremendous benefit to hospitals with a decentralized phlebotomy function because they coach less-experienced phlebotomists through the process, including selecting the correct container and taking the right specimen amounts. Because it's a real-time system, showing immediately when a specimen has been drawn, it keeps providers from "resticking" a patient because they viewed stale data.

Level 4 BPOC systems produce true eMARs that comply with legal requirements and produce verifiable evidence for any member of the health care team to view. While other levels verify if it is appropriate to administer a given dose, Level 4 systems produce a layer of administrative oversight.

Level 4 systems can remind clinicians to take vital signs and perform other checks, verify correct identification of lab samples, and calculate the amount of blood needed for all tests to avoid having to draw additional samples later.

Going Wireless at the Point of Care

PDAs give providers access to important information when they are not physically located within the walls of their organization. PDAs no longer simply complement larger workstations; they are getting powerful enough to replace them.

Some important tasks your PDA can handle include capturing documentation of clinical interventions and initiating processes that you later finalize on a full-sized computer workstation. You can also use your PDA to create audio recordings to send remotely to a transcriptionist using the PDA's wireless transmission features—or you can later use the speech recognition program on another computer to transcribe the PDA recording. (Because current PDAs have limited processing power, most do not allow speech to be transcribed as it is spoken into the PDA.)

BOX 7-5

PDAs Help Manage Information Overload

It has been estimated that, for each medical specialty, more than 6000 articles relevant to evidence-based medicine appear in the biomedical literature annually. Furthermore, the volume of material being published in specialty journals means that every specialist would need to read 17 articles a day to stay current. Information in health care becomes outdated so fast, it's very difficult for providers to keep up in their discipline or specialty. And when critical new diagnostic or treatment information emerges, years can transpire before it reaches everyone who needs it.

Personal digital assistants (PDAs), pocket-sized portable computers, have the ability to carry all kinds of material needed by health care providers, including information compendia that can be updated daily. This is powerful, because it allows you to honestly answer a question with, "Rather than give you an answer off of the top of my head, let's see if anything changed while we slept last night."

Source: References 11 and 12.

Uses and Benefits of PDAs

PDAs make data entry relatively fast and easy and bring updated patient information to health professionals throughout the facility. When PDA technologies are wirelessly connected, needed information can be accessed quickly. Key tasks that can be handled via PDA include:

1. Updating patient vital signs, intake and output information such as family and social histories, and information about laboratory specimen collection.
2. Entering or clarifying prescription orders.
3. Checking whether a drug is on the formulary and covered by insurance programs.
4. Checking prescriptions for interactions with a patient's existing medications.
5. Therapeutic substitution.
6. Authorizing refill renewals.
7. Reporting on patient adherence to medication regimens.
8. Making notes on a patient's problems with specific medication regimens or dosage forms.
9. Instant messaging with other members of the health care team (when connection speed is high enough).
10. Accompanying questions about specific medications with a product photograph.
11. Transmitting batches of work in real-time.
12. Accessing electronic medical records.
13. Accessing a health care organization's intranet.

BOX 7-6

PDA Cautions and Caveats

1. PDA users, whether onsite or off, must be authorized to access health information remotely so all users have a login procedure to follow.
2. Typically, a software authentication tool known as virtual privacy network (VPN) represents an additional layer of security that allows PDA users more highly authenticated access to closed systems.
3. Special software called middleware can be used to reformat information in existing record-keeping software and transfer it to a PDA. The technology company that designs the middleware should confirm in writing that state and federal policies regarding prescription transmission, security, patient confidentiality, and necessary data encryption have all been met.
4. Careful consideration should be given to how information will be reformatted onto a PDA environment from larger workstations. Since decision making that affects life-and-death outcomes is being made from a small screen, clinicians need to feel comfortable that the display of information is appropriate to their practice needs.

PDA Adoption

When considering adopting PDAs in a health care practice, it's important to analyze how they will save time and increase productivity. Selecting the best solution for an individual practice increases the likelihood that it will be used consistently. It is really important to try to capture a vision for all the possible uses of a technology. Some people start with the problems they are trying to solve. Others examine how they have used similar technology such as computers and then look for similar features in the more portable PDA technology. The PDA produced today can replace most functions that full-sized notebook and desktop computers perform. Doing a Google search to find how experts use their PDAs and even writing to a discussion forum about the questions you have is a good way to get a picture of PDA options.

BOX 7-7

Master Your PDA

This checklist presents the things you should know how to do to get the most from your PDA. If you're mystified by any of these functions, consult your users' manual or do a Google search to see how more experienced users solve PDA problems.

- Assemble the synchronization cradle included with every PDA purchase.
- Install the software on your personal computer that complements the initial software housed on your PDA.
- Set the formats and time/date settings.
- Install new files.
- Set the synchronization custom features that determine what kind of information you wish to synchronize.
- Create new information on the desktop to synchronize with the PDA.
- Select external content to synchronize with the PDA such as AvantGo, a customizable news, sports, weather, and professional information Web site.
- Adjust the contrast and brightness of the PDA screen.
- Determine alternative ways to charge the PDA.
- Set preferences for display screens on the PDA.
- Enter text using these approaches:
  - touch sensitive input for selection
  - drawing with the stylus
  - on-screen keyboard

continued on page 181

BOX 7-7 *continued*

- letter recognition
- voice recorder
- accessory keyboards
- Categorize and organize applications by logical grouping.
- Use multitasking capabilities (when present).
- Use soft reset and hard reset features.
- Know how to use personal organizer features:
  - calendar
  - address book or contacts
  - task list or to do list
  - notes or memos
  - calculator
- Use pull-down menus for special functions within applications.
- Digitize or align screen calibration.
- Adjust clock features to time zones.
- Use alarm features.
- Beam applications, appointments, contacts, notes, files, tasks, and business cards to other PDA devices.
- Use categories to organize sets of information.
- Use various calendar views for planning and appointments.
- Create recurring appointments and appointments without time (all day).
- Create, prioritize, sort, and delegate tasks.
- Convert, download/synchronize and edit documents in Microsoft Word, Excel, and PowerPoint.
- Convert, download/synchronize, and edit multimedia assets such as images, sound files, and movies.
- Beam between Pocket PC and Palm OS PDAs.
- Manage external/extended memory.
- Use word completer features that suggest a complete typing of a word after you enter the first two letters.
- Identify and select of PDA accessories:
  - cases
  - keyboards
  - memory/storage
  - modems
  - PC connectivity and cables
  - wireless features

continued on page 182

BOX 7-7   continued

- Understand Bluetooth peripherals that allow wireless communications between your PDA and other devices such as computers, printers, and bar code devices.
- Print from Bluetooth or infrared printers.
- Troubleshoot PDA problems.
- Understand PDA return policies.
- Set security of the PDA and/or files on a PDA.
- Know proper cleaning procedures for a PDA.
- Identify appropriate Web resources for the PDA.
- Establish methods for keeping up with new PDA technologies.

ACTIVITY 7-1

PDA Practice

Using the checklist in Box 7-7, try out at least 10 tasks you are not already familiar with. Identify three sources on the Web to help you make the most of your PDA's functionality.

Enhanced Outcomes Through Point of Care Technology

It is now possible to perform many types of laboratory testing at the point of care, including blood gas measurement, blood glucose, blood pressure, and pulmonary function. Using peripheral attachments, PDAs and other portable appliances can perform reliable testing in examination rooms or directly at the bedside. Proper interfaces can even transfer interview data directly into the patient's medical record.

Diagnostic procedures and physical assessments can be supplemented by PDA-based stethoscopes, electrocardiograph attachments, etc. Bar code scanners that connect with PDAs can help eliminate transcribing errors and verify that products about to be administered to patients match those that were intended. The PDA has the ability to capture data generated by physical assessment and receive results sent electronically from remote locations, analyze and manipulate those data, and help clinicians interpret results.

Using a PDA and clinical information systems designed to run in a wireless environment you can check for drug allergies and receive results seamlessly from all available sources of clinical data. As transactions take place, inventory can be adjusted and com-

> Bar code scanners that connect with PDAs can help eliminate transcribing errors and verify that products about to be administered to patients match those that were intended.

municated to an enterprise database so the wholesaler can re-place products. When consultations are required, an intercom system built into the local area network (LAN) can allows nurses, physicians, pharmacists, and other personnel to communicate through voice-activated "badges" with capabilities integrated into their PDAs—making it easy to make the most of colleagues' ex-pertise. Cameras built into PDAs can transmit images, such as to a dermatologist who can verify wound healing, for example. In a completely integrated environment that incorporates the latest technology and good information flow, the opportunity to achieve positive patient outcomes is greatly enhanced.

BOX 7-8

Challenges to Information Transfer

The following obstacles can impede the performance of point of care technology:

1. Hardware and software are not integrated and standardized throughout each health care enterprise.
2. Physician practices, in an effort to be progressive, purchase office-based software such as EMRs and order entry systems that were never intended to integrate with hospital-based patient records.
3. In hospitals, data from the laboratory, ambulatory clinics, radiology, nursing, and pharmacy are contributed to the hospital information system in different flavors (protocols, formats, and hardware platforms).
4. Individual practitioners carry different information appliances, such as laptops and PDAs, with different display capabilities.
5. Providers at the point of care think and write notes in language that is not standardized, saying, for example, "hypertension" in one instance and "high blood pressure" in another. Right now, because of nonstandard terminology, a patient's life could be threatened by something as simple as a progress note misinterpreted by a machine analysis.

Standards-setting organizations such as the American Health Information Management Association are attempting to address the challenges listed above. The health care informatics field is so dynamic and the standard-setting process so laborious, however, that change usually outstrips our ability to standardize information.

Extensible markup language (XML) is gaining traction as a promising solution for standardizing data transfer. XML uses the connectivity of the Internet and the simplicity of a browser to define data fields and send information, allowing the Web to become a bridge between existing software applications and newer approaches.

Charge Capture at the Point of Care

Recording charges and documenting services as they are performed reduces data entry effort by increasing speed and accuracy, eliminates paperwork, and makes data immediately accessible to the accounting department so billing (and therefore reimbursement) can take place faster.[13] The lag time between the physician performing a service in a clinic and the medical coder receiving the paperwork necessary to begin the coding and reimbursement process can exceed 12 hours. Point of care systems not only automate and speed up billing, but they cut down on charges that are "lost" or overlooked in manual systems. Often, the potential to capture charges and improve cash flow is the impetus for investing in point of care technology.

Clinical Data Repositories (CDR)

Traditionally, clinical data repositories (CDR) have been paper storehouses containing test results, medication information, discharge summaries, progress notes, and other individual patient information. Now a growing number of organizations are setting up electronic CDRs so that providers have available complete information about each patient—thus improving safety and cutting down on the possibility of duplicate tests and treatments.

The IOM's *To Err Is Human* report[5] described the impact of missing information at the point of care, noting, for example, that physicians are not aware of four out of every 10 prescriptions a patient takes when they prescribe a new therapy and that one out of seven hospital admissions is directly correlated to information missing in the emergency room. One out of five deaths can be prevented, authors of the report state, by having better information available at the point of care.

CDR Data

Today's CDRs are real-time databases that consolidate information from a variety of clinical sources to provide a unified view of a single patient. Typical kinds of data in a CDR include:

- Clinical laboratory test results
- Patient demographics
- Pharmacy information
- Radiology reports and images
- Pathology reports

- Dates of hospital admission, discharge, and transfer
- ICD-9 codes
- Discharge summaries
- Progress notes

A CDR stores and makes available at the point of care clinical information about individual patients. If kept up to date, these data can provide longitudinal, historical information on demand. However, the primary goal of CDR is to facilitate patient management, not to identify a population of patients with common characteristics or to aid in managing a clinical department.

Today's CDRs are real-time databases that consolidate information from a variety of clinical sources to provide a unified view of a single patient.

CDR Implementation Issues

Before selecting a CDR vendor and investing in a CDR system, you must consider issues in these areas:

- Organizational. Does the CDR support the entire enterprise?
- Financial. Are all transactions related to clinical care contained in the database?
- Implementation. When will paper-based data become digital for input into the CDR?
- Governance. Who will determine the structures and policies required for access to the CDR?
- Provider relations. How will interfaces be managed between vendor systems?
- Communication. Once launched, how will troubleshooting take place during unscheduled downtime?
- Legal and regulatory. How will the data be secured to comply with legal and regulatory requirements?

Because many organizations and providers can contribute to a CDR, they must decide beforehand whether to have a loose confederation or a fiduciary partnership and must budget the direct and indirect costs of participating in this data-sharing arrangement. Also needed is a schedule for updating the technology necessary to maintain and communicate with the CDR.

Contributors to the CDR may include:

- Health systems that obtain data in acute care settings.
- Private and public clinics.
- Pharmacies, which can provide drug profile information for

all prescriptions used by the patient. This profile can list the prescription medications being used by the patient as well as, in some cases, medication regimen compliance data, reports of patient education issues, and records of herbal or over-the-counter medicine use.

- Physicians in the community from every medical specialty who can offer data relevant to the patient's ambulatory care.
- Health plans, which can contribute eligibility and formulary information.

There are many other implementation issues related to CDRs, including:

- Making decisions about information that should be available to share with each discipline and specialty. Mental health data could be supplied to some, for example, while oncology data would be relevant to others.
- Setting format standards that allow data to be transmitted and received with appropriate data integrity.
- Identifying training issues for existing users and new hires.
- Deciding who will operate the CDR—a separate organization or one member group who acts as the "keeper" of the data?
- Determining whether to allow patients to see their own information through a Web-based connection, typically called community health information networks (CHINs) and, more recently, electronic health records (EHRs).
- Ensuring data integrity so that what was sent is what was received.
- Maintaining confidentiality so patients' expectations of privacy are maintained.
- Making data available to those with a bona fide "need to know" for achieving positive patient outcomes.
- Launching procedures to prohibit unauthorized access, detecting when unauthorized access is being attempted, blocking that access, and identifying and pursuing offenders electronically.

Evidence-Based Guidelines at the Point of Care

Incorporating evidence-based clinical practice guidelines into everyday decision making should improve the quality of care, reduce practice variation to reasonable levels, and maximize use of the most appropriate interventions. It is common knowledge that simply publishing guidelines on either paper or the Internet creates little change in the way clinicians provide care; instead, guidelines need to be instantly available at the point of care. They also must be up-to-date and seamlessly integrated into the workflow of busy health care practitioners.

Some health systems require providers to follow practice guidelines and protocols while rendering care so as to overcome the limits of human memory and reduce conjecture in selecting interventions and evaluating outcomes. Because many clinical guideline systems automate documentation and associated paperwork, an additional benefit is that they yield more time for patient care.

BOX 7-9

Veterans Administration Case Study

The Veterans Health Administration (VHA) probably provides the best example of a comprehensive point of care system. Working with EDS, the VHA developed the new Bar Code Medication Administration (BCMA) system, which runs on a laptop PC and uses a standard bar code scanner, either wired or cordless. BCMA uses wireless local area network (WLAN) technology to display real-time information for each patient, such as medications that need to be administered at a certain time.

A physician enters the patient's medication order electronically with a workstation or PDA input device. This action can take place from just about anywhere: at the bedside, from an office across town, from a restaurant. The order is routed to the pharmacy, where it is staged in the pharmacy management software for the pharmacist to verify before being dispensed.

A nurse scans the patient's wristband to confirm that the patient's identity matches the designated recipient of the medication. Next, she scans the bar code for each medication to ensure that the patient will receive the right medications at the right dose at the right time by the right route. All these checks are done in real-time through a wireless network allowing communication with the pharmacy system. When everything is correct, an auditory beep and a green light is activated. If any of the checks results in a negative match, a description of the problem and procedures for resolving it are displayed on the screen of the bar code device. The software offers a comprehensive package of management and accountability tools including site- and user-specific parameters and defaults, patient medication log, and paperless medication administration history.

continued on page 188

BOX 7-9   *continued*

BCMA has a continuous, real-time connection to VHA hospital information system databases through 2.4 gigahertz wireless network devices. Because the devices use spread-spectrum technology, which spreads transmissions over a wide band of frequencies, they are extremely secure and do not suffer interference with devices using other frequencies. The engineering department usually performs a spectral analysis to eliminate the likelihood that unwanted radiation from other devices could create errors in medication systems.

VHA's wireless network allows it to build additional robust mobile systems—medical records and telecommunication systems, for example—that improve multidisciplinary team interactions. The systems can also connect to the community to virtually "follow" patients home. Because the wireless technology is in accordance with industry standards, other applications such as radiological imaging systems can run on the same hardware, thus leveraging the investment beyond BCMA. Together, the wireless network and industry-standard technology allow laptop users to move throughout their work environment with uninterrupted access to BCMA and other VHA information systems.

Source: Reference 14.

ACTIVITY 7-2

Point of Care Technology for You

1. Identify the major point of care functions and technologies already available in your practice.
2. List some of the problems and challenges associated with your current point of care technology. Are there any frustrations associated with its use? Are any key functions missing?
3. Describe the ideal system to support your needs as a practitioner. What would you most like to be able to do using real-time, point of care technology?

References

1. Colkin Cuneo E. Universal's wireless network frees up staff, improves care, and cuts costs. InformationWeek Web site. Available at: www.informationweek.com/story/showArticle.jhtml?articleID=17701265. Accessed July 27, 2004.

2. 16th Annual Leadership Survey: Trends in Healthcare Information Technology. Chicago: Healthcare Information Management and Systems Society; 2005. Available at www.himss.org/2005survey/healthcareCIO_home.asp. Accessed August 15, 2005.

3. Koppel R, Metlay JP, Cohen A, et al. Role of computerized physician order entry systems in facilitating medication errors. *JAMA*. 293(10):1261-3.

4. Rabinovitz J. Computers vital to reducing medical errors, doctor says. *Stanford Report*. March 9, 2005. Available at: http://news-service.stanford.edu/news/2005/march9/med-bates-030905.html Accessed August 1, 2005.

5. Kohn LT, Corrigan JM, Donaldson MS, eds. *To Err Is Human: Building a Safer Health System.* Washington DC: National Academy Press; 1999.

6. American Society of Health-System Pharmacists. *Patient Concerns National Survey Research Report.* Bethesda, MD: American Society of Health-System Pharmacists; September 1999.

7. Davis K, Schoenbaum S, Collins K, et al. *Room for Improvement: Patients Report on the Quality of Their Health Care.* New York: Commonwealth Fund; April 2002.

8. Barker KN, Flynn EA, Pepper GA, et al. Medication errors observed in 36 health care facilities. *Arch Intern Med*. 2002;162:1897-903.

9. Bates DW, Cullen DJ, Laird N, et al. Incidence of adverse drug events and potential adverse drug events. *JAMA*. 1995;274:29-34.

10. Grotting JB, Yang M, Kelly J, et al. The Effect of Barcode-Enabled Point-of-Care Technology on Patient Safety. Available at: www.bridgemedical.com/pdf/whitepaper_barcode.pdf Accessed July 7, 2004.

11. Arndt KA. Information excess in medicine. Overview, relevance to dermatology, and strategies for coping. *Arch Dermatol*. 1992;128:1249-56.

12. Davidoff F, Haynes B, Sackett D, et al. Evidence based medicine. *BMJ*. 1995;310:1085-6.

13. ADL Data Systems, Inc. web site. New Technology: Point-of-Care. Available at: www.adldata.com/NewTech/PointOfCare.html. Accessed July 27, 2004.

14. Electronic Data Systems Corporation web site. Veterans Health Administration Case Study. Available at: www.eds.com/services/casestudies/veterans_health.aspx. Accessed July 27, 2004.

Selected Readings on Point of Care Technology

Alexander PT. Selected readings on point of care technology. Timely information is key to critical care. *Health Manag Technol*. 1999;20(11):32.

Andrew WF. Applied information technology: a clinical perspective: the continuum of interoperability. *Comput Nurs*. 1995;13(1):38-40.

Aymard S, Fieschi D, Volot F, et al. Towards interoperability of information sources within a hospital intranet. [Proceedings]. AMIA Annual Symposium 1998:638-42.

Blumenfeld B. Integrating knowledge bases at the point of care. *Health Manag Technol*. 1997;18(7):44-6.

Brigl B, Ringleb P, Steiner T, et al. An integrated approach for a knowledge-based clinical workstation: architecture and experience. *Methods Inf Med*. 1998;37(1):16-25.

Chin TL. Gathering clinical data. *Health Data Manag*. 1998;6(11):44-57.

Ebell M. Information at the point of care: answering clinical questions. *J Am Board Fam Pract*. 1999;12(3):225-35.

Evans J. Systems integration at a higher level. *Health Manag Technol*. 1998;19(11):22-4.

Fuller SS, Ketchell DS, Tarzy-Hornoch P, et al. Integrating knowledge resources at the point of care: opportunities for librarians. *Bull Med Libr Assoc*. October 1999;87(4):393-403.

Gadd CS, Baskaran P, Lobach DF. Identification of design features to enhance utilization and acceptance of systems for internet-based decision support at the point of care. [Proceedings]. AMIA Annual Symposium 1998:91-5.

Geissbuhler A, Randolph AM. Distributing knowledge maintenance for clinical decision-support systems: the "Knowledge Library" model. [Proceedings]. AMIA Annual Symposium 1999:770-4.

Gillepsie G. A pillar of support. *Health Data Manag.* 1999;7(8):58-65.

Hagland M. IT and point-of-care decision support. *Health Manag Technol.* 1998;19(11):10-4, 69-70.

Hanka R, Karel F. Information overload and "just-in-time" knowledge. *The Electronic Library.* 2000;18(4):279-84.

Klein MS, Ross FV, Adams DL, et al. Information at the point of care: effect on patient care and resource consumption. *J Healthc Inf Manag.* 1999;13(1):489-95.

Lowe HJ. Multimedia electronic medical record systems. *Acad Med.* 1999;74(2):146-51.

Lucier RE, Matheson NW, Butler KA, et al. The knowledge workstation: an electronic environment for knowledge management. *Bull Med Libr Assoc.* 1988;76(3):248-55.

McCormack J. The missing link. *Health Data Manag.* 1999;7(9):72-82.

McDonald CJ, Overhage JM, Tierney WM, et al. The regenstrief medical record system: a quarter century experience. *Int J Med Inform.* 1999;54(3):225-53.

McDonald CJ. The barriers to electronic medical record systems and how to overcome them. *J Am Med Inform Assoc.* 1997;4(3):213-21.

McGowan K. Adopting mobile technology to enhance patient care: issues and status of nursing use and attitudes. Available at: www.rnpalm.com/issues_and_attitudes.htm.

McGrath F, Morgenweck L. Rebuilding the clinical workstation with spider's silk of the web. *Bull Med Libr Assoc.* 1999;87(4):387-92.

Medical Records Institute. Medical Records Institute's Survey of Electronic Health Record Trends and Usage [Web site/survey]. Available at: www.medrecinst.com/survey/2005/index.asp.

Melles RB, Cooper T, Peredy G, et al. User interface preferences in a point-of-care data system. [Proceedings]. AMIA Annual Symposium 1998:86-90.

Overhage JM, Tierney WM, McDonald CJ, et al. Design and implementation of the Indianapolis network for patient care and research. *Bull Med Libr Assoc.* 1995;83(1):48-56.

Sandrick K. Information management systems: the "Real World" in 1999. *Health Manag Technol.* 1999;20(2):10-3.

Schmalhofer FJ, Tschaitschian B. Cooperative knowledge evolution: a construction-integration approach to knowledge discovery in medicine. *Methods Inf Med.* 1998;37(1):491-500.

Sherter AL. Providing easier access to clinical data. *Health Data Manag.* August 1997:33-7.

Silverman BG, Moidu K, Clemente BE, et al. HOLON: A web-based framework for fostering guideline applications. [Proceedings]. AMIA Annual Symposium 1997:374-8.

Spreckelsen C, Spitzer K. Formalising and acquiring model-based hypertext in medicine: an integrative approach. *Methods Inf Med.* 1998;37(3):239-46.

Thiel F. Convergence in the post-PC era: point of care devices speed data to hospital and laboratory information systems. *Health Manag Technol.* 2000;21(2):24.

Tuttle MS, Cole WG, Sherertz DD, et al. Navigating to knowledge. *Methods Inf Med.* March 1995;34:214-31.

Van de Velde R. Framework for a clinical information system. *Int J Med Inform.* 2000;57(1):57-72.

Wingarde FJ, Sun Y, Harary O, et al. Linking multiple heterogeneous data sources to practice guidelines. [Proceedings]. AMIA Annual Symposium 1998:391-5.

Literature Retrieval 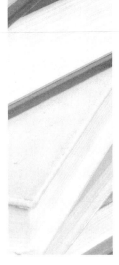 8

Margaret R. Thrower

Chapter Objectives

After completing this chapter, you should be able to:

■ Use the modified systematic approach when approaching a clinical question.

■ Frame a clinical question using the PICO method.

■ Determine when to use primary, secondary, or tertiary literature.

■ Retrieve relevant literature to answer clinical questions effectively and efficiently.

■ Perform a search on a biomedical database using Boolean operators AND, OR, and NOT.

Retrieving information effectively and efficiently is critical to any field in health care. Using the right tools and methods can drastically improve information retrieval to help you solve problems and answer questions from patients, other health care providers, and colleagues. Health care professionals are bombarded with information every day; far too much to read, let alone evaluate and incorporate into practice. This chapter helps you answer clinical questions by breaking the approach into steps.

As a rule of thumb, when looking for information you should start with general (tertiary) literature and get more specific as needed. If you have more time or seek key details you may need to go to original research (primary literature). See Box 8-1 for definitions of the three levels of literature.

BOX 8-1

Primary, Secondary, and Tertiary Literature Defined

- Primary literature presents results of original research and clinical trials, usually in the form of articles in journals such as the *Journal of the American Medical Association*, the *New England Journal of Medicine*, and *Pharmacotherapy.*
- Secondary literature consists of databases that index primary literature and make the search for original research more efficient. Examples include Medline, CINHAL, and International Pharmaceutical Abstracts.
- Tertiary literature summarizes available information. It includes medical and drug information textbooks, reference texts, clinical practice guidelines, review articles, full-text computer databases, and compendia. Most of the health information on the Internet is tertiary literature.

The Modified Systematic Approach to Drug Information

The "systematic approach"[1] for responding to drug information requests was developed as a teaching tool for pharmacy students—a five-step process made up of the following: 1. Classifying the request; 2. Obtaining background information; 3. Systematic search; 4. Response; and 5. Reclassification. In 1987, a drug information specialist modified this approach so any clinician can use it to tackle clinical problems, answer questions, or prepare for professional consultations. The modified systematic approach improves accuracy, effectiveness, and efficiency in answering questions and is applicable regardless of the type of medication or health question. After you've used this approach several times, the steps become automatic and you don't even have to think about them.

As detailed in Figure 8-1, the modified systematic approach involves seven steps. In discussing these steps, we assume that the person looking for the information (the receiver) is not the same person as the one who needs it (the requestor). However, even if you are seeking information to answer your own questions, the same process applies.

1. Receive the clinical question from the requestor.
2. Expand your knowledge. Gather pertinent background information.
3. Classify the question into a category (diagnosis information, prognosis information, disease information, adverse drug reaction, general drug information, etc).
4. Search for the information in the best resources.
5. Evaluate literature for accuracy and relevance.
6. Formulate a response.
7. Communicate information and follow up.

FIGURE 8-1

The modified systematic approach to answering clinical questions.

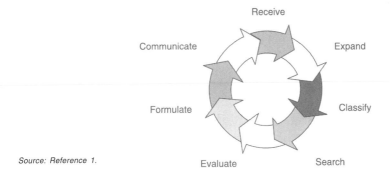

Source: Reference 1.

Receive a Question

The modified systematic approach begins by identifying or receiving a clinical question. Identifying a clinical question sounds like an easy step, but in the biomedical field, questions are rarely straightforward. Furthermore, the question can change as the receiver finds out more information. For example, "What is the maximum dose of acetaminophen?" is a question that requires clarification. Does it refer to a healthy adult? A patient with severe liver dysfunction? A pediatric patient?

When questions are generated—during patient encounters, phone calls, academic meetings, medical rounds, etc.—you should try to frame the question as specifically as possible and obtain such key information as the requestor's name, the patient's name (if the question is patient specific), and the requestor's phone number, pager, or fax number.

Expand the Background

The background data you gather should clearly tell you, Why is this patient or provider asking this question?

Next, collect patient-specific data such as age, height, weight, past medical history, and a complete medication list to get a feel for how the requestor is going to use the information provided. The background data you gather should clearly tell you, "Why is this patient or provider asking this question?" This the most important part of the modified systematic approach—and the most challenging, because requestors don't always ask straightforward questions. What they ask may not be what they really want to know. When this step is done properly, you— the receiver of the question—generally ask more questions than the requestor.

Classify the Question

Classifying a question simplifies the research process and helps you select the best references to use. For instance, if you receive a question about the pharmacology of a drug, a textbook such as Goodman & Gilman's *The Pharmacological Basis of Therapeutics* would be a good first choice to help narrow and define your search.

Search the Literature

In most cases, you should consult at least two references. If the first two references disagree, consult a third source. Remember to consider important factors, such as time of publishing, the accuracy and validity of information in the references, and relevance to the clinical situation.

Evaluate the Source

Evaluate the source based on appropriate criteria. For example, if you use primary literature, evaluate it based on criteria in Chapter 10. If it is tertiary literature, use Box 8-4 on page 199.

Formulate a Response

How you formulate your response depends on how the requesting party wants the information communicated. Most answers in health care are spoken, but written information is sometimes necessary. The advantage of writing is that the response and documentation are completed at the same time. For busy clinicians, documenting all that is said and done on behalf of patients is a constant challenge, but it is important both for planning future care and for reducing legal liability.

Communicate the Response

In this step, you give your answer to the requestor. At this point, you sometimes find that requestors have uncovered additional information they didn't know, or thought was unimportant, when they made their initial inquiry. If this happens, you must consider the relevance of the new information and, if necessary, do more research.

Part of the communication step is following up to verify the response's correctness and completeness, especially when important new information enters the equation. For example, if tests reveal a change in the patient's kidney or liver function that could affect the elimination or metabolism of certain drugs, you would need to follow up immediately to let the requestor know how this new information could change the original recommendation. Follow-up also serves a "quality assurance" function to ensure that information was appropriately provided and used.

Telephone is a common medium for follow-up, but in some health care settings it's easy to do in person. Follow-up via e-mail has increased drastically in the last 10 years and will continue to grow.

ACTIVITY 8-1

The Modified Systematic Approach ✓

1. At his annual check-up, a patient asks you if vitamin E is "good for you." What questions would you ask him to gather more information?
2. A colleague asks you what you usually prescribe for gout. What additional questions would you want to ask her?
3. During a checkup, a patient asks if any of her medications could be causing her hot flashes. The patient is currently taking Premarin, Provera, Prozac, Lipitor, hydrochlorothiazide, and bupropion. What additional information would you want to ask this patient?

The PICO Method for Framing a Clinical Question

In the medical field, a method commonly used to frame a clinical question is called PICO (Population, Intervention, and Clinical Outcomes).[2] Using the PICO method during the first step of the systematic approach helps you define the clinical question effectively. Under the PICO method, the receiver determines answers to three key questions, as listed in Box 8-2.

BOX 8-2

Three Key Questions to Answer in the PICO Method

1. The population. Who are the relevant patients?
2. The intervention or exposure. What diagnostic tests, foods, lifestyle changes, medications, surgical procedures, etc., will be needed?
3. The clinical outcome. What results could come about from the intervention that are relevant to the patient?

For example, suppose you are a family practitioner and a physician colleague asks you, "When treating hypertension, what target blood pressure should we aim for?"

This is a very broad question, and the requestor fails to give any detail about the first question in the PICO method—the population. The benefits of tight blood pressure control differ in diabetic versus nondiabetic patients and in patients with impaired versus healthy renal function. You need additional information, such as whether the patient has diabetic complications and what degree of nephropathy exists, before you can go further. Such information will determine whether the patient's diastolic goal is < 75 mmHg, < 80 mmHg, or < 90 mmHg.

After speaking with the physician further, you determine that the patient is a 64-year-old African American woman with type 2 diabetes mellitus, hypertension, hyperlipidemia, and proteinuria (2 grams protein/24 hours). Her recent fasting blood glucose readings have been within goal for many months. She is on glipizide 10 mg every morning and Lipitor 10 mg daily for her hyperlipidemia. For hypertension, she takes 12.5 mg of hydrochlorothiazide every morning. Over the last 5 months, her blood pressure has been very consistent at 160/90 mmHg.

With this added information, you can now organize the information into an improved, specific clinical question that addresses issues regarding the population, management strategy, and patient-specific factors.[3,4] A PICO analysis would look like this:

1. **Patient population:** Hypertensive, hyperlipidemic, type 2 diabetic with complications of nephropathy.
2. **Interventions:** Antihypertensive agent that controls blood pressure to a goal of < 125/75 mmHg.
3. **Outcome:** If blood pressure can be lowered to < 125/75 mmHg then risk of stroke, myocardial infarction, and cardiovascular death is reduced.

Using and Evaluating Tertiary Literature

Tertiary literature—reference books and the like—is used the most, mainly because it is so accessible and offers comprehensive information in a single source. Well-prepared tertiary references, most often written by experts in the field, review the literature on a topic and provide a concise, easy-to-use overview. Many clinical questions can be answered using tertiary literature alone, and it also provides helpful background information.

Tertiary literature can usually answer questions about indications for a medication, simple pharmacology, pharmacokinetics (absorption, distribution, metabolism, and elimination), warnings, cautions, contraindications, adverse drug reactions, overdose information, dosage, storage, and patient information, and it provides basic disease state information such as pathophysiology, epidemiology, risk factors, and treatment overview. Box 8-3 details some examples of when to use tertiary literature. Table 8-1 summarizes the advantages and disadvantages of tertiary literature.

> Well-prepared tertiary references, most often written by experts in the field, review the literature on a topic and provide a concise, easy-to-use overview.

BOX 8-3

Examples of When to Use Tertiary Literature

- To obtain general information
- To refresh your knowledge or learn about a subject
- For background information regarding a disease or treatment
- For information regarding the gold-standard diagnosis or treatment algorithm for a particular disease or condition

---

Many practitioners rely on clinical practice guidelines, which combine available evidence, to help them make decisions about treating a disease or condition.

Clinical practice guidelines, which combine available evidence, are an example of a highly useful form of tertiary literature in the health care field. Many practitioners rely on such guidelines to help them make decisions about treating a disease or condition. Guidelines often use the letters A, B, or C to "grade" the level of evidence, with "A" indicating strong evidence supporting using a certain intervention and "C" indicating weak evidence. To reflect the balance between benefits and risks of therapy, guidelines may also use a numbering system of 1, 2, or 3, with "1" indicating benefit clearly outweighs risk and "3" indicating no clear risk/benefit ratio. A 1A recommendation, for example, means that there is clear risk/benefit ratio and a high level of evidence supporting use in most patients.[2]

TABLE 8-1

Advantages and Disadvantages of Tertiary Literature

Advantages	Disadvantages
Usually written by experts	May not be timely
Compiled from many literature sources	May not answer the question
Easy to use	May be incomplete or inaccurate
Convenient, concise, and compact	May be biased

A problem with tertiary literature is the lag time from writing to publishing, which may reduce its currency. Or the information included in the source may be incomplete due to the author's lack of knowledge or an insufficient search strategy. In addition, there is a potential for bias introduced by an unbalanced interpretation of available literature

Reference works should be clear, concise, and easy to use.[5] Before using a piece of tertiary material, evaluate it. Check the publication date, references cited, author's credentials, peer review process (or absence thereof), and relevance. Box 8-4 highlights key steps for evaluating tertiary literature.

Timeliness is Key

The resource's date of publication, together with the dates of works cited in the references, gives you an idea of how current the information is. Usually you want to consult the latest edition of a resource rather than an older version. You can easily check the Internet to find out if new editions or updates have been released.

Consider whether information has been published that could change or influence recommendations made within the source. To find out, perform a primary literature search in a secondary biomedical database using the appropriate key words. See the "Searching the Secondary Literature" and "Search Strategy" sections in this chapter for more information on how to do this.

BOX 8-4

Evaluating Tertiary Literature

When checking the quality of tertiary literature, ask yourself the questions below.

Date of publication
- Is the resource current?
- Is it the most recent edition?
- Could recently published information influence or change the recommendations made within the resource?
- Could additional information be obtained from the primary literature that is not included in this resource?

References
- Does the resource provide references throughout?
- Were the references timely when the resource was published?

Credentials and experience in field of authors and editors
- Does the author have sufficient experience and expertise?
- Are the claims that the author makes supported in the biomedical literature?
- Could there be selection bias regarding the references included?

Relevance
- Does the reference contain relevant information on the subject?

Peer review
- Is there evidence of a peer review process?

Ease of use
- Is the reference clear and concise?
- Is the reference easy to use?

Source: References 5 and 6.

The resource's bibliography is a good starting point for determining the time lapse between the publication date of information on which the resource is based and the release of new information.

The resource's bibliography is a good starting point for determining the time lapse between the publication date of information on which the resource is based and the release of new information. Using the bibliography, you can find a source, retrieve it, and evaluate it in more detail. You can also tell by the bibliography how thoroughly the author searched the literature, which helps you determine whether the work is useful or not credible.

Expert Sources

Ideally, tertiary resources should be written by experts in the field. However, even experts can turn out poorly written or incomplete chapters, so it's a good idea to verify "big picture" statements an author makes to ensure they are supported in the biomedical literature.

Be alert to the possibility of selection bias in the references cited. For example, if the author cites works by himself or colleagues many times when a host of other applicable material is available, it should raise your suspicions. To investigate the possibility of bias, perform a literature search to find other sources on the topic. Has any relevant work performed by other authors been omitted that was available at the time the reference was published?

Peer review of tertiary literature is becoming a necessity to ensure high quality.[5] Sometimes, books print the names of each person who peer-reviewed the material, which allows you to verify that reviewers have credentials in the topic area.

ACTIVITY 8-2

Types of Literature

Complete the following exercises regarding types of literature:

1. Locate the most current treatment guidelines on a disease state of your choice from an Internet source.
2. Establish a personalized algorithm or guidelines to help you retrieve primary literature effectively and efficiently.
3. Using Medline (www.ncbi.nlm.nih.gov/entrez/query.fcgi) locate a full-text review article on a disease state of your choice.
4. Using a search engine, find three health-related Web sites that contain information on treating Alzheimer's disease (or a disease state of your choice). Evaluate the site according to the evaluation criteria in Chapter 10, page 231.

Searching the Secondary Literature

Secondary databases help you locate primary literature such as original research articles, editorials, letters to the editor, and commentaries. They can also help you find tertiary literature and clinical practice guidelines. In most cases, secondary literature consists of electronic databases such as Medline, although a few paper resources still exist. Electronic search capabilities have greatly improved the effectiveness and efficiency of searching for literature.

Regardless of what database you use, online tutorials and Help functions can be quite useful. You should consult them initially when using a new database and check regularly for updates.

When researching a clinical question, consult at least two databases to prevent missing a significant piece of work on the subject. Because references and journals indexed in databases overlap only minimally, search results can yield significant differences. For example, Embase (an expansive international biomedical database) and Medline have only about a 40% overlap of information.

In addition to using multiple databases, you should choose the appropriate database for researching a given question. Chapter 9 contains additional information on specific secondary databases.

Search Strategy

Your search strategy is almost more important than the search itself. When using a new database, familiarize yourself with its language by using the online tutorial or Help function. Secondary databases use several languages. For example, the National Library of Medicine (NLM) uses MeSH (Medical Subject Headings), a controlled vocabulary with a specific database "language," for indexing articles in Medline. MeSH provides a consistent way to retrieve information that may use different terminology for the same concepts.

Secondary databases such as IDIS (Iowa Drug Information Service) use a "Thesaurus" to improve the quality of searching. The Thesaurus cross references all valid drug, disease, and descriptor terms to their synonyms, drug trade names, or similar concepts. You can use the Thesaurus to determine the valid IDIS term for searching within the basic or advanced search.

Boolean operators, such as AND, OR, and NOT, are routinely used to broaden or narrow a search by combining terms.[7] They are named after George Boole, a British mathematician who invented these operators as part of a system of logic in the mid-1800s. For example, apples AND oranges narrows the search to information about both apples and oranges, while apples OR oranges expands

Secondary databases help you locate primary literature such as original research articles, editorials, letters to the editor, and commentaries, as well as tertiary literature and clinical practice guidelines.

the search. The NOT operator prevents the word after it from appearing in items resulting from your search, such as orange NOT color. Be careful when using NOT because it decreases the results of a search, which can potentially eliminate useful articles. Box 8-5 gives an example of searching strategies. Figure 8-2 graphically illustrates how Boolean operators broaden or narrow a search.

FIGURE 8-2

Boolean operators; the black portion indicates the breadth of the search.

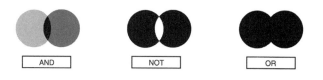

AND   NOT   OR

BOX 8-5

Case Example: Searching Strategy

Suppose you see a lot of patients with psoriasis and follow treatment guidelines published in 1997. Recently, you've been wondering if these guidelines are still valid or if new evidence has changed them. Your patients with moderate to severe psoriasis have had good luck when treated with methotrexate or cyclosporine, and you'd like to know which agent is best. And what about the new drugs for psoriasis your patients have been asking about? You want to understand how they fit into the picture. In this example, you have just framed two clinical questions:

1. Is methotrexate or cyclosporine more effective in treating moderate to severe psoriasis?
2. How do new agents compare to the standards of treatment in terms of efficacy and safety?

After pulling a few review articles and checking some reputable Internet sites, you determine that these resources do not address your specific questions. You need to check primary literature.

Go to the Medline database, which is available free online through PubMed (www.ncbi.nih.gov/entrez/query.fcgi) and combine several keyword terms such as methotrexate AND cyclosporine AND psoriasis to see what the search yields. You can also check Medline to see if valid guidelines have been updated or published since 1997 by typing methotrexate AND cyclosporine AND psoriasis AND guidelines, or omit the last "AND guidelines. If no guidelines come up, you can search by combining names of new drugs to see if valid efficacy trials have been performed against the "standard agents."

In addition to the most commonly used operators—AND, OR, and NOT—some databases use the terms WITH or NEAR. You can consult the Help function of the database to determine which terms the database recognizes and how they are used.

Limiting Searches

Due to the enormous amount of biomedical literature, sometimes a search produces too many "hits" to sort through. If you obtain more than 50 to 100 results from a search, consider limiting your search and asking the question, "Am I sure what it is I want to know?"

You can make a search more specific by using limiting factors or terms, such as age ranges, language, human studies only, review articles, randomized controlled trials, clinical trials, or practice guidelines. To correctly apply limitations, however, you must know the specific clinical question you want to answer. Without taking the important step of defining exactly what you're looking for, you will spend a lot of time sifting through information that may not be useful.

The most commonly used limitations are English language and the type of studies, such as review articles or randomized controlled trials. However, the English language is quickly becoming less of a barrier, because many search engines are now equipped with a translator function. Figure 8-3 shows an example of how to limit searches on PubMed.

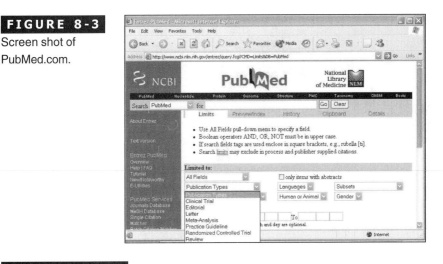

FIGURE 8-3

Screen shot of
PubMed.com.

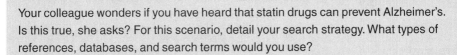

ACTIVITY 8-3

Search Strategy

Your colleague wonders if you have heard that statin drugs can prevent Alzheimer's. Is this true, she asks? For this scenario, detail your search strategy. What types of references, databases, and search terms would you use?

Retrieving Literature

The Free Medical Journals site (www.freemedicaljournals.com), which promotes free Internet access to medical journals, has a collection of approximately 1300—some free as soon as they are published, others free after a specified time has passed after publication.

After you identify the best articles to answer your clinical question, you can begin to retrieve them. The Internet has made retrieving and accessing medical information much easier. Medline and other databases offer links to many full-text references. It is important to select the *best* references, not just articles that are available online by full text. Box 8-6 outlines useful steps for retrieving literature.

Sometimes you can get access to full-text articles free through the Web site of the journal in which the article is published. The Free Medical Journals site (www.freemedicaljournals.com), which promotes free Internet access to medical journals, has a collection of approximately 1300—some free as soon as they are published, others free after a specified time has passed after publication, such as 6 months or 1 year. For example, the prestigious *New England Journal of Medicine* requires Web site registration but makes articles available for free if they are at least 6 months old. Figure 8-4 shows a screen shot from Free Medical Journals.

BOX 8-6

Systematic Steps to Retrieving Literature

If you need to retrieve a specific piece of primary literature, it's useful to follow a systematic, step-by-step process—or algorithm—to find it. The steps you follow may depend on your work setting. For example, a professor of medicine may be able to retrieve just about everything through the school's library, while a physician in private practice may not have access to anything except free sources. An example of an algorithm follows. Note that free sources are highly sought after and appear first, whereas pay-per-view articles are last.

- Is the article available free in full text through the PubMed version of Medline (www.ncbi.nlm.nih.gov/entrez/query.fcgi)?
- Is the article available from www.freemedicaljournals.com?
- Is the article free on the Web site of the journal's publisher?
- Does my institution have any full-text databases such as EBSCO, Ingenta, or Embase that provide access to the article?
- Does my institution have an affiliation with a library where I can get access to the article?
- Can I get access to the article through a nearby library?
- Can I pay a fee (usually by credit card) to access and download the article over the Internet?

If your lack of knowledge about these resources limits you, librarians can help you find articles and give you pointers for effective searching.

FIGURE 8-4

Screen shot of
FreeMedicalJournals.com.

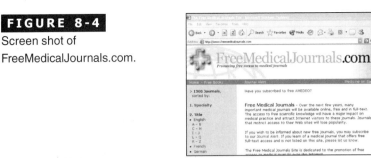

Primary Literature

Primary literature consists of original research published in more than 20,000 biomedical journals. You would have to read 6000 articles each day to keep up,[9] so it's no wonder many health care professionals feel overwhelmed by the massive amount of information available.

Primary literature represents the most current information available. It provides details of research methodology and, if it contains important new findings, can have a significant impact on therapeutic decisions. Disadvantages include the thousands of studies to sift through and the fact that some studies are published even though they lack quality or validity. Box 8-7 suggests when you should consult primary literature.

BOX 8-7

Examples of When to Use Primary Literature

- When researching a new medication or a new indication for a medication.
- When a therapeutic controversy exists between two agents.
- When treatment options appear to have similar efficacy.
- When tertiary literature does not provide the answer.
- When you need to know key details.

In the past, health care professionals subscribed to several journals to "keep up." They would skim each table of contents for relevant articles, a method that has become outdated because so few articles published in core medical journals—less than 10%, by some estimates—are useful and of high quality.[2]

If you use primary literature you must be able to determine whether a study's conclusions are sound based on the study design, patient population, and results. You also need to be able to evaluate the literature for validity and applicability to clinical situations, which is discussed in Chapter 10.

ACTIVITY 8-4

Literature Review ✓

Identify which type of literature would be most helpful in answering the following questions or handling these scenarios:

1. When should I hospitalize a patient with pneumonia?
2. When is a serum pregnancy test necessary, instead of using a urine pregnancy test?
3. A patient is on Premarin, Provera, Prozac, and Lipitor. Do any of these medications cause hair loss?
4. What are the target blood glucose levels for a diabetic woman who is pregnant or planning on becoming pregnant?
5. Is a Lyme test indicated in a patient who has one or two supporting symptoms?
6. Are there any experimental drugs that have shown effectiveness in preventing multiple sclerosis?

Source: Reference 11.

References

1. Host TR, Kirkwood CF. Computer-assisted instruction for responding to drug information requests [abstract]. Presented at the 22nd Annual ASHP Midyear Clinical Meeting; December 1987; Atlanta, GA.

2. Guyatt G, Rennie D. *Users' Guides to the Medical Literature: A Manual for Evidence-Based Clinical Practice*. Chicago IL: American Medical Association Press; 2002.

3. Haynes RB. Loose connections between peer reviewed clinical journals and clinical practice. *Ann Intern Med*. 1990;113:724-8.

4. Oxman AD, Sackett DL, Guyatt GH. Users' guides to the medical literature, I: how to get started. *JAMA*. 1993;270:2093-5.

5. Kier KL, Malone PM, Mosdell KW. Drug Information Resources. In: *Drug Information: A Guide for Pharmacists*. 2nd ed. New York, NY: McGraw-Hill; 2001:56-7.

6. Harper ML. Clinical study design and literature evaluation. In: *Pharmacotherapy Self-Assessment Program*. Vol 5. 4th ed. Kansas City, MO: American College of Clinical Pharmacy; 2002:217.

7. Anderson PO. How to get started with computerized literature searches. *Am J Hosp Pharm*. 1994;51:2303-7.

8. Oxman AD, Cook DJ, Guyatt GH. Users' guides to the medical literature. Part VI: how to use an overview. *JAMA*. 1994;272:1367-71.

9. Lowe H.J, Barnett GO. Understanding and using the medical subject headings (MeSH) vocabulary to perform literature searches. *JAMA*. 1994;271:1103-8.

10. Arndt KA. Information excess in medicine. Overview, relevance to dermatology, and strategies for coping. *Arch Dermatol*. 1992;128:1249-56.

11. Alper BS, Stevermer JJ, White DS, et al. Answering family physicians' clinical questions using electronic medical databases. *J Fam Pract*. November 2001;50:11. Available at: www.jfponlin.com/content/2001/11/jfp_11-1_09600.asp. Accessed March 20, 2003.

Finding Resources Electronically ❾

Margaret R. Thrower

Chapter Objectives

After completing this chapter, you should be able to:

■ Locate and use electronic sources of tertiary information.

■ Locate and use electronic secondary databases that can help you find relevant original research (primary literature).

■ Locate Internet sources of health and drug information designed for you to use in your daily practice.

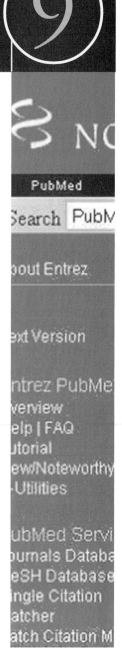

The Medline database is known as the "gold standard" of biomedical databases.

As you apply health care informatics—the science of using information to improve health care—to researching a clinical question, the most important step is identifying what you are trying to answer. Reducing your clinical scenario to an answerable question (a process addressed in Chapter 8) is the best way to begin, followed by classifying and identifying resources that will let you search most efficiently. This chapter helps you in those latter steps by familiarizing you with databases and other electronic resources that ease your search for original studies, review articles, and clinical practice guidelines. Increasingly you can use the Internet, which contains mostly tertiary literature (summaries of available information), to help with your research.

Secondary Sources

As noted in Chapter 8, secondary literature consists of databases that index and simplify the search for primary literature: original research articles, editorials, letters to the editor, commentaries, and the like. Secondary literature can also help you find tertiary literature: medical and drug information textbooks, reference material, clinical practice guidelines, review articles, full-text computer databases, and other resources that summarize available information. This section highlights some secondary sources most useful to health care professionals.

Medline: www.ncbi.nlm.nih.gov/entrez/query.fcgi

The Medline database is known as the "gold standard" of biomedical databases. Although many versions exist, perhaps the most widely known is PubMed, a free service of the National Library of Medicine available over the Internet. PubMed, which

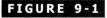

FIGURE 9-1

PubMed version of Medline home page.

covers more than 4800 journals, provides access to more than 15 million Medline citations dating back to the mid-1960s.[1] Figure 9-1 on page 208 shows a screen shot of the PubMed home page.

Cumulative Index to Nursing and Allied Health Literature: www.cinahl.com

The Cumulative Index to Nursing & Allied Health is a comprehensive database with primary journals indexed from the following fields: cardiopulmonary technology, physical therapy, emergency service, health education, radiologic technology, technology therapy, social service/health care, medical records, surgical technology, and occupational therapy. This database is available only by subscription.[2]

Current Contents Connect: www.isinet.com/products/cap/ccc

Current Contents Connect is a production of the Thomson ISI company, a well-known publisher of medical information. Updated daily, this searchable database provides tables of contents and records from approximately 7500 journals and 2000 books. In addition, its sites link to more than 4000 Web sites that have been evaluated for quality of content and 440,000 full-text Web documents. Because Current Contents Connect is expensive, its typical subscribers are organizations, not individuals. A good way to gain access is through your local medical library.[3]

International Pharmaceutical Abstracts: www.thomsonscientific.com/products/ipa/

The goal of International Pharmaceutical Abstracts is to be the world's most comprehensive pharmacy and pharmaceutical science database. In addition to publishing abstracts (in English) of articles from pharmacy journals, the database includes abstracts from meetings such as the American Society of Health-System Pharmacists, Midyear Clinical Meeting. The main subscribers of this pricey but useful resource are institutions such as universities, the pharmaceutical industry, and hospitals.

Iowa Drug Information Service: www.uiowa.edu/~idis/idistday.htm

The Iowa Drug Information Service (IDIS) database is a bibliographic indexing service for 200 high-quality, peer-reviewed English-language medical and pharmaceutical journals. The database's primary goal is to provide references for drug therapy.

The goal of International Pharmaceutical Abstracts is to be the world's most comprehensive pharmacy and pharmaceutical science database.

Among areas covered are pharmacy and pharmacology, general and internal medicine, infectious disease and immunology, transplantation, cardiovascular medicine, rheumatology, microbiology, geriatrics, and endocrinology. The advantage of this database is that it is full text from 1997 to the current year. Furthermore, you can download portable document format (PDF) files for immediate use. Articles published before 1997 are available in full text on microfiche. Because of IDIS's cost, its primary subscriber base is institutions.

Cochrane Library: www.cochrane.org

The Cochrane Library, a collection of seven databases, is produced by the Cochrane Collaboration, an international nonprofit organization composed mainly of volunteer health care professionals. Dedicated to making up-to-date, accurate information about the effects of health care readily available worldwide, the Cochrane Collaboration produces and disseminates systematic reviews of health care interventions and promotes the search for evidence in the form of clinical trials and other studies of interventions.

The Cochrane Library, published four times a year (January, April, July, and October, both on CD and on the Internet), provides information and evidence to support health care decisions and to inform people receiving care. Figure 9-2 shows the Cochrane Library home page.[4]

Like the Cochrane Collaboration, the Cochrane Library is known for rigorous quality standards.[4] Five of its databases deal directly with the effects of interventions in health care, or "evidence-based medicine," and two are devoted to providing information on research methodology. The Cochrane Database of Systematic Reviews, discussed in more detail on page 225, is the Collaboration's major product. The Cochrane Library databases are:

- The Cochrane Database of Systematic Reviews (CDSR)
- The Database of Abstracts of Reviews of Effects (DARE)
- The Cochrane Central Register of Controlled Trials (CENTRAL)
- The Cochrane Database of Methodology Reviews (CDMR)
- The Cochrane Methodology Register (CMR)
- The Health Technology Assessment Database (HTA)
- The NHS Economic Evaluation Database (NHS EED)

Dedicated to making up-to-date, accurate information about the effects of health care readily available worldwide, the Cochrane Collaboration produces and disseminates systematic reviews of health care interventions and promotes the search for evidence in the form of clinical trials and other studies of interventions.

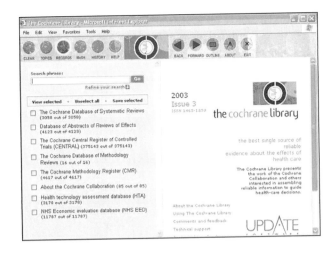

FIGURE 9-2

The Cochrane Library home page.

Embase: www.embase.com

Embase, which covers roughly 4500 journals, is thought of as an international Medline. The contents in Embase and Medline overlap by about 40%. Embase provides one of the most comprehensive databases to help you search the biomedical literature, but because subscriptions are expensive, most often it is available through medical school libraries or hospitals associated with large teaching institutions. You can visit the Embase home page and click on "about Embase" to sign up for a 1-month free trial.[5] Figure 9-3 shows the Embase home page.

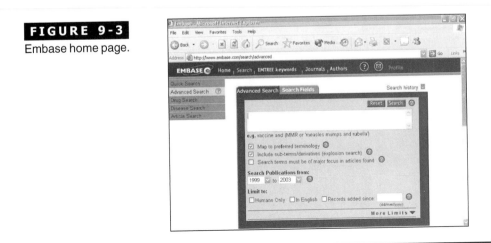

FIGURE 9-3

Embase home page.

Tertiary Sources

The following reference materials are respected, well-known sources of medical and health information and clinical guidelines.

Physicians' Desk Reference: www.pdr.net

Probably one of the most recognizable of all medical sources, the *Physicians' Desk Reference* (PDR) presents pharmaceutical manufacturers' package information approved by the Food and Drug Administration (FDA). Companies purchase their space in this resource, which provides no evaluation of information or comparison with other agents. Most health care professionals are familiar with the paper version of the *Physicians' Desk Reference,* available free to physicians, nurse practitioners, physician assistants, medical students, and residents in the United States. Information from the printed reference is also available through the Micromedex online package, described below. The PDR Web site includes information contained in the PDR, drug interaction information, and a downloadable drug information program for your personal digital assistant (PDA).

Micromedex: www.micromedex.com

Micromedex publishes clinical decision support databases and tools. The Micromedex Healthcare Series Databases, comprehensive sources tailored for health care professionals, include information related to drugs, acute care, toxicology, and patient education. The cost of subscriptions tends to limit subscribers to large medical institutions or those affiliated with them.[6] Names and descriptions of Micromedex databases available as of January 2005 are listed below and denoted with an (M).

(M) **AltCareDex System.** Contains peer-reviewed, referenced patient education on complementary and alternative medicines. Designed to answer patients' questions with easy-to-understand information, the database has documents in three categories: dietary supplements, disease state/medical conditions, and therapies. Dietary supplement monographs cover indications, dosage, storage, interactions, side effects, and warnings associated with popular complementary and alternative medicines, including vitamins and minerals. The disease state/medical condition materials cover medical conditions and potential complementary treatments as well as causes, signs and symptoms, and prevention and wellness

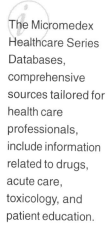

The Micromedex Healthcare Series Databases, comprehensive sources tailored for health care professionals, include information related to drugs, acute care, toxicology, and patient education.

recommendations. The therapy documents give information on treatments for certain ailments, including biofeedback, aromatherapy, and acupuncture.

(M) **AltMedDex System.** Part of the Micromedex *Complementary & Alternative Medicine Series* of peer-reviewed, evidence-based dietary supplement information, AltMedDex has two parts:

■ Alternative Medicine Evaluation monographs, published in a standardized format for quick reference. These include dosing information, synonyms for names of supplements, pharmacokinetic properties, contraindications, side effects and drug interactions, place in therapy, mechanism of action, clinical uses, and comparative efficacy.
■ Alternative Medicine Consults provides information on FDA warnings, pregnancy risk categories, dosing guidelines, and product efficacy for herbal medicines and other dietary supplements.

(M) **AltMedDex Protocols.** Peer-reviewed, referenced, comprehensive information for health care professionals on the efficacy and use of complementary and alternative therapies to treat medical conditions.

(M) **AltMedDex Points System.** Offers brief highlights of herbals, vitamins, minerals, and other dietary supplements, including dosing, indications, contraindications, side effects, drug interactions, therapeutic class, pregnancy, and lactation. Great for providing an overview, this resource is linked to more in-depth information in the AltMedDex Evaluations.

(M) **AltMed-REAX for the Patient.** Peer-reviewed information in easy-to-understand consumer language about drug interactions involving dietary supplements. It includes information on drug-supplement, supplement-supplement, food-supplement, and alcohol-supplement interactions.

(M) **ClinicalPoints System.** Contains brief highlights and key information about diagnosing and treating various conditions; linked to more comprehensive information in the DISEASEDEX Clinical Review documents.

(M) **Current Concepts Program.** A continuing education (CE) program in which Thomson Micromedex offers online modules that can be completed for CE credit. Although intended for pharmacists, any health care professional may participate. The CE available through Current Concepts is approved by the American Council on Pharmaceutical Education. Each module is approved for 1 hour of continuing education credit, or 0.1 CEUs.

(M) **DISEASEDEX General Medicine.** Supports diagnostic and therapeutic decisions in outpatient and in-patient settings, helping clinicians manage diseases more effectively and efficiently. The documents highlight key information on management, background, diagnosis, treatment, complications, special circumstances, when to consult or refer, prognosis, advice for the patient, follow-up, prevention, and screening.

(M) **DISEASEDEX Emergency Medicine.** Previously named EMERGINDEX, this resource includes three different products:

■ **Emergency and Acute Care Summaries**, which provides a succinct overview of emergency conditions, including diagnosis and treatment.
■ **Clinical Reviews**, which presents information necessary to diagnose and treat emergency clinical situations.
■ **Pre-Hospital Care Protocols**, which contains treatment guidelines that factor in patient history, signs, and symptoms. It covers issues such as stabilizing the patient, base contact, and special considerations. The abstracts portion reviews the literature on a broad scope of topics.

(M) **DRUGDEX System.** Includes FDA-approved medications as well as investigational, nonprescription, and foreign drugs. Topics include dosage, pharmacokinetics, cautions, interactions, clinical applications, and comparative drug efficacy. The DRUGDEX system contains three different modules:

■ **Drug Evaluations**, which contains comprehensive monograph information.

- **Drug Consults**, which provides patient consultation cases involving FDA-approved drugs, investigational drugs, international drugs, and nonprescription products.
- **The Product Index**, a helpful resource containing medication trade names, manufacturers, and dosage forms.

Ⓜ **DrugPoints System.** An abbreviated and more efficient form of DRUGDEX that presents a summary of the most important facts about of medications, including dosing, drug interactions, adverse effects, pregnancy warnings, indications, cautions, therapeutic class, and brand information. An advantage of this system is that it links directly with the more comprehensive DRUGDEX system to provide more complete information when it is needed.

Ⓜ **Drug-REAX System.** Allows health care professionals to check for drug interactions, their effects, and their clinical significance. It provides drug-drug, food-drug, drug-disease, and drug-ethanol interactions. Unique to this database is users' ability to build a patient profile by choosing drugs from the database and then check for drug interactions. You can check for a variety of interactions, such as all severities or only those that are major. Information on drug interactions can also be filtered based on documentation surrounding the drug interaction, including excellent, good, fair, poor, and unlikely.

Ⓜ **Herbal Medicines: A Guide for Health-Care Professionals.** The electronic counterpart of the print resource published by the Pharmaceutical Press, the publications division of the Royal Pharmaceutical Society of Great Britain. It contains more than 140 referenced herbal supplement monographs and gives information on species, safety, efficacy, uses, common doses, pharmacology, side effects, toxicity, contraindications, and warnings.

Ⓜ **IDENTIDEX System.** Useful when you need to identify a tablet or capsule from the imprint code. This database includes nonprescription and prescription products, both brand name and generic, and also contains color and shape information and contact information for the product's manufacturer. International drugs and street drugs are included, as is an extensive index of drug-related slang terms.

The Drug-REAX System allows health care professionals to check for interacting drug ingredients, their effects, and their clinical significance.

Ⓜ **Index Nominum.** An international drug directory with information for 45 countries; covers more than 5300 substances and derivatives, 12,800 synonyms for drug names, and 41,800 trade names. Information is organized into monograph format containing a medication's name, synonyms (both official and unofficial), and chemical structure (including diagram). It also has a list of worldwide manufacturers, including addresses.

Ⓜ **IV INDEX System with Trissel's Tables.** Provides information from the well-known *Trissel's Tables of Physical Compatibility*. This database contains more than 35,000 test results for combinations of two drugs in three different infusion solutions, covering 145 common parenteral medications, specifically for Y-site application. You can use this information to check for the compatibility of IV medications.

Ⓜ **Martindale: The Complete Drug Reference.** The electronic equivalent of the print version of *Martindale: The Complete Drug Reference,* published by the Pharmaceutical Press, contains information on drugs available worldwide including some investigational, veterinary, and herbal medicines. Vaccines, radiopharmaceuticals, diagnostic agents, medicinal gases, recreational drugs and drugs of abuse, and toxic substances are covered as well. Overall, this comprehensive resource includes more than 70,000 brand name products from 17 countries, 5300 drug monographs, and information from approximately 6000 manufacturers. More than 5000 herbal products and 200 herbal medicine monographs are included, as are more than 600 reviews on diseases and the drugs used to treat them.

Ⓜ **Material Safety Data Sheets (MSDS) from USP.** Provides access to more than 1000 Material Safety Data Sheets (MSDS) written by the U.S. Pharmacopeial Convention, Inc. These electronically available sheets let you quickly find drug and chemical information including health hazards, handling procedures, and government regulations. Each sheet contains the following information about hazardous substances: hazardous ingredients, physical and chemical characteristics, physical hazards, health hazards, special protection information, special precautions, and spill/leak procedures.

(M) **mobileMICROMEDEX System.** This version of Micromedex, available for download onto a PDA, is free for subscribers to Micromedex. Refer to the Point of Care Resources section, on page 222 of this chapter, for more details.

(M) **Patient Education: The Care Notes System, Aftercare Instruction & Drug Leaflets.** This database, designed to improve patient education at the point of care, lets practitioners produce and print information for patients. The Care Notes System includes both CareNotes documents and DrugNotes documents. Care Notes, written at a 4th- to 6th-grade reading level, can be customized to provide facility- or clinician-specific data. DrugNotes, with information for patients on approximately 1000 drugs prescribed most often, covers medication use, warnings, and food and drugs to be avoided while taking medications.

(M) **P&T QUIK Reports.** Presents valuable formulary information on drugs, which is useful to pharmacy and therapeutics committees or other decision-making entities.

(M) **Physicians' Desk Reference.** Gives efficient electronic access to three different sources: the PDR, the PDR for Nonprescription Drugs and Dietary Supplements, and the PDR for Ophthalmic Medicines, all covering current FDA-approved prescription drugs, common prescription drugs, and specialized ophthalmic pharmaceuticals in monographs identical to those in the print version described on page 212.

(M) **POISINDEX System.** Contains hundreds of thousands of commercial, pharmaceutical, and biological substances—ranging from nonprescription products to household cleaners and cosmetics. Mainly used to identify ingredients and appropriate actions when someone ingests these products.

(M) **REPRORISK System.** Presents information on the effect of substances on human reproduction and development, including prescription, nonprescription, illicit, and recreational drugs.

(M) **TOMES System.** Helps health care professionals manage medical and environmental issues associated with almost any chemical.

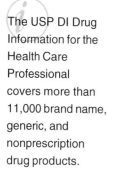

The USP DI Drug Information for the Health Care Professional covers more than 11,000 brand name, generic, and nonprescription drug products.

(M) **ToxPoints System.** The summary version of POISINDEX; covers clinical effect, treatment, and range of toxicity and links directly to the full POISINDEX System if you need detailed information.

(M) **USP DI Drug Reference Guides.** Made up of two products: the USP DI Drug Information for the Health Care Professional and the USP DI Advice for the Patient. Together, these resources represent the consensus of 35 expert USP Advisory Panels made up of more than 800 volunteer health care professionals. The guides are recognized by the federal government under Medicare and Medicaid as a source for drug use review (DUR), patient education, and reimbursement for uses not on the drug's labeling. The USP DI Drug Information for the Health Care Professional covers more than 11,000 brand name, generic, and nonprescription drug products. The USP DI Advice for the Patient provides medication information in language that patients can easily understand. The electronic format of these resources lets you print drug information for patients right at the point where you are delivering care.

Stat!REF: www.statref.com

Stat!REF is an electronic medical library you can access online or by CD-ROM and DVD, in PDA format, or for use via intranet. The company's Web site offers a free trial of the product, which contains electronic versions of general and specialty resources that are most often found only in print. You can tailor the references to fit your practice setting. Box 9-1 lists the references available at the time this book went to press.[7]

Point of Care Resources

Point of care technologies can help you be more efficient in your everyday practice because they offer quick access to key information while you are delivering patient care. Some of these technologies, such as desktop computers, are stationary, but others—laptops and notebook computers, for example—are portable, and some, such as PDAs, are small enough to fit in the palm of your hand, making them versatile tools for looking up information on drugs and diseases, finding diagnostic aids, and checking literature references on pharmacy and medical topics. Thanks to Internet access, these devices can even retrieve patient-specific data from remote databases, and wireless networks give you the flexibility to use them while you interact with patients or move from place to place.[8]

BOX 9-1

Items Available Through Stat-Ref

Stat-Ref (www.statref.com) lets you pick and choose references to include in an online library customized for a particular setting or discipline. At press time, Stat-Ref offered the following references on CD-Rom and Online. (Note: an * indicates only available online.)

ACP Medicine
ACP's PIER—Physicians Information and Education Resource*
ACS Surgery: Principles & Practice*
Adams & Victor's Principles of Neurology*
AHFS Drug Information
AJCC Cancer Staging Handbook*
An@tomy.tv
Basic & Clinical Pharmacology
Brunner & Suddarth's Textbook of Medical-Surgical Nursing*
Color Atlas & Synopsis of Clinical Dermatology
Current Critical Care Diagnosis & Treatment
Current Diagnosis & Treatment in Cardiology
Current Diagnosis & Treatment in Gastroenterology
Current Diagnosis & Treatment in Infectious Diseases*
Current Diagnosis & Treatment in Orthopedics
Current Emergency Diagnosis & Treatment
Current Medical Diagnosis & Treatment
Current Obstetric & Gynecologic Diagnosis & Treatment
Current Pediatric Diagnosis & Treatment
Current Surgical Diagnosis & Treatment
Davis's Drug Guide for Nurses*
DeGowin's Diagnostic Examination
Delmar's Guide to Laboratory and Diagnostic Tests*
Delmar's Fundamental and Advanced Nursing Skills*
Dictionary of Medical Acronyms and Abbreviations
Diseases and Disorders: A Nursing Therapeutics Manual*

continued on page 220

219

BOX 9-1 *continued*

DSM-IV-TR: Diagnostic and Statistical Manual of Mental Disorders
Emergency Medicine: A Comprehensive Study Guide
Family Medicine: Principles & Practice
Geriatric Medicine: An Evidence-Based Approach
Goldfrank's Toxicologic Emergencies
Goodman & Gilman's The Pharmacological Basis of Therapeutics*
Griffith's 5 Minute Clinical Consult
Harrison's Principles of Internal Medicine*
Holland-Frei Cancer Medicine*
Hurst's The Heart*
The ICU Book
Infectious Diseases: The Clinician's Guide*
Ingenix ICD-9-CM VOLS 1&3 and CPT with RVUs Data Files
Internal Medicine
Medical Immunology
Medical Letter on Drugs and Therapeutics*
Merck Manual of Diagnosis and Therapy
Mosby's Drug Consult
Natural Standard*
Nurse's Guide to Cancer Care*
Nurses' Pocket Guide: Diagnoses, Interventions, and Rationales*
Nursing Diagnosis in Psychiatric Nursing*
Nursing Diagnosis Reference Manual*
Pediatric Nursing: Caring for Children and Their Families*
Primary Care for Physician Assistants: Clinical Practice Guidelines*
Principles of Critical Care*
Principles of Surgery
Red Book: 2003 Report of the Committee on Infectious Diseases*
Review of General Psychiatry
Review of Medical Physiology
Rosen & Barkin's 5 Minute Emergency Medicine Consult
Rudolph's Pediatrics
Smith's General Urology
Stedman's Medical Dictionary
Taber's Cyclopedic Medical Dictionary*
Trauma
Treatments of Psychiatric Disorders
USP DI Vol. I: Drug Information for the Health Care Professional
USP DI Vol. II: Advice for the Patient
Williams Obstetrics

PDA Applications

To get the most current information via your PDA, it's best to use programs that are updated frequently, even daily, whenever possible. Publishers have started having their PDA drug information programs clinically evaluated, but this process is complicated because databases are updated constantly and there is no certification board that oversees quality of content of PDA resources. The evaluations give publishers valuable feedback to help them improve their products. Here are highlights of some leading PDA programs.

> To get the most current information via your PDA, it's best to use programs that are updated frequently, even daily, whenever possible.

ePocrates RX:
www2.epocrates.com

ePocrates RX, updated daily, includes comprehensive drug information, including alternative medicines. Its region-specific formulary information helps clinicians select products covered by the patient's insurance. Epocrates has products to suit many practitioners, from free drug information to comprehensive packages that contain multiple databases.[9] Figure 9-4 shows the main menu of ePocrates RX Pro.

Lexi-Complete: www.lexi.com/web/index.jsp

Lexi-Complete, known for its PDA applications, is published by the well-respected Lexi-Comp. A comprehensive source of

FIGURE 9-4

Epocrates RxPro PDA program, main menu.

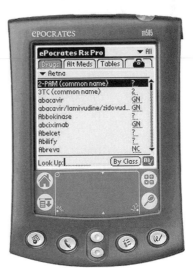

drug and health information, Lexi Complete combines 15 databases (listed below).[10] Some practitioners have commented that Lexi-Comp information is the most clinically dependable and offers the greatest breadth of information; however the product has undergone drastic revisions since those opinions were published. Updated evaluations comparing this product to others would be needed to validate breadth and clinical dependability.[11] Figure 9-5 shows a display for the drug gemifloxacin.

FIGURE 9-5

Lexi-Comp Platinum showing a display for gemifloxacin.

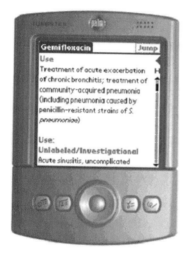

- Lexi-Drugs
- Pediatric Lexi-Drugs
- Griffith's 5-Minute Clinical Consult
- Lexi-Natural Products
- Lexi-Poisoning & Toxicology
- Lexi-Infectious Diseases
- Lexi-Lab & Diagnostic Procedures
- Lexi-Interact
- Dental Lexi-Drugs
- Nursing Lexi-Drugs
- Medical Abbreviations
- Lexi-Pharmacogenomics
- LEXI-PALS Patient Advisory Leaflets
- Stedman's Medical Dictionary—Concise
- Nuclear Biological and Chemical (NBC) Exposure Database

*mobile*Micromedex: www.micromedex.com/products/ mobilemicromedex/mobileinstructions.html

*mobile*Micromedex provides reliable, unbiased clinical information to help support and confirm treatment decisions at the point of care. Free for all health care professionals associated with a facility that subscribes to the Micromedex Health Care Series Databases, *mobile*Micromedex offers the following information:

- **Drugs**—search more than 3200 drugs for information on adult dosage, pediatric dosage, dose adjustments, administration, monitoring, dosage forms, indications (separated into "FDA labeled" and "non-FDA labeled"), contraindications, precautions, adverse effects (separated into "common" and "serious"), drug interactions, pregnancy category, and breastfeeding safety.

- **Alternative medicines**—search more than 300 of the most popular herbal and other dietary supplements for information on class, adult dosage, pediatric dosage, administration, availability, indications, contraindications, adverse effects, drug interactions, pregnancy category, and breastfeeding safety.
- **Acute care**—concise information for more than 320 common emergency conditions, including information about treatment, diagnosis, and key points.
- **Toxicology**—information explaining how to manage more than 200 of the most common poisonings, including information about clinical effects, treatment, and range of toxicity.[6]

Clinical Practice Guidelines

The Agency for Health Care Research and Quality's National Guideline Clearinghouse (NGC) at www.guidelines.gov is a compilation of evidence-based clinical practice guidelines, which gives health care professionals and health systems a convenient and efficient way to obtain objective, detailed guidelines.

For a guideline to be included in the NGC it must adhere to strict criteria, listed in Box 9-2.[12,13] Figure 9-6 shows the NCG home page.

FIGURE 9-6

National Guideline Clearinghouse Web site available at www.guidelines.gov.

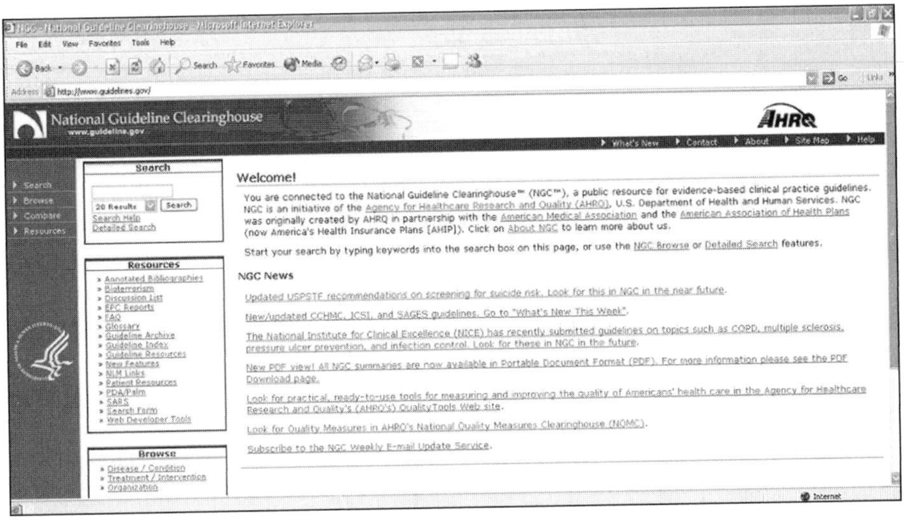

BOX 9-2

Criteria for Including Clinical Practice Guidelines in the National Guideline Clearinghouse (NGC)

For a clinical practice guideline to be included in the NGC, all criteria below must be met.

- The guideline must contain systematically developed statements that include recommendations, strategies, or information to help physicians, other health care practitioners, and patients make decisions about appropriate health care for specific clinical circumstances.
- The guideline must be produced under the auspices of medical specialty associations, relevant professional societies, public or private organizations, government agencies at the federal, state, or local level, or health care organizations or plans. The guideline cannot be developed and issued by an individual not officially sponsored or supported by one of the above types of organizations.
- There must be corroborating documentation available to verify that scientific literature published in peer-reviewed journals was systematically searched and reviewed while the guideline was being developed. If a guideline has gaps in scientific evidence for some of its recommendations the guideline is not necessarily excluded from the NGC, but the gaps must be documented.
- The guideline must be current, in English, and the most recent version produced, and must have been developed, reviewed, or revised within the last 5 years, as verified by documented evidence.

Systematic Reviews

In a systematic review—a term commonly used in this era of evidence-based medicine—the results of primary investigations addressing a specific topic or problem are critically evaluated and synthesized and the studies included in the review are systematically identified. Although Chapter 11, Tools for Bringing Evidence into Practice, discusses systematic reviews in more detail, they are mentioned here because health care professionals commonly seek them to research questions.

The article "Drug Treatment of Hyperlipidemia in Women," which appeared in the *Journal of the American Medical Association* in 2004, gives an example of an appropriately performed systematic review.[14] The authors searched Medline, the Cochrane Database, and the Database of Abstracts of Reviews of Effectiveness for articles published from 1966 through December 2003, examined bibliographies for other relevant articles, and consulted content experts For a study to be included in the review, it had to include trials involving outpatients treated for hyperlipidemia for at least 1 year, assess the impact of lipid lowering on clinical outcomes, and report results by sex. Outcomes evaluated included total mortality, coronary heart disease (CHD) mortality, nonfatal myocardial infarction, revascularization, and total CHD events. For the review, the authors calculated statistics for patients with and without a previous history of cardiovascular disease to determine whether outcomes were actually linked to the presence of hyperlipidemia.

The Cochrane Database of Systematic Reviews, discussed earlier on page 210, contains reviews of health care interventions that are based on the highest level of evidence and relevance. In compiling the reviews, the Cochrane Collaboration examines the evidence for and against the effectiveness and appropriateness of treatments (medications, surgery, education, etc.) in specific circumstances.[4]

The Internet

Thousands of Web sites are available to help health care professionals give patients information about their diseases and treatments. In 2002, almost 93 million Americans (about 80% of adult Internet users) used the Internet to look for health information.[15] Anyone, regardless of educational background or credentials, can publish a Web site, so the quality of Internet health care information varies widely—and health care practitioners need to know how to evaluate it. Specific skills health practitioners should have to assess usefulness, accuracy, and quality are outlined in Chapter 10, Evaluating the Literature.

The following list describes Web sites where you can find clinical information. Some are specifically designed for health care practitioners and others are oriented toward consumers.

> In 2002, almost 93 million Americans (about 80% of adult Internet users) used the Internet to look for health information.

Centers for Disease Control and Prevention: www.cdc.gov

Redesigned in 2004 and easier to navigate, the U.S Centers for Disease Control and Prevention Web site specializes in the treatment and prevention of infectious diseases. Among hot topics the site covers are bioterrorism, immunizations, SARS, and travel medicine. The site gives information on A to Z health topics and women's health and hosts some journals oriented toward health professionals, including *Emerging Infectious Diseases Journal,*

Morbidity and Mortality Weekly Report (MMWR), and *Preventing Chronic Disease Journal.*[16]

Food and Drug Administration: www.fda.gov

The FDA Web site is so comprehensive it can be overwhelming to sift through when searching for information. The authority for new product approvals and drug and food recalls, a major strength of the site is its current updates. An easy-to-use feature helps users find information about FDA-approved drug products.[17]

Center for Drug Evaluation and Research: www.fda.gov/cder

The Center for Drug Evaluation and Research (CDER), responsible for evaluating new drugs before they can be sold to consumers, reviews applications for new drugs, both prescription (including new brand names and generics) and nonprescription, for safety and efficacy. In addition, it reviews information provided to physicians and patients so that medications can be used in the most appropriate manner.[18]

National Institutes of Health: www.nih.gov

The National Institutes of Health, directed at the health care professional, also has a comprehensive drug information library for consumers and links to Medline Plus, the consumer version of Medline. Highlights of this enormous site include links to information about health conditions, drugs, bioterrorism, alternative medicine, clinical trials, volunteering for NIH research studies, and health statistics.[19]

American Heart Association: www.americanheart.org

The American Heart Association's Web site contains a comprehensive library of practice guidelines, free for downloading. Useful for both practitioners and consumers, the site focuses on cardiovascular disorders such as stroke and heart attack.[20]

American Diabetes Association: www.diabetes.org

The American Diabetes Association's Web site is helpful for both health care practitioners and patients with diabetes. One of its most important features is a posting of the most recent practice guidelines for the treatment of diabetes, available free for downloading.[21]

Clinical Trials: www.Clinicaltrials.gov

Practitioners fielding questions from patients regarding new or emerging therapies will find this a good source for current clinical trial information.[22]

Medscape from WebMD: www.medscape.com

Medscape is a popular source for health care professionals worldwide: more than 2 million are registered for the service. Medscape provides clinical information that is helpful for patient care as well as continuing medical education, online coverage of medical conferences, access to more than 100 medical journals, and medical news.[23]

ACTIVITY 9-1

Searching for Information

This chapter describes resources you can use to answer different types of questions. To become familiar with these resources—including how they operate and what they can offer—you must use them. Using resources discussed in this chapter (or your preferred resources) answer the questions below. Alternatively, substitute questions that came up recently in your practice.

1. Is vitamin E (tocopherol) effective in preventing heart disease?
2. Can you mix gentamicin and cimetidine in the same IV bag?
3. Is there any evidence to support the benefit of megestrol acetate in an 80-year-old male nursing home patient who has abdominal cancer and has lost 30 pounds over the last 3 months?

ACTIVITY 9-2

Comparing PubMed and Medline Plus

Pick a term to search on both the PubMed version of Medline and on Medline Plus. Note the differences and similarities in results. Which site should a patient or consumer use?

ACTIVITY 9-3

Organizing Your Personal Medical Library

Establish a strategy for organizing your personal medical library articles, Internet sites, online reference books, and secondary databases.

References

1. PubMed Web site. National Library of Medicine. Available at: www.ncbi.nlm.nih.gov/entrez/query.fcgi. Accessed January 28, 2005.

2. Cinahl Web site. Available at: www.cinahl.com/. Accessed November 3, 2003.

3. Current Contents Connect Web site. Available at: www.isinet.com/cap/ccc. Accessed January 30, 2005.

4. Cochrane Library Web site. Available at: www.cochrane.org/reviews/clibintro.htm. Accessed January 30, 2005.

5. Embase Web Site. Available at: www.embase.com. Accessed January 30, 2005.

6. Thomson Micromedex Healthcare Series Vol. 119. Available at: www.micromedex.com and http://micromedex.duc.auburn.edu/mdxdocs/knowbase.htm#altcaredex. Accessed January 27, 2005.

7. Stat-Ref Web site. Available at: www.statref.com/. Accessed January 30, 2005.

8. Felkey B, Fox BI. Emerging technology at the point of care. *J Am Pharm Assoc.* 2003;43(5 Suppl 1):S50-1.

9. Epocrates Web site. Available at: www.epocrates.com. Accessed January 30, 2005.

10. Lexi-Comp Web site. Available at: www.lexi.com/web/index.jsp. Accessed January 14, 2005.

11. Enders SJ, Enders JM, Holstad SG. Drug-information software for Palm operating system personal digital assistants: breadth, clinical dependability, and ease of use. *Pharmacotherapy.* August 2002;22(8):1036-40.

12. National Guideline Clearinghouse Web site. Available at: www.guidelines.gov. Accessed January 19, 2004.

13. National Guideline Clearinghouse Web site. Inclusion Criteria. Available at: www.guidelines.gov/about/inclusion.aspx. Accessed January 19, 2004.

14. Walsh JME, Pignone M. Drug treatment of hyperlipidemia in women *JAMA.* 2004;291:2243-52.

15. Fox S, Fallows D. Internet Health Resources: Health searches and email have become more commonplace, but there is room for improvement in searches and overall Internet access. Pew Internet and American Life Project, July 2003. Available at: www.pewinternet.org/reports/pdfs/PIP_Health_Report_July_2003.pdf. Accessed August 22, 2003.

16. Centers for Disease Control and Prevention Web site. Available at: www.cdc.gov. Accessed March 7, 2004.

17. Food and Drug Administration Web site. FDA Launches New Easy-to-Use Drug Information Web Site. Available at: www.fda.gov/bbs/topics/NEWS/2004/NEW01031.html. Accessed March 7, 2004.

18. CDER Web site. Frequently asked Questions About the CDER. Available at: www.fda.gov/cder/about/faq/default.htm. Accessed January 15, 2005.

19. National Institutes of Health Web site. Available at: www.nih.gov. Accessed March 13, 2004.

20. American Heart Association Web site. Available at: www.americanheart.org. Accessed January 4, 2004.

21. American Diabetes Association Web site. Available at: www.diabetes.org. Accessed June 13, 2004.

22. Clinical trials.gov Web site. Available at: http://clinicaltrials.gov. Accessed February 2, 2004.

23. Medscape Web site. Available at: www.medscape.com. Accessed January 27, 2005.

Evaluating the Literature ⑩

Margaret R. Thrower

Chapter Objectives

After completing this chapter, you should be able to:
- ■ Evaluate literature found on the Internet.
- ■ Evaluate clinical practice guidelines.
- ■ Evaluate primary literature.
- ■ Understand the basics of study designs.

Literature evaluation skills are essential for health care professionals, allowing you to identify beneficial treatments for patients, become aware of options that may be harmful, and respond to patients' questions when they ask about information they "saw on the news last night" or "found on the Internet."

When you need to interpret important clinical information and apply it—often for a specific patient in the clinical setting—it's not unusual to feel overwhelmed. So much information is available, how do you make sense of it and put it to good use? This chapter presents key techniques for evaluating the literature. No single technique will serve you best in all situations. Instead, you will likely come to rely on a hybrid of the methods presented here.

Literature evaluation skills are essential for health care professionals, allowing you to identify beneficial treatments for patients, become aware of options that may be harmful, and respond to patients' questions when they ask about information they "saw on the news last night" or "found on the Internet." Because an estimated 40% to 50% of studies found in the medical literature have serious limitations in trial design, statistical analysis methods, and conclusions, being able to critically evaluate clinical trials is important so that correct information can be given to patients.[1,2]

The information in this chapter addresses Web sites, clinical practice guidelines, and primary—or original—research, such as clinical trials. How to evaluate systematic review articles, sometimes referred to as meta-analyses, is covered in Chapter 11, Tools for Bringing Evidence into Practice.

Information on the Internet

Thousands of health care information Web sites are available to patients. Inevitably, your patients will ask you about something they read on the Internet regarding their health. One source reported that, by the end of 2002, almost 93 million Americans (about 80% of adult Internet users) had used the Internet to look for health information.[3] Because anyone can publish a Web site, regardless of educational background or credentials, the quality of health care information on the Internet varies widely. Consequently, you need skills to evaluate the usefulness, accuracy, and validity of information. Box 10-1 identifies characteristics of credible, reliable information. Table 10-1 lists criteria for evaluating the quality of Web sites.

How to Evaluate Web Content

Before you use health care Web sites, you must evaluate them for reliability and validity. The criteria for your evaluation fall into several categories: ownership, authorship, review process,

BOX 10-1

Evaluation Criteria for Web Sites

Because anyone can publish Web sites, you must evaluate their credibility. Following is a list of areas to examine to determine whether you can rely on a Web site's information.

- **Ownership.** Who owns the site? This can help you determine whether there may be a commercial bias.
- **Authors.** Who are the authors of the material? Names of authors should be readily available on the site, either on each piece of information or in the "About Us" section. To establish their credibility, sites that have qualified staff say so.
- **Review.** What is the review process? Determining the answer to this question gives you an idea of how particular the site is about its postings. Preferably the site uses a peer-review process for each document.
- **Timeliness.** Is the last update on each page clearly noted? Being able to see the date lets you know how current the information is.
- **Believability.** Are claims believable? If the site makes claims or presents information that doesn't seem believable, beware. As the old saying goes, "If it sounds too good to be true, it probably is."
- **Support.** Can you find support for the information? If no other source, such as other Web sites or articles, confirms information found on the site, the site may not be accurate.
- **References.** Is the material referenced? Proper use of references on the site is a good indicator that the information it provides is supported in the literature.

TABLE 10-1

Characteristics of Credible Health Care Web Sites

Characteristic	What It Means
Accurate	Information is error-free.
Reliable	Information can be depended on.
Current	Information reflects the latest evidence available.
Complete	Information contains all the important facts.
Economical	Access to the information is free or low cost.
Relevant	Information is important to the user.
Simple	Information is not overly complex.
Timely	Information is delivered when it is needed.
Verifiable	Information can be checked in another source for correctness.
Accessible	Information can be obtained easily in the right format and when needed.
Secure	Information access is limited to authorized users.

Source: Adapted from Reference 4.

If someone is promoting a commercial product, which is characteristic of Web sites whose address ends in ".com," the information could be biased in favor of the product.

date of last update, believability, support by biomedical literature, and references. The following paragraphs detail criteria to consider when evaluating credibility (also described briefly in Box 10-1 on page 231).

Ownership

Who *owns* the Web site? Answering this question can help you determine whether there is any potential for commercial bias. If someone is promoting a commercial product, which is characteristic of Web sites whose address ends in ".com," the information could be biased in favor of the product. However, some .com sites actually do provide good information, therefore demanding further evaluation. Look for warning signs such as one-sided information and failure to mention alternatives.

Authors

Identifying the *authors* of material can help you determine its credibility. The authorship information should be readily available and easy to find on the site. Typically, sites that have qualified content developers are upfront about this because the authors' credentials establish the site's credibility with readers.

Sometimes it is hard to determine the actual authors of individual articles, so look for clues that the site is maintained and edited by experts in the field. Although Web sites vary, the most obvious place to look for author information, if it is not posted on each individual article, is in the "About Us" section. Be leery of sites that do not post this information in an easily accessible spot, for they may have something to hide.

Review

What review process is content on the Web site subjected to? Is information about the review process clearly stated and easy to access? Generally this information is in the "About Us" section. Knowing the site's review process gives you an indication of how particular the site is about information it posts. Each document on the highest-quality sites has been subjected to a *peer-review process*, in which peers of the authors—professionals with equal qualifications—review and edit the content.

Timeliness

How *timely* is the information? Internet sites can be continually updated, which is good if new information is posted as soon as it is available and outdated material is deleted. Unfortunately, you don't always know how current the information on a Web site actually is. When a site displays a "last updated" notice, you get a sense of its timeliness, but it's possible that not all the content was updated on the date listed. Therefore you must critically evaluate the information for accuracy and validity.

If you are using the Web page content to address a question from a patient, it's a good idea to print out the page and attach it to the documentation you save when communicating the response to the patient. Given the Web's continuous changes, a paper backup helps you assess whether the information is still accurate and find current updates.

In general, before you rely on a piece of information— found on the Internet or anywhere—you should confirm it in at least one other source. Information that is credible and believable is usually available in many places.

Believability and Support

Another critically important area for evaluating information is *believable and evidence-based* claims. If the information on a site does not sound believable—such as, "this is the only product of its kind"—the doubts it raises in your mind should prompt you to verify the information. Can you find other credible sources, such as citations in the medical literature, that confirm the information on the site? In general, before you rely on a piece of information—found on the Internet or anywhere— you should confirm it in at least one other source. Information that is credible and believable is usually available in many places.

A related question to consider: Is the information *consistent with other sources of biomedical information?* If the material contains references from pertinent, credible, and up-to-date sources, it gives you key evidence that the information is credible. For further proof or more detailed information, you can easily refer to the primary source. It's always a good idea to evaluate references for validity, credibility, and relevance to the subject. Appropriate referencing is generally considered a good indication that the information is supported in the biomedical literature.

Standards for Internet Content

Regulating and controlling the quality of content on the Internet has been difficult. However, some organizations have developed criteria for development of health Web sites in an attempt to guide consumers and health care practitioners. The two groups described below serve to improve the quality of health information available on the Internet.[5] Even so, it can be a challenge to find quality health care information on the Web, so you and your patients need evaluation skills.

Health On the Net Foundation: www.hon.ch

The Health On the Net Foundation (HON), a Swiss organization, has taken steps to set ethical standards for Web site developers. In keeping with its mission to guide consumers and health care practitioners to useful, reliable information, the foundation developed a HON Code of Conduct (HONcode). Medical and health Web sites must follow a set of eight principles before they can display the HONcode logo on the site (see Figure 10-1). The foundation also has a "site checker" to help you determine whether a Web site follows the principles of the HONcode.

Box 10-2 lists the ethical principles established by the HONcode organization for Internet-based health information. If the Web site meets criteria from a review process conducted by the HONcode organization and is granted permission, it may display the HONcode logo. HON conducts annual reviews of all accredited Web sites.[6]

URAC is an independent, nonprofit organization that provides accreditation and certification to many types of health care services, including setting standards with which Web sites must comply.

FIGURE 10-1

HONcode seal from the Health On the Net Foundation.

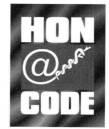

URAC: www.urac.org

Another organization, URAC, offers a certification seal (see Figure 10-2) for Web sites that meet extensive criteria and pay a fee of $5000 annually to be reviewed. The organization was originally incorporated under the name Utilization Review Accreditation Commission.

URAC is an independent, nonprofit organization that provides accreditation and certification to many types of health care services, including setting standards with which Web sites must comply. Some of these standards—there are more than 50— deal with disclosure of information, health content, editorial processes, links the site contains, privacy, accountability, and policies and procedures. A Web site must comply with all the standards to receive accreditation.

URAC has a quality oversight committee responsible for performing a full, formal review of each Web site annually.

FIGURE 10-2

URAC logo for Web sites that have been shown to comply with rigorous standards.

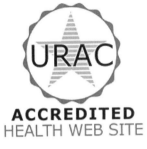

ACCREDITED
HEALTH WEB SITE

BOX 10-2

HONcode's Ethical Principles for Internet-Based Health Information

Principle 1: Authority
Any medical or health advice provided and hosted on this site will only be given by medically trained and qualified professionals unless a clear statement is made that a piece of advice offered is from a non–medically qualified individual or organization.

Principle 2: Complementarity
The information provided on this site is designed to support, not replace, the relationship between a patient/site visitor and his/her existing physician.

Principle 3: Confidentiality
Confidentiality of data relating to individual patients and visitors to a medical/health Web site, including their identity, is respected by this Web site. The Web site owners undertake to honor or exceed the legal requirements of medical/health information privacy that apply in the country and state where the Web site and mirror sites are located.

continued on page 236

BOX 10-2 *continued*

Principle 4: Attribution

Where appropriate, information contained on this site will be supported by clear references to source data and, where possible, have specific HTML links to that data. The date when a clinical page was last modified will be clearly displayed (e.g., at the bottom of the page).

Principle 5: Justifiability

Any claims relating to the benefits/performance of a specific treatment, commercial product, or service will be supported by appropriate, balanced evidence in the manner outlined above in Principle 4.

Principle 6: Transparency of Authorship

The designers of the Web site will seek to provide information in the clearest possible manner and provide contact addresses for visitors that seek further information or support. The Webmaster will display his/her e-mail address clearly throughout the Web site.

Principle 7: Transparency of Sponsorship

Support for this Web site will be clearly identified, including the identities of commercial and noncommercial organizations that have contributed funding, services, or material for the site.

Principle 8: Honesty in Advertising and Editorial Policy

If advertising is a source of funding, it will be clearly stated. A brief description of the advertising policy adopted by the Web site owners will be displayed on the site. Advertising and other promotional material will be presented to viewers in a manner and context that facilitates differentiation between it and the original material created by the institution operating the site.

Source: Reference 6.

ACTIVITY 10-1

Evaluating a Web Site

Locate a health care Web site dealing with a disease state of your choice and evaluate it according to the criteria in Box 10-1.

Clinical Practice Guidelines

Developed to help practitioners and patients make informed decisions about health care for specific diseases and conditions, clinical practice guidelines explain what has worked in clinical trials and what has not worked as well. The goal of properly developed and implemented guidelines is to increase the quality of care in the following ways:

- Improving the frequency of appropriate care.
- Reducing unnecessary or inappropriate care.
- Improving patient outcomes.
- Enhancing the continuity of care and improving communication when multiple providers are involved.

In 1989, the Agency for Health Care Policy and Research—now called the Agency for Healthcare Research and Quality (AHRQ)—was created specifically to respond to the United States' need for knowledge about health care. The AHRQ provides recommendations regarding evidence-based guideline development.

Ideally, properly constructed guidelines improve the quality of health care and decrease costs. For example, the guidelines provided in the Seventh Report of the Joint National Committee on Prevention, Detection, Evaluation, and Treatment of High Blood Pressure, published in 2004, provide an evidence-based approach to identifying and managing hypertension, which aims to saves lives and reduce costs from disorders linked to high blood pressure, such as myocardial infarction and stroke.

The Agency for Healthcare Research and Quality (AHRQ) provides recommendations regarding evidence-based guideline development.

Barriers to Adopting Guidelines

Although guidelines can help in clinical decisions, practitioners often do not know that specific guidelines exist for their clinical situation—or maybe they are aware of the guidelines, but don't know them well. Health care providers may resist changing their practice to bring it in line with the guidelines for a wide range of reasons, including:

- Disagreeing with the guidelines.
- Thinking the guidelines will not bring about the necessary outcomes.
- Seeing no reason to change approaches that have "worked so far."
- Patients' resistance to change.

■ Increased cost to the patient (for example, a new preventive medicine that the patient must purchase to decrease risk of illness).

■ Lack of time to implement the change.

■ No monetary incentive for the health care provider to change approach.

■ Incompatibility between approaches the guideline recommends and the way things are done in the practice setting.

To surmount some of these barriers, practitioners need to be alerted to new guidelines and taught about their potential impact and usefulness by other respected health care professionals.

BOX 10-3

Common Approaches to Developing Clinical Practice Guidelines

To properly evaluate, interpret, and implement guidelines—and to have confidence that you can rely on them—you must be familiar with the methods used to develop them.

■ **Informal Consensus:** The least rigorous and common of the three primary ways to develop guidelines, informal consensus is the quickest, easiest, least inexpensive approach. Consensus is gathered by a panel of experts that has an open discussion and reaches agreement, sometimes in a single meeting. Often the guidelines provide only the recommendation, with little information on evidence incorporated or methodology used by the group. This method makes it difficult for readers to verify accuracy of the recommendation and it produces guidelines of questionable quality.[7]

■ **Formal Consensus:** Developed through a more rigorous, labor-intensive, and expensive process than informal consensus, this is an efficient method, but the quality of the recommendations can be questionable, lacking explicit methods and varying widely in the amount of evidence supporting them. For this approach, an expert panel is convened to discuss the topic, reach agreement, and make recommendations—a process exemplified in the NIH Consensus Development Program.[8] All health care disciplines should be actively involved in this process so important issues are not missed. Bias can be introduced if the guidelines are not backed by specific evidence, a multidisciplinary approach is not used, or there are conflicts of interest among panelists.

■ **Evidence-Based Approach:** Also called the explicit approach, this method incorporates the best scientific evidence available into the guidelines process, stressing extensive documentation of methods and evidence used to make recommendations. This is the most rigorous approach to developing guidelines, but it is extremely time- and labor intensive. Sometimes years and millions of dollars are invested in the process.

Evaluating Guidelines

Guidelines should be one of the first sources clinicians seek when starting to research a clinical question. However, validity and practical relevance can vary widely, so you need evaluation skills to know when and how to use guidelines in making health care decisions. Box 10-3 on page 238 helps you assess clinical guidelines by explaining the common ways they are developed.

> Guidelines should be one of the first sources clinicians seek when starting to research a clinical question.

Checklists

Checklists are an evaluation approach that some health professionals prefer for the sake of simplicity; they become so familiar with the checklist that a quick glance tells them whether they forgot to consider something critical. The AHRQ, formerly in charge of writing clinical practice guidelines, now provides guidance on the guideline development process and recommends eight characteristics all clinical practice guidelines should adhere to. (See Box 10-4.)

BOX 10-4

Eight Desirable Characteristics of Clinical Practice Guidelines

1. Validity
- Estimated outcome: are objectives met? This can include both health and cost outcomes.
- Strength of evidence: is the relationship between evidence and recommendations provided, and is the rationale for the judgment behind them clear?

2. Reliability/Reproducibility
- Are the guideline recommendations reproducible and are they the same that others, given the same literature, would give?
- Given that guidelines are used by multiple practitioners, can the guideline be interpreted and applied consistently by all practitioners?

3. Clinical Applicability
- In the evidence presented, are the patient populations representative and explicitly stated so readers can determine whether the guidelines are applicable to their patients?

4. Clinical Flexibility
- Does the guideline identify known or expected exceptions to its recommendations and discuss how to deal with them?

5. Clarity
- Are the guidelines written clearly, are terms defined, and is the material presented in an easy-to-understand format?

continued on page 240

BOX 10-4 *continued*

6. Multidisciplinary Process
■ Did the guideline preparation involve a variety of health care providers so that the final result is complete and easy to apply?
7. Scheduled Review
■ Has the entity responsible for releasing the guideline specified a time for review and a way to determine whether revisions are needed when new evidence becomes available?
8. Documentation
■ Have the methods been described and documented that were used to develop the guidelines, involve participants, apply the evidence, accept assumptions and rationales, and conduct the analysis?
Source: Reference 9.

Categories

Sackett and colleagues have developed another method for evaluating clinical practice guidelines in which you must consider three main categories: validity, usefulness, and application to practice.[10] See Box 10-5 for an example of a clinical practice guidelines worksheet that applies to this method.

BOX 10-5

Evaluation Worksheet for Determining Validity of Guidelines

Are the recommendations in this guideline valid?
1. Were all important decision options and outcomes clearly specified?
2. Was the evidence relevant to each decision option identified, validated, and combined in a sensible and explicit way?
3. Are the relative preferences that key stakeholders attached to the outcomes of decisions (including benefits, risks, and costs) identified and explicitly considered?
4. Is the guideline resistant to clinically sensible variations in practice?

Is this guideline or strategy potentially useful?
1. Does this guideline offer an opportunity for significant improvement in the quality of health care practice?
2. Is there a large variation in current practice?

continued on page 241

BOX 10-5 *continued*

3. Does the guideline contain new evidence (or old evidence not yet acted on) that could have an important effect on management?
4. Would the guideline affect the management of so many people, or concern individuals at such high risk, or involve such high costs, that even small changes in practice could have major effects on health outcomes or resources (including opportunity costs)?

Should this guideline or strategy be applied in your practice?
1. What barriers exist to its implementation?
2. Can these barriers be overcome?
3. Can you enlist the collaboration of key colleagues?
4. Can you meet the educational, administrative, and economic conditions that are likely to determine the success or failure of implementing the strategy?

Source: Reference 10.

ACTIVITY 10-2

Evaluating a Treatment Guideline

Locate the most current treatment guideline on a disease state of your choice from a source on the Internet. A good starting place is www.guidelines.gov. Evaluate the guideline using the characteristics in Box 10-4 on page 239.

Primary Literature

One approach for evaluating primary literature—a simple technique you might call "the basics"—is useful for screening an article quickly to determine its validity and relevance to your practice. Although a good starting point, this technique does not provide all the information or evaluation items you may need. A more comprehensive approach to evaluating primary literature breaks down articles section by section, which helps you simplify ideas and considerations.

Technique One: Simple Evaluation

The Users' Guides to the Medical Literature: A Manual for Evidence-Based Clinical Practice by Guyatt and Rennie[11] identifies four fundamental categories of clinical trials in the medical field: therapy, harm, diagnosis, and prognosis. If you are evaluating therapy studies—which determine a treatment's effect on patient outcomes such as quality of life, mortality, morbidity—Guyatt and Rennie recommend several main questions to address, listed in Box 10-6. Understanding clinical trial design, discussed in Box 10-7, is important for answering the questions in Box 10-6.

BOX 10-6

Evaluating Therapy-Related Primary Literature

In *The Users' Guides to the Medical Literature: A Manual for Evidence-Based Clinical Practice*, Guyatt and Rennie present the following questions to consider when you are evaluating studies involving medical therapies.[11]

1. Are the results valid?
2. Did experimental and control groups begin the study with similar patient populations?
3. Were patients randomized?
4. Was randomization concealed (blinded or masked)?
5. Were patients analyzed in the groups to which they were randomized?
6. Were patients in the treatment and control groups similar with respect to known prognostic factors?
7. Did experimental and control groups retain similar patient populations throughout the study?
8. Were patients aware of group allocation?
9. Were clinicians aware of group allocation?
10. Were outcome assessors aware of group allocation?
11. Was follow-up complete?
12. What were the results?
13. How large was the treatment effect?
14. How precise was the estimate of the treatment effect?
15. How can I apply the results to patient care?
16. Were the study patients similar to my patient?
17. Were all clinically important outcomes considered?
18. Are the likely treatment benefits worth the potential harm and costs?

Source: Reprinted with permission from Reference 11.

BOX 10-7

Understanding Study Design

To evaluate the results of a clinical study you must understand some basics of clinical trial design. Each type of design has advantages and disadvantages, and situational factors often dictate the design used.

- **Randomized controlled trials (RCT)** are the best study design for determining cause and effect. In this type of study, patients are randomized to a treatment group or a placebo group and are followed forward in time to determine whether they have a particular outcome, such as improved bone density.

    Figure 10-3 shows an RCT with a parallel design, in which each group is given only one intervention or treatment, and Figure 10-4 shows a crossover design, in which patients serve as their own control and are exposed to two or more different treatments with a washout period between each treatment. When the treatment is a medication, the washout period should equal 5 to 7 half-lives of the medication in question. Otherwise, effects seen may be from the previous drug or a synergistic effect between the two treatments.

    Although RCTs sometimes identify potential harm from a therapy, that is not usually their general purpose. The number of participants needed, ethical issues, time, cost, and other factors make it impossible to conduct RCTs to investigate every hypothesis.

- **Observational studies** generally supply weaker evidence than RCTs because they cannot determine a cause-and-effect relationship, but are useful for detecting harm from a therapy. They fall into two main categories: cohort studies (see Figure 10-5) and case-control studies (see Figure 10-6). In a cohort study, patients can be followed after exposure to factors of interest—vitamin E supplements or secondhand smoke, for example—to see whether they have a particular outcome. In a case-control study, people with a particular disease are compared to a similar group of people without it to define risk factors that may have led to the disease, such as levels of exposure to radiation or chemicals.

- **Diagnostic trials** follow a study design in which a diagnostic test is compared with the known and accepted "gold standard" test for diagnosing the particular disease or condition. Figure 10-7 shows the design of a diagnostic trial.

- **Prognosis studies** are used to follow people at risk of a particular event (see Figure 10-8). A patient population is identified, such as women with gestational diabetes, and followed to see whether they experience the outcome of interest, such as the diabetes persisting after the baby is born or complications occurring that are associated with diabetes, such as a myocardial infarction.

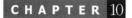

FIGURE 10-3

Randomized clinical trial: parallel design.

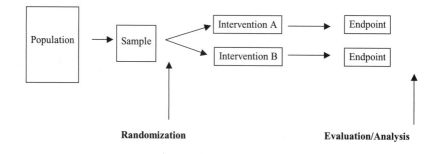

FIGURE 10-4

Randomized clinical trial: crossover design.

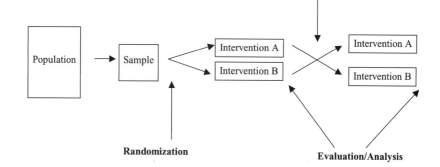

FIGURE 10-5

Randomized clinical trial: cohort study.

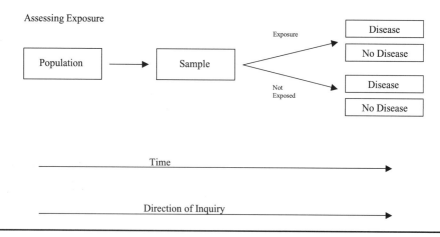

FIGURE 10-6

Observational study: case-control study.

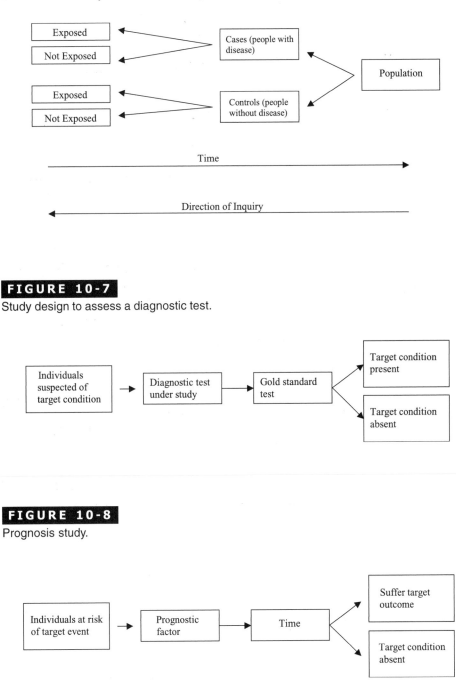

FIGURE 10-7

Study design to assess a diagnostic test.

FIGURE 10-8

Prognosis study.

CHAPTER 10

Technique Two: Advanced Literature Evaluation

The abstract should summarize the purpose of the study, the methods used, and the results.

Advanced literature evaluation requires you to scrutinize a piece of primary literature closely, section by section, asking yourself key questions along the way. The questions appear in Box 10-8.

Abstract

First, read the abstract to determine the relevance of the study to your question before you retrieve a full-text version of the article. The abstract should summarize the purpose of the study, the methods used, and the results. You can't rely on it entirely, however, because sometimes words or important details are left out to meet word count limits, or numbers or words are inaccurately transferred from the full-text article to the abstract. Biased language can appear in abstracts. Pay careful attention to phrases such as "trended toward significance" or "close to significance," which mean that the end points did not reach significance. Also, be aware of end points highlighted that were not the primary focus of the trial.

BOX 10-8

Questions to Consider When Conducting an Advanced Literature Evaluation

Abstract
- Is the title consistent with the information in the abstract and free from bias?
- Does the abstract accurately reflect the purpose, methods, and results of the study?
- Are any data present that are not included in the text of the manuscript?
- Is any biased language present in the abstract?

Article Introduction
- Do the researchers appear to have appropriate qualifications for conducting the study?
- Was the research conducted in an appropriate setting?
- Is appropriate background provided, stating important reasons that prompted the study to be conducted?
- Who sponsored the study? Could that lead to bias?
- Are the objectives and hypotheses clearly defined and free from bias?

Methods Section
- Was the study design clearly stated and described, and was it appropriate for the hypothesis?

continued on page 247

BOX 10-8 *continued*

- Was the study sample large enough and were the subjects representative of the general population to which the results will be applied?
- Were inclusion and exclusion criteria appropriate and clearly stated?
- Were subjects randomly assigned to groups?
- Were controls adequate and appropriate?
- Were blinding procedures appropriate and adequate?
- In drug studies, were appropriate doses and regimens used for the disease state under study?
- Was the length of the study observation period adequate?
- If crossover design was used, was the length of the washout period adequate?
- Was patient adherence monitored and assured?
- Were the measurements and assessments used both appropriate and sufficient?
- If there were multiple observers, how was variation among their observations minimized, measured, or both?
- Were measurements or assessment of effects made at the appropriate times and with the appropriate frequency?
- Were measurements reproducible and precise?
- Were statistical tests chosen before the data were gathered and were they appropriate?
- Was the significance level chosen before the study was started?
- Was a power analysis performed?

Results Section
- Are the data presented in an appropriate and understandable format?
- Are standard deviations and confidence intervals shown, along with mean values?
- Are data presented in a way that allows you to conduct an independent analysis?
- Are all subjects enrolled in the study accounted for, including dropouts?
- Are adverse events reported in sufficient detail, along with rates of occurrence?
- Are there any missing data or discrepancies between the presentation and evaluation of data?

Discussion and Conclusion
- Is the discussion an appropriate representation of the results and free from bias?
- Are the conclusions supported by the data, or could some factor other than the treatment have resulted in the observed outcomes?
- Are the conclusions based on the results, which were statistically and clinically significant?
- Are the data extrapolated by the author to situations or populations not adequately addressed in the study?
- Are study limitations adequately discussed?

Source: Reference 12.

Introduction

The introduction of an article generally contains key information to bring readers unfamiliar with the topic up to speed, including prior work done in the field and background on the study's importance. The investigators should be qualified to undertake the study and should conduct it in an appropriate research setting. If these conditions are not met, it is difficult to determine whether the results can be extended to real-world environments. The study's objectives and hypotheses should be clearly stated so you can decide for yourself whether the investigators accomplished what they set out to do.

The sponsor of the study is important to note, but keep in mind that sponsorship by a commercial company does not necessarily discredit the results. Pharmaceutical companies, for example, are among the few entities with the money, incentives, and resources to conduct large-scale studies.

Methods

The easiest way to tell if the study sample was large enough is to look for the author's commentary on how the sample size was calculated.

The methods section, generally regarded as the most important part of an clinical research report, contains details such as trial design, inclusion criteria, and exclusion criteria, which help you determine the study's validity and relevance to your clinical question. The trial's design should be clearly stated so its appropriateness can be evaluated: for example, although a randomized controlled trial can determine cause and effect, in some situations it would be unethical or inappropriate, such as comparing a standard drug to a placebo even though the standard is known to be superior to placebo. Comparing a promising new drug to the standard therapy, however, is appropriate.

Sample size gives you an idea of the real-world application of the results. If the sample is too small, you probably can't extend the findings to the general population. The easiest way to tell if the study sample was large enough is to look for the author's commentary on how the sample size was calculated. The inclusion and exclusion criteria help you determine whether patients represent those in real life and whether they reflect the population in your clinical practice.

In addition to clarifying how they estimated the sample size, the authors should state their target power and whether it was achieved for the primary outcome. Power is the ability to detect a statistical difference between study groups. You need to consider power especially carefully when the results show no difference between groups. Power depends on sample size; a power of $\geq 80\%$ is generally considered acceptable.

Randomizing patients enhances the likelihood that the groups will be equal. A control group sometimes involves comparing the investigational agent with a placebo, but in other cases the investigational agent is compared with an "active control"—a drug with known efficacy in treating a condition.

Both patients and investigators are subject to study bias: if they know they are being observed, they may act differently. Blinding can minimize the chance of bias. In double-blinding, neither investigators nor patients know who is in the active study drug group and who is in the control group.

The drug being studied should be dosed appropriately. When an active control is used it should be compared with appropriate doses of the investigational drug; regular doses of the investigational drug should never be compared with subtherapeutic doses of the active control, for example, because it may falsely appear that the investigational drug is more effective.

The study's duration is important when considering outcomes. In a study involving a slow-growing cancer, for example, a mortality end point at 6 months would not be appropriate. Equally useless would be the effect on mortality at 3 months of an anticancer drug to treat a slow-growing cancer. If a randomized controlled trial with a crossover design is used to assess a medication, the washout period should be equal to 5 to 7 half-lives of the medication in question. Otherwise, effects seen may be from the previous drug or a synergistic effect between the two drugs.

The importance of participants' adherence to the treatment regimen is arguable when you are evaluating a clinical trial. Some trials are preceded by a "run-in period" of several weeks during which participants demonstrate their adherence. Those who do not adhere are dropped before the study begins, which likely gives better results about the efficacy of the treatment. The downside is that this approach does not mimic adherence rates in an actual patient population and thus may overstate real-world efficacy.

Any measurements or outcomes should be appropriate for the desired end point, and outcomes should reflect reliable methods or tests so they are accurate, reproducible, and representative of true clinical practice. If the measurements are too rigorous, they're unlikely to be reproduced in practice and the results will be invalid. The frequency and timing with which the participants are monitored to determine outcomes is equally important.

Any measurements or outcomes should be appropriate for the desired end-point, and outcomes should reflect reliable methods or tests so they are accurate, reproducible, and representative of true clinical practice.

When multiple study sites are used, variation among observations is more likely because different practitioners are performing the observations. It is important for the study to use specific training or criteria to minimize these variations. Also, observations between the sites should be monitored to detect differences, which should be explained in the methods section of the study report.

You should assess the researchers' choice of statistical tests and verify that they decided which test to use before they started gathering data. The level of significance, which is conventionally $p < 0.05$, should also be decided before tests are performed and data gathered.

Results

The results section details what happened in the study and includes important information about patient demographics. A key consideration is whether the patient population reflects real life. If the clinical trial involves a medication, this section should discuss adverse effects of treatment. Also, any reasons why patients dropped out of the study should be noted.

In the results section, each objective or end-point presented in the methods section should be addressed. In presenting their data, authors should choose a way that most accurately represents what occurred in the study. If results are presented that were not clearly defined as an objective in the methods section, be wary.

Discussion and Conclusion

In these sections the authors should discuss clearly and thoroughly what the study means in application to clinical practice. They also should compare and contrast their results with those of similar clinical trials and clearly define any limitations of their study.

Documenting the Literature Searched

It is becoming common for authors to document how they searched for background literature to prepare their articles, including databases used, such as Medline; limitations, such as English language only; dates searched; and keywords. Increasingly they also state how they selected the most appropriate, pertinent literature. Where authors put this information depends on the journal; sometimes it's in the abstract, but more commonly you find it in the methods section.

ACTIVITY 10-3

Evaluating a Clinical Trial

Locate a full-text clinical trial on memantine and Alzheimer's disease (or a therapy topic of your choice) and evaluate it according to the questions in Box 10-6 on page 242.

ACTIVITY 10-4

Randomized Controlled Trial Designs

1. List the strengths and limitations of a randomized controlled parallel trial. Include examples of what could appropriately be studied by this method.
2. List the strengths and limitations of a randomized controlled crossover trial. Include examples of what could appropriately be studied by this method.

References

1. Glantz SA. Biostatistics: how to detect, correct and prevent errors in the medical literature. *Circulation.* 1980;61:1-7.

2. Thorn MD, Pulliam CC, Symons MJ, et al. Statistical and research quality of the medical and pharmacy literature. *Am J Hosp Pharm.* 1985;42:1077-82.

3. Fox S, Fallows D. Internet Health Resources: Health searches and email have become more commonplace, but there is room for improvement in searches and overall Internet access. Pew Internet and American Life Project, July 2003. Available at: www.pewinternet.org/reports/pdfs/PIP_Health_Report_July_2003.pdf. Accessed August 22, 2003.

4. Stair RM. An Introduction to Information Systems. In: *Principles of Information Systems: A Managerial Approach.* 2nd ed. Danvers, MA: Boyd & Fraser Publishing Company; 1996:7.

5. URAC Web site. URAC's Health Web Site Check-Up Service and Accreditation Program. Available at: www.urac.org. Accessed February 14, 2004.

6. Health On the Net Foundation Web site. HONcode of Conduct for medical and health Web sites and HONcode membership application. Available at: www.hon.ch/. Accessed September 17, 2003, and March 3, 2004.

7. Woolf SH. Practice guidelines: a new reality in medicine. II. Methods of developing guidelines. *Arch Intern Med.* 1992;152:946-52.

8. Perry S. The NIH consensus development program. A decade later. *N Engl J Med.* 1987;317:485-8.

9. Field JM, Lohr KN, eds. *Guidelines for Clinical Practice: From Development to Use.* Washington DC: National Academy Press; 1992.

10. Centre for Evidence-Based Medicine Website. Oxford Centre for Evidence-Based Medicine. Evaluation of Guidelines worksheets. Available at: www.cebm.net/downloads/worksheets.pdf. Accessed June 10, 2004.

11. Guyatt G, Rennie D. *Users' Guides to the Medical Literature: A Manual for Evidence-Based Clinical Practice.* Chicago, IL: American Medical Association Press; 2002.

12. Smith GH, Mays DA. Clinical study design and literature evaluation. In: *Pharmacotherapy Self-Assessment Program.* 4th ed. Kansas City, MO: American College of Clinical Pharmacy; 2002:206.

Tools for Bringing Evidence into Practice

11

Margaret R. Thrower

Chapter Objectives

After completing this chapter, you should be able to:

- Define evidence-based medicine.
- Discuss misconceptions about and barriers to implementing evidence-based medicine.
- Research a clinical question using either a set of Web sites you have bookmarked or other research tools identified in this chapter.
- Discuss the five-step method of evidence-based medicine to find an answer to your clinical question.
- Locate two meta-analyses and critique them using tools in this chapter.
- Select Patient-Oriented Evidence that Matters (POEMs) from among a variety of types of evidence.

Clinical Question: In infan purchasing infant carrier, u

Are the results of this sys
1. Did the review addres: clearly focused question?
2. How likely is it that th search strategy would hav missed eligible trials?
3.1 Are the inclusion crit clearly stated?
3.2 Are the inclusion crit relating to population, intervention, and compari groups and outcome appropriate?
4. How likely is it that th conclusions are valid (i.e. the included studies good quality randomized, conti trials)?
5. If a meta-analysis was performed, were the inclu studies sufficiently homogeneous to make it appropriate to pool data?

Are the valid results of this
Translate odds ratios to nu
The numbers in the body o
corresponding odds ratios a
expected event rate (PEER

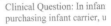

		0.9	0.85
	.05	209[1]	139
	.10	110	73
)l	.20	61	40
	.30	46	30
	.40	40	26
)	.50[3]	38	25
	.70	44	28
	.90	101[4]	64

Thanks to the Internet and its global connectivity, evidence-based medicine (EBM) has evolved quickly in recent years. EBM improves access to evidence critically needed at the point of care, helps practitioners better explain evidence to patients, and facilitates shared therapy decisions between practitioner, health care team, and patient.

One popular definition describes EBM as the "conscientious, explicit, and judicious use of current best evidence in making decisions about the care of individual patients."[1] This sounds like something every medical professional strives for, yet supporters of EBM meet a surprising amount of resistance. This chapter introduces resources, tools, and methods to help you integrate the best evidence into your practice. First, however, it explores common arguments against EBM.

Misconceptions and Barriers

A common myth is that EBM uses only objective evidence and neglects patient values. On the contrary, EBM requires combining clinical expertise, evidence, and an intimate knowledge of the individual patient's situation, beliefs, priorities, and values.[2] For instance, when a physician who practices EBM is deciding which antihypertensive to select for a patient with hypertension, he should not only consult the Seventh Report of the Joint National Committee on Prevention, Detection, Evaluation, and Treatment of High Blood Pressure (JNC 7), but also consider the patient's comorbid conditions, allergies, values, and economic resources to be sure the treatment is in line with best practices and is something the patient will stick with.

In recent years, the focus has shifted from whether to teach EBM to how best to teach it.[3] Given the increase in EBM training over the last 10 years, you might say that recent health profession graduates "grew up on" EBM. It's true that EBM is diffusing through health care, especially among practitioners with recent training, but some remain strongly opposed to EBM.

For example, in December 2002 the *British Medical Journal* published an attack by the Clinicians for the Restoration of Autonomous Practice (CRAP) Writing Group titled "EBM: unmasking the ugly truth." The paper's clear message—despite its humorous presentation—is that EBM is "cookbook" medicine, based on blind faith in methodology.[4]

In a 2000 commentary in the *Canadian Medical Association Journal*,[3] Straus and McAlister listed common misconceptions of EBM cited in the literature, including the time it takes to learn new skills for searching out, retrieving, and evaluating literature and clinicians' lack of interest in learning these skills. Surveys suggest, however, that literature searching and critical evaluation can be taught at any level of training and that these skills can be integrated into grand rounds, seminars (undergraduate, graduate, or postgraduate), and other learning environments without adding significant time to training.

Some critics of EBM point to the limited time and money available to busy health care professionals, who work in a field already faced with a shortage of practitioners in many disciplines. How can they take on a new practice approach? The quick answer to this question is that it doesn't take long to develop a working knowledge of where to locate resources, how to retrieve them, and how to apply the information to practice situations. Electronic searching of databases and journals has improved to the point where much information is at your fingertips, and summaries of medical evidence are available in a single source, easily printed at the point of care—often free or discounted.

Data are limited regarding whether EBM improves patient outcomes, which is unlikely to change, unfortunately, because these kinds of studies have inherent ethical problems with blinding and randomization.[3] Without clear proof of improved outcomes, some practitioners resist EBM. Some regard EBM as threatening—feeling unsure how to incorporate it or fearing that they are not technologically proficient enough. Others simply refuse to change, having practiced a particular way their entire career. It's not uncommon to hear, "I've done it this way for 25 years and haven't had any problems—why should I change now?"

Resistance is understandable, because change requires motivation, time, and effort. Entire fields of study focus on changing behaviors—a topic beyond the scope of this book. Suffice it to say that often the greatest barrier to change is the person, not the tool being introduced.

Three common misconceptions are that EBM completely ignores clinical expertise, ignores patients' values,[5] and promotes cookbook medicine.[6,7] However, the true definition of EBM includes patients' values and supplements clinical expertise by emphasizing data from sound evidence such as randomized controlled trials.

Surveys suggest that literature searching and critical evaluation can be taught at any level of training and that these skills can be integrated into grand rounds, seminars, and other learning environments without adding significant time to training.

The true definition of EBM includes patients' values and supplements clinical expertise by emphasizing data from sound evidence such as randomized controlled trials.

Others argue that EBM is only a cost-cutting tool. However, research regarding statin drugs for lowering cholesterol in patients with high cholesterol suggests otherwise. Because statin use has been shown to decrease mortality (i.e., decreased incidence of cardiovascular death) and morbidity (i.e., decreased incidence of myocardial infarction), it is now widely accepted therapy—despite the expense of these drugs. This demonstrates that EBM holds patient outcomes, not cost, as first priority.

Some critics call EBM an "ivory tower" concept that doesn't work in the real world—a misconception refuted by practicing clinicians who use EBM daily.[8] Others think EBM is limited to conducting clinical research, not *using* clinical research, but the truth is that few practitioners who use EBM—which is strictly a method for providing patient care—are also researchers.[3]

Another misconception is that only randomized trials or systematic reviews constitute the "evidence" in EBM and that these methods ignore the basic sciences.[9,10] Although EBM does rely heavily on randomized controlled trials, a design that can detect cause and effect, each study's design and outcomes should be scrutinized by the end user.

The health care profession has learned the hard way that just because pathophysiology or etiology suggests a certain outcome, it doesn't mean that outcome will occur. For example, it was once thought that some antiarrhythmic agents, such as encainide,

BOX 11-1

Five Steps to Using EBM

According to experts, EBM involves five linked activities to guide the decision-making process regarding the therapy, prognosis, and diagnosis.

1. Convert information needs into a clearly defined, answerable clinical question.
2. Conduct a systematic search for the best available evidence regarding the problem.
3. Evaluate the validity and applicability of the evidence.
4. Prepare a synthesis or summary of the evidence for decision making. Consider patient-specific information, including the patient's values, and integrate this information with your clinical expertise before implementing the decision in practice.
5. Evaluate performance and follow up on any areas needing improvement.

Source: Reference 13.

flecainide, and moricizine, would decrease mortality because electrocardiograms showed they decreased premature ventricular contractions. However, later evidence from the Cardiac Arrhythmia Suppression Trials (CAST) showed that these classes of anti-arrhythmic agents actually increased mortality.[11,12]

Background on EBM Tools

It would be helpful to have studies clearly refuting the misconceptions, but the best proof of EBM's value is intuitive: it makes sense that practitioners who stay up to date, can read the literature critically, and know how to distinguish strong from weaker evidence will choose therapies that offer a better chance of positive outcomes for patients. The pages that follow introduce you to tools that can help you make the most of EBM in your practice. A summary of the basic activities involved in performing evidence-based medicine appears in Box 11-1 on page 256.

> It makes sense that practitioners who stay up to date, can read the literature critically, and know how to distinguish strong from weaker evidence will choose therapies that offer a better chance of positive outcomes for patients.

ACTIVITY 11-1

Using Five Steps of EBM ✓

Thinking back to questions that arose in your practice today—or using a question you often encounter—follow the five-step method of EBM (listed in Box 11-1) to find an answer to your question.

Levels of Evidence

One of the most important concepts in EBM is levels of evidence. When you search for answers to a clinical question you have framed (a process described in Chapter 8), you want to find the highest level of evidence. Unfortunately, not everything has been studied, and even when studies are conducted, they may not have been designed in a way that provides the level of evidence you want.

The lowest level of evidence, commonly referred to as an "N of 1" randomized controlled trial, involves one patient taking a target treatment during one period and a placebo or standard therapy for another period. Such trials are simple and often feasible to perform, and they can provide valuable data.[14,15]

Some EBM authorities have argued that N of 1 trials offer the highest level of evidence because you see benefit directly in the patient for whom you are providing care. Although it's true that these trials provide definitive evidence of benefits such as efficacy and safety in individual patients,[16] you can't extrapolate results beyond the single patient without large-scale clinical trial data. Benefit and risk should be determined on a large scale before a therapy is used for patient care.

Box 10-7 in Chapter 10 gives an overview of key clinical trial designs, including randomized controlled trials (RCT), cohort observational studies, and case-control observational studies. Observational studies rank below RCT in the levels of evidence hierarchy, shown in Figure 11-1, because they cannot determine a cause-and-effect relationship. Meta-analyses and systematic reviews, discussed below, fall above or below RCTs in the hierarchy depending on the quality of the studies they include.

FIGURE 11-1

Hierarchy of clinical evidence.

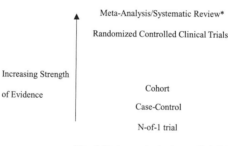

Meta-Analysis/Systematic Review*

Randomized Controlled Clinical Trials

Increasing Strength
of Evidence

Cohort

Case-Control

N-of-1 trial

*May fall below randomized controlled clinical trials, depending on the quality of studies they include.

Reviews and Meta-Analyses

The ideal review article should include all recent, relevant studies about a specific drug therapy or disease.

Just as a study's design determines the level of evidence it provides, the methodology used in preparing and writing a review article determines where the evidence it provides fits into the answer for your clinical question.

The primary purpose of a review article is to help practitioners make therapy decisions. Therefore, the ideal review article should include all recent, relevant studies about a specific drug therapy or disease. In the past this did not always happen, but now, with the advent of "systematic reviews," it is becoming the norm.

Traditional review articles, written by experts in the field, include literature the authors deem relevant. Such reviews, still frequently published, have their place when you search the medical literature, but they have disadvantages. Authors of traditional reviews do not routinely define how studies were included in the review—nor are they expected to. And because their conclusions are supported by the evidence provided,[17] failure to search the literature systematically could bias their results—under- or overestimating the treatment effects—and could cause important issues dealing with safety (side effects, adverse effects, etc.) to be ignored, underreported, or overreported.

The concept of systematic reviews was developed in the 1970s to help avoid subjectivity and problems with validity.[18] Using a systematic process, a systematic review assembles, critically evaluates, and synthesizes results of primary investigations that address a specific topic or problem. These types of reviews are also known as *qualitative* systematic reviews.

Meta-analyses also assemble, evaluate, and synthesize results of primary investigations to address a specific topic or problem, but they add additional steps—statistically combining results from previously conducted studies, summarizing them, and making a conclusion. These types of meta-analyses are also known as *quantitative* systematic reviews.[19,20]

The Cochrane Collaboration (www.cochrane.org/reviews/clibintro.htm), discussed in Chapter 9, is a worldwide organization established to promote the development, maintenance, and dissemination of health care meta-analyses and systematic reviews.

For all these types of reviews, limitations on usefulness and validity are the same: What if the author did not conduct a thorough literature search? Were important studies that would change the conclusion missed?

The systematic review, a concept developed to help avoid subjectivity and validity problems, assembles, critically evaluates, and synthesizes results of primary investigations that address a specific topic.

Meta-Analysis in EBM

Using meta-analyses that include rigorous studies is one of the best ways to practice EBM because of the high quality of evidence they provide to answer your clinical question. Meta-analyses combine many pieces of primary literature in an easy-to-understand format with summaries and conclusions. Rather than reading 25 articles to make a conclusion, you can read one article and digest the results efficiently. And meta-analyses have the ability to combine findings from small trials to obtain results that are more precise and are, therefore, a higher level of evidence.

The quality of a meta-analysis is limited by biases and flaws of incorporated studies. Among sources of bias are:

■ Including extreme results—evidence of extreme benefits or harm—which tend to be found in small studies and studies that are stopped early.

■ Sensitivity to publication bias. Although the general body of original research is plagued by publication bias (that is, trials that have favorable results are the ones usually published), meta-analyses tend to be particularly sensitive to it because they combine *published* trials, potentially overestimating the treatment effect of those results.

Authors conducting a meta-analysis should use funnel plots to assess the presence of publication bias by plotting the summarized effect size for the outcomes of interest versus the inverse of the variance of an individual study effect size.[17] When you look in the statistics section of the article, the plotted points should form a symmetrical funnel shape indicating that no publication bias is present.[17]

Just like original research, meta-analyses begin with planning. Authors must generate a focused, answerable clinical question, without which you—the clinician—would have a hard time determining whether the results of a meta-analysis are relevant to

---

BOX 11-2

Important Criteria for Including a Study in an Analysis

In the book *Evaluating Drug Literature: A Statistical Approach*, author John Devlin identifies four questions to help investigators decide whether or not to incorporate a study into an analysis. It is important for clinicians to recognize whether an analysis was done properly so they can assess whether it overestimates results.

1. Were patients randomly assigned to treatment?
2. Was follow-up sufficiently thorough and were all patients accounted for?
3. Were patients analyzed according to the groups in which they were randomly assigned?
4. Did proper concealment and blinding occur between control and experimental groups?

Source: Reference 17.

---

your needs. In their planning, authors of a meta-analysis must decide on criteria for including and excluding trials and define these factors:

- **Design** (e.g., randomized, controlled, double blind).
- **Population** (e.g., 18–65-year-olds with familial hyperlipidemia who had never had a cardiac event).
- **Exposure** (was the subject exposed to the intervention).
- **Control group** (placebo or standard of care).
- **Outcome** (e.g., all cause mortality, cardiovascular disease, myocardial infarction).

Grades in Systematic Reviews

As shown in Table 11-1, recommendation grades can be used to characterize the strength of data when developing systematic reviews and guidelines. Guyatt and Rennie, who developed these grades, discuss their use and implications in the 2002 American Medical Association monograph *Users' Guides to the Medical Literature*.[20] Although the Canadian Task Force on the Periodic Health Examination proposed the first taxonomy of levels of evidence, Guyatt and Rennie modified the framework—taking into consideration that clinical practice guidelines must focus on systematic reviews that incorporate only the best evidence from individual studies. Guyatt and Rennie assign both letter and number grades to studies, with letters reflecting methodologic strength and numbers reflecting the balance between benefits and risks. Their letter grades are defined like this:

- **A** represents the most rigorous methodology—generally reserved for a methodologically sound, randomized controlled trial.
- **B** is assigned to a randomized controlled trial that has some methodological flaws—therefore considered weaker evidence than grade A.
- **C** is assigned to observational studies, since this study design cannot confirm a cause-and-effect relationship.

As for the numbers, they are applied in the following way:

- **1** is assigned if benefit clearly outweighs the risk.
- **2** is assigned if benefit does not clearly outweigh the risk.

Guyatt and Rennie assign both letter and number grades to studies, with letters reflecting methodologic strength and numbers reflecting the balance between benefits and risks.

TABLE 11-1

Grading Treatment Recommendations Based on Systematic Reviews of Relevant Evidence

Recommendation Grade	Clarity of Risk/Benefit	Strength of Evidence	Implications/Strength of Recommendation
1A	Clear	Randomized controlled trials (RCTs) without critical flaws	Strong recommendations; can apply to most patients
1B	Clear	RCTs with important flaws	Strong recommendations; can most likely apply to most patients
1C+	Clear	No RCTs that directly answer the question; no overwhelming evidence from observational trials	Strong recommendations; applies to most patients under most circumstances
1C	Clear	Observational studies	When stronger evidence is available, may change
2A	Unclear	RCTs without critical flaws	Intermediate strength; decision may depend on patient circumstances or values
2B	Unclear	RCTs with critical flaws	Weak recommendations; alternative approach should be considered for some patients
2C	Unclear	Observational studies	Very weak recommendations; other alternatives may be equally reasonable

Source: Reference 18.

Evaluating Meta-Analyses

Evaluating studies and meta-analyses goes hand-in-hand with practicing EBM. A meta-analysis is a rich source of information because it combines data from many studies into one publication. For meta-analyses, evaluation techniques assess the exhaustiveness of the search strategy, study inclusion and exclusion criteria, quality of included studies, and whether studies and results are similar. A useful tool for evaluating these features of a meta-analysis is the checklist, an example of which is presented in Box 11-3.

BOX 11-3

Key Points to Consider When Critically Appraising a Meta-Analysis

This checklist, published in *Annals of Internal Medicine* in 1997, is a popular tool for evaluating a meta-analysis. As you read the meta-analysis you can quickly answer the eight questions to determine validity and usefulness to your practice.

1. Was an important, well-focused question described that includes people, exposure, control group, and outcome?
2. Were the inclusion and exclusion criteria clear and logical?
3. Was the search strategy sensible, thorough, and clearly reported?
4. Did the authors retrieve data from more than just Medline?
5. How did the studies compare in terms of rigor, heterogeneity between the studies, and applicability to clinical practice?
6. Were results from individual studies graphically displayed using a common scale to allow for visual examination of heterogeneity?
7. What model was used? To combine data, a fixed-effects model is preferable in most cases to a random-effects model, unless significant heterogeneity is detected because the fixed-effects model preserves randomization.
8. Was a thorough sensitivity analysis done to assess the robustness of combined estimates with regard to different assumptions and inclusion criteria?

Source: Adapted from Reference 21.

Some health care professionals prefer to use a comprehensive worksheet rather than a checklist to evaluate information. Figure 11-2 shows a completed worksheet that is useful for evaluating information systematically.[22] Sackett and colleagues developed another useful method that revolves around four key questions (below). The format of the worksheet in Figure 11-2 helps users arrive at the answers by providing specific subquestions to answer.

1. Are the results of this systematic review of therapy valid?
2. Are the valid results of this systematic review important?
3. Can you apply this valid, important evidence from a systematic review in caring for your patient or patients?
4. Should you believe an apparent qualitative difference in the efficacy of therapy in some subgroups of patients?

For meta-analyses, evaluation techniques assess the exhaustiveness of the search strategy, study inclusion and exclusion criteria, quality of included studies, and whether studies and results are similar.

FIGURE 11-2

Systematic review of therapy, completed worksheet.

Clinical Question: In infants with colic, do behavioral interventions (e.g., responding rapidly to crying, purchasing infant carrier, using a dummy, etc.) reduce crying?

Are the results of this systematic review of therapy valid?	
1. Did the review address a clearly focused question?	Yes. Population < 6 months with crying/colic. Outcome = reduced crying
2. How likely is it that the search strategy would have missed eligible trials?	Not very likely. Searched Medline, Embase, and CCTR, and checked references. Did not look at nursing journals or contact authors
3.1 Are the inclusion criteria clearly stated?	Yes. Infants < 6 months with colic. Outcome: reduction in crying
3.2 Are the inclusion criteria relating to population, intervention, and comparison groups and outcome appropriate?	Yes
4. How likely is it that the conclusions are valid (i.e., are the included studies good-quality randomized, controlled trials)?	Likely. There were 2 reviews with defined criteria. Consensus obtained. Included studies have variable quality (see table)
5. If a meta-analysis was performed, were the included studies sufficiently homogeneous to make it appropriate to pool data?	Yes. Did not test for homogeneity but only combined studies of similar interventions. Studies weighted according to quality

Are the valid results of this systematic review important?
Translate odds ratios to numbers needed to treat (NNT).
The numbers in the body of the table are the NNTs for the corresponding odds ratios at that particular patient's expected event rate (PEER).

		Odds Ratios (OR)								
		0.9	0.85	0.8	0.75	0.7	0.65	0.6	0.55	0.5
	.05	209[1]	139	104	83	69	59	52	46	41[2]
	.10	110	73	54	43	36	31	27	24	21
Control	.20	61	40	30	24	20	17	14	13	11
Event	.30	46	30	22	18	14	12	10	9	8
Rate	.40	40	26	19	15	12	10	9	8	7
(CER)	.50[3]	38	25	18	14	11	9	8	7	6
	.70	44	28	20	16	13	10	9	7	6
	.90	101[4]	64	46	34	27	22	18	15	12[5]

Can you apply this valid, important evidence from a systematic review in caring for your patient?	
Do these results apply to your patient?	
1. Are my patients so different from those in the review that there are likely to be important differences in treatment effect?	No
2. Is the intervention in the studies in the review sufficiently similar to the treatment that I am considering?	Yes
3. Are the outcome measures documented an adequate reflection of the outcomes of importance to my patients?	Yes
4. How great would the potential benefit of therapy actually be for your individual patient?	
Method 1: In the table, find the intersection of the closest odds ratio from the overview and the CER that is closest to your patient's expected event rate if receiving the control treatment (PEER)	No evidence of benefit
Method 2: To calculate the NNT for any OR and PEER: $$NNT = \frac{1 - \{PEER \times (1 - OR)\}}{(1 - PEER) \times PEER \times (1 - OR)}$$	
Are your patient's values and preferences satisfied by the regimen and its consequences?	
Do your patient and you have a clear assessment of his or her values and preferences?	Yes
Are they met by this regimen and its consequences?	No. No evidence that it works

Should you believe apparent qualitative differences in the efficacy of therapy in some subgroups of patients? Only if you can say "yes" to all of the following:
1. Do they really make biologic and clinical sense?
2. Is the qualitative difference significant both clinically and statistically?
3. Was this difference hypothesized before the study began (rather than the product of dredging the data), and has it been confirmed in other, independent studies?
4. Was this one of just a few subgroup analyses carried out in this study?

[1]The relative risk reduction (RRR) here is 10%.
[2]The RRR here is 49%.
[3]For any OR, NNT is lowest when PEER = .50.
[4]The RRR here is 1%.
[5]The RRR here is 9%.

Additional Notes:
In behavior studies, reduced stimulation rather than increased stimulation is more effective.
Studies references 34, 35, and 36: 95% CI of treatment effect all include 0 so not statistically significant
Study 35: treatment effect = -0.37 (95% CI -0.69 to -0.05) i.e., Placebo better

Source: Adapted from the Centre for Evidence-Based Medicine.

ACTIVITY 11-2

Evaluating a Meta-Analysis

1. Locate a meta-analysis by searching with PubMed (www.ncbi.nlm.nih.gov/entrez/query.fcgi).
2. Evaluate the meta-analysis using these two methods: the checklist in Box 11-3 and the worksheet in Figure 11-2.
3. Describe clinical situations in which one method may be preferable to the other.

Evidence-Based Clinical Guidelines

In the late 1990s a survey in the United Kingdom found that the best way to shift practitioners to EBM is through the use of evidence-based practice guidelines,[23] tools that help you make decisions regarding diseases and treatments. To promote EBM practice in everyday care in the United States, the Agency for Health Care Research and Quality (AHRQ) is urgently seeking evidence-based research through its Evidence-Based Practice Program, which it established in 1997.

This program awards 5-year contracts to 12 institutions in Canada and the United States that serve as Evidence-Based Practice Centers, charged with reviewing relevant biomedical literature on clinical, behavioral, financial, and health care organization and delivery issues, especially those that are common, expensive, or significant to the Medicare and Medicaid populations. The centers produce and translate evidence reports, technology assessments, and research on methodologies and efficacy of implementation. This program has allowed AHRQ to become a "science partner" with both public and private organizations in their efforts to improve the quality, effectiveness, and appropriateness of clinical care and translate evidence-based research findings into clinical practice.[24] You can find more information on the AHRQ Web site at www.ahrq.gov/clinic/epc.

> The best way to shift practitioners to EBM is through the use of evidence-based practice guidelines, tools that help you make decisions regarding diseases and treatments.

Tools for EBM in Clinical Practice

This section introduces tools to help you find the best evidence regarding your clinical questions. You may want to take the time to preview them and bookmark them as "favorites" for later use. If you don't have the time or desire to look for resources, you can benefit from searchable databases—which usually charge a subscription fee but are fast and convenient.

POEMs and DOEs

POEMs ("patient-oriented evidence that matters") and DOEs ("disease-oriented evidence") encourage outcomes-based research and help practitioners manage the amount of information thrown at them every day. The terms were coined by David C. Slawson, MD, professor of family medicine at the University of Virginia and Allen F. Shaughnessy, PharmD, clinical professor of family medicine at Tufts University, for approaches that help practitioners master important clinical information.

POEMs refer to literature that addresses questions you face as a health care professional—measuring endpoints such as mortality, morbidity, decreased hospitalizations, and quality of life.

POEMs refer to literature that addresses questions you face as a health care professional—measuring endpoints such as mortality, morbidity, decreased hospitalizations, and quality of life. POEMs, which represent randomized controlled trials, have the potential to change the way you practice because they focus on outcomes you and your patients care about. Slawson and Shaughnessy encourage you to read only POEMs and to discard DOEs: studies that are based on pathophysiology and etiology.[25,26]

InfoPOEMs: The Clinical Awareness System (www.infopoems.com) is an electronic database to help answer your clinical questions on the spot. It identifies, reviews, and summarizes articles from top medical journals to provide only the most valid and applicable evidence (POEMs) for use in clinical practice. The InfoPOEM database is quick and convenient, packaging many POEMs in one spot and summarizing them. For example, here's part of an InfoPOEM in the database:

Clinical Question: Does knee taping decrease pain and disability in patients with knee osteoarthritis?

Bottom Line: Rigid taping by physical therapists, applied above the knee and, when necessary, below the knee, significantly decreased pain and disability, which lasted 3 weeks after taping was stopped. LOE = 1c.

The item (found at www.infopoems.com/productInfo/samplePOEM.cfm) then goes on to give the reference, study design, setting, and synopsis.

Two other products available through this service are DailyPoems—e-mail alerts of POEMs identified in the literature—and the InfoRetriever database, which can be downloaded to a personal digital assistant (PDA), used on a desktop computer, or accessed online. InfoRetriever allows you to search the POEMs database; six other evidence-based databases—including Cochrane Systematic Review abstracts; more than 200 decision rules, 2000 predictive calculators, and 700 summarized evidence-based practice guidelines; and the popular program 5-Minute Clinical Consult. Other benefits of the InfoPOEM system include an ICD-9 lookup function for help in determining payment coding, guided Medline searches, and a link to patient education materials available on the Internet.[26]

ACTIVITY 11-3

Differentiating POEMs and DOEs

Go to the Web site of a major medical journal publisher, such as *The New England Journal of Medicine* (www.nejm.org) or *British Medical Journal* (www.bmj.com). Scan the most recent table of contents and abstracts. Try to identify from the abstracts which are POEMs and which are DOEs. Hint: Look for endpoints or outcomes of morbidity, mortality, or quality of life for POEMs versus studies based on etiology and pathophysiology for DOEs.

CATs

Critically appraised topics (CATs) are an evidence-based tool for teaching and learning based on the five steps to using EBM listed in Box 11-1 on page 256. Each CAT is a structured, one-page document that translates needs into answerable questions and incorporates the best evidence to answer them.

Using CATs, you critically evaluate evidence for validity and applicability, integrate the evidence with clinical expertise, apply it to practice, and evaluate performance. For an example of how a CAT can be used in clinical practice, see Box 11-4.

BOX 11-4

Sample Scenario: Constructing a Critically Appraised Topic (CAT)

You learn that a 54-year-old man with non–insulin-dependent diabetes mellitus (NIDDM) whose myocardial infarction (MI) you treated 6 months ago has died suddenly at home. Wondering whether you could have done more for him, you review his notes and confirm that he, in fact, was at low risk for a MI and had no complications. His blood sugar was elevated on admission (13 mmol/L) but decreased within 3 days. In view of the success that has been shown with "tight control" of insulin-dependent diabetes mellitus in preventing or postponing retinopathy and neuropathy, you wonder if a more aggressive treatment of his NIDDM might have postponed his untimely death.

On the other hand, you recall how one of your profs back in medical school insisted that insulin was atherogenic, saying you should back off insulin doses when diabetics developed angina pectoris.

continued on page 268

BOX 11-4 *continued*

You Form the Clinical Question

You ask the librarian at your local postgraduate center to help you with this question: "Among patients with NIDDM who are having MIs, does tight control of blood sugar reduce their risk of dying?" With her assistance you do a computerized literature search using the Medical Subject Headings (MeSH) terms "diabetes mellitus" and "myocardial infarction," limited by "publication type = randomized controlled trial." You find a possibly useful article: Malmberg K et al.: Randomized trial of insulin-glucose infusion followed by subcutaneous insulin treatment in diabetic patients with acute myocardial infarction (DIGAMI Study). *J Am Coll Cardiol.* 1995;26:57-65.

By applying the appropriate users' guides for evidence on therapy, you decide that the study's results and conclusions are both valid and potentially important. The study's number needed to treat (NNT) was only 11. That is, you would only have to treat 11 patients with high-intensity insulin therapy for at least 3 months to prevent one death. You generate a one-page CAT summarizing your patient and this evidence, and add it to your file of CATs.

You Use the CAT to Support Decision Making

The following month, while you're rounding, a patient with NIDDM is admitted with characteristic chest pain, and despite thrombolysis he goes on to have a myocardial infarction. At the post-take rounds you raise the question of whether he should be started on an intensive insulin regimen. Your teammates are skeptical, but you make a copy of your previously constructed CAT and show it to them. They are sufficiently impressed that they urgently study the full article. They agree with your appraisal, and within hours the patient is begun on an intensive insulin regimen.

Source: Reference 27. Used with permission of the Oxford Centre for Evidence-Based Medicine.

Cochrane Database of Systematic Reviews: www.cochrane.org

EBM is the primary focus of this database (discussed in more detail in Chapter 9). The Cochrane Database of Systematic Reviews contains reviews of health care interventions that are based on the highest level of evidence and relevance.

TRIP Database: www.tripdatabase.com

Started in 1997, the TRIP Database was one of the first resources to combine evidence-based materials with full-text access, all in one place. (TRIP is an acronym for Turning Research into Practice.) The database was developed in response to the vast amount of medical information made available by the Internet.

By combining all information in one place, the TRIP Database attempted to lower the barrier busy practitioners face of not having enough time to implement EBM.

The TRIP Database is now obsolete and has been replaced by TRIP Plus, which includes such improvements as direct searching of PubMed and a feature called TRIPwire that allows you to focus your searches more appropriately by clicking on suggested additional search terms. The TRIP Plus Database is updated monthly. Although the original TRIP Database was free, TRIP Plus allows a limited number of free searches for those without paid subscriptions.[28] Figure 11-3 shows an image of the database.

FIGURE 11-3

An image of the Trip Plus Database.

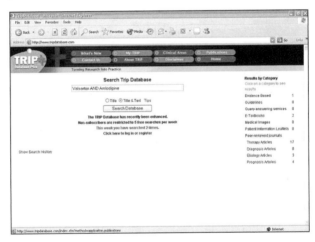

Web Sites that Support Evidence-Based Practice and Skills

Users' Guides to the Medical Literature: www.cche.net/usersguides/main.asp

This Web site provides access to the complete set of well-known *Users' Guides to the Medical Literature* that were published serially in the *Journal of the American Medical Association* (*JAMA*). The site is produced by the Centre for Health Evidence, a nonprofit organization in Canada that helps promote evidence-based practice. This site once contained tools associated with the guides, such as calculators, worksheets, and additional educational materials, but these are now at a new interactive Web site (www.usersguides.org) accessible only by subscription through *JAMA*.[29]

Centre for Evidence-Based Medicine: www.cebm.net

The Centre for Evidence-Based Medicine Web site is associated with the University Department of Psychiatry, Warneford Hospital, Headington, in Oxford, England. Its goal is to promote evidence-based health care and provide users with support and resources. The easy-to-use home page is separated into four areas: learning EBM, doing EBM, teaching EBM, and the EBM toolbox. Figure 11-4 shows a view of this Web site.[27]

FIGURE 11-4

A view of the Centre for Evidence-Based Medicine Web site.

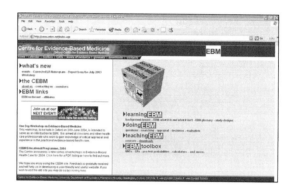

New Zealand Guidelines Group: Tools for Guideline Development and Evaluation: www.nzgg.org.nz/tools/htm

The New Zealand Guidelines Group plays a key role in leading the movement toward high-quality, evidence-based health and disability services in New Zealand. Through its Web site, it shares information about EBM practice, promotes collaborative practice in guideline development and implementation, and trains clinicians, providers, consumers, and researchers to find, evaluate, and use evidence.[30] Figure 11-5 shows an image from this Web site.

FIGURE 11-5

The Web site of the New Zealand Guidelines Group.

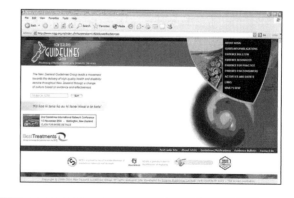

ACP Journal Club:
www.acponline.org/journals/acpjc/jcmenu.htm

The American College of Physicians (ACP) publishes the *ACP Journal Club*, a bimonthly journal affiliated with McMaster University. More than 100 journals are reviewed for articles that meet *ACP Journal Club's* explicit criteria, listed in Box 11-5.

This publication selects articles from the biomedical literature that are important and relevant for physicians who want to keep up with internal medicine topics, including cause, course, diagnosis, prediction, prevention, treatment, and economics of medical conditions that internists or related specialists would see in clinical practice.

Other topics covered include quality improvement and continuing medical education intervention trials in internal medicine. The literature, including original research and systematic reviews, is summarized in structured abstracts and includes comments from experts. The ACP strives to distribute these summaries as quickly as possible to internists and others. This service is available in print and online for a fee.[31]

BOX 11-5

ACP Journal Club Criteria for Abstracting

All articles in a journal issue are considered for abstracting by the *ACP Journal Club* if they meet the following basic and category-specific criteria.

Basic Criteria for Original or Review Articles
- In English.
- About adult humans.
- About topics important to the clinical practice of general internal medicine and its subspecialties, other than descriptive studies of prevalence.
- Analysis of each article is consistent with the study question.

Additional Criteria for Studies of Prevention or Treatment
- Random allocation of participants to comparison groups.
- Follow-up (end point assessment) of at least 80% of those entering the investigation.
- Outcome measure of known or probable clinical importance.

continued on page 272

BOX 11-5 *continued*

Additional Criteria for Studies of Diagnosis

■ Inclusion of a spectrum of participants, some but not all of whom have the disorder of interest.

■ Objective diagnostic ("gold") standard (e.g., laboratory test not requiring interpretation) OR current clinical standard for diagnosis (e.g., a venogram for deep venous thrombosis), preferably with documentation of reproducible criteria for subjectively interpreted diagnostic standard (i.e., report of statistically significant measure of agreement beyond chance among observers).

■ Each participant must receive both the new test and some form of the diagnostic standard.

■ Interpretation of diagnostic standard without knowledge of test result.

■ Interpretation of test without knowledge of diagnostic standard result.

Additional Criteria for Studies of Prognosis

■ Inception cohort of individuals, all initially free of the outcome of interest.

■ Follow-up of at least 80% of patients until the occurrence of a major study end point or to the end of the study.

Additional Criteria for Studies of Etiology

■ Exploration of the relation between exposures and putative clinical outcomes.

■ Prospective data collection with clearly identified comparison groups for those at risk for the outcome of interest (in descending order of preference from randomized controlled trial, quasi-randomized controlled trial, nonrandomized controlled trial, cohort studies with case-by-case matching or statistical adjustment to create comparable groups, to nested case-control studies).

■ Masking of observers of outcomes to exposures (criterion assumed to be met if outcome is objective, i.e., all-cause mortality, objective test).

Additional Criteria for Studies of Quality Improvement or Continuing Education

■ Random allocation of participants or units to comparison groups.

■ Follow-up of at least 80% of participants.

■ Outcome measure of known or probable clinical or educational importance.

Additional Criteria for Studies of the Economics of Health Care Programs or Interventions

■ The economic question addressed must be based on comparison of alternatives in real patients.

continued on page 273

BOX 11-5 *continued*

- Alternate diagnostic or therapeutic services or quality improvement activities must be compared on the basis of both the outcomes produced (effectiveness) and resources consumed (costs).
- Evidence of effectiveness must be from a study (or studies) of real (not hypothetical) patients, which meets the above-noted criteria for diagnosis, treatment, quality improvement, or a systematic review article that also meets criteria.
- Results should be presented in terms of the incremental or additional costs and outcomes of one intervention over another.
- Where uncertainty exists in the estimates or imprecision in the measurement, a sensitivity analysis should be done.

Additional Criteria for Studies of Clinical Prediction Guides
- The guide must be generated in one or more sets of real (not hypothetical) patients (training set).
- The guide must be validated in another set of real (not hypothetical) patients (test set) and must deal with treatment, diagnosis, prognosis, or etiology.

Additional Criteria for Studies of Differential Diagnosis
- A cohort of patients who present with a similar, initially undiagnosed but reproducibly defined clinical problem.
- Clinical setting, including the referral filter, is explicitly described.
- Ascertainment of diagnosis for 80% of patients using a reproducible diagnostic workup strategy for all patients and follow-up until patients are diagnosed or follow-up of 1 month for acute disorders or 1 year for chronic or relapsing disorders.

Additional Criteria for Systematic Review Articles
- An identifiable description of the methods indicating the sources and methods for searching for articles.
- Statement of the clinical topic and the inclusion and exclusion criteria for selecting articles for detailed review.
- At least one article in the review must meet the above-noted criteria for treatment, diagnosis, prognosis, clinical prediction, etiology, quality improvement, economics of health care, or differential diagnosis.

Source: Reference 31.

Bandolier: www.jr2.ox.ac.uk/bandolier

Bandolier's purpose is to find evidence of effectiveness (or lack of it) and put the results forward as simple bullet points indicating what worked and what did not.

Bandolier is an independent journal about evidence-based health care. The journal began in 1994 with a print version written by Oxford University scientists, and a year later the popular Web site was introduced, attracting more than one million visitors per month. Most users are health care professionals, but the site also contains information for patients and caregivers.

Bandolier's purpose is to find evidence of effectiveness (or lack of it) and put the results forward as simple bullet points indicating what worked and what did not. *Bandolier* personnel search PubMed and the Cochrane Library each month for recent systematic reviews, meta-analyses, randomized controlled trials, and high-quality observational studies, which are reviewed, evaluated, and discussed in the print version before appearing on the free Web site 3 months later. Sometimes *Bandolier* conducts systematic reviews as well.[32]

PedsCCM and IntensiveCare.com: Resources for Practicing Evidence-Based Medicine: pedsccm.wustl.edu/EBJ/EB_Resources.html

This Web site provides resources and links for practicing EBM. Among topics covered are critical appraisal of the literature, statistics and trial design, systematic reviews, EBM in critical care, EBM groups on the Web, EBM databases, online journal clubs, and teaching resources and tutorials. This site is maintained by the Multidisciplinary Intensive Care Unit, Department of Anesthesia, at Children's Hospital and Harvard Medical School and the Departments of Anesthesiology and Pediatrics at St. Louis Children's Hospital and Washington University School of Medicine. Although its primary focus is pediatric EBM, this is a great general source to get started with.[33]

ACTIVITY 11-4

Getting Familiar with EBM Sites

1. Explore all the EBM Web sites mentioned in this chapter and, in the "Favorites" or "Bookmarks" section of your browser, save links to the ones that will be most useful to you.
2. For each site, list three features that you like and state why.

References

1. Sackett DL, Rosenberg WM, Gray JA, et al. Evidence-based medicine: what it is and what it isn't. *BMJ.* 1996;312:71-2.

2. Moores KG. Evidence-Based Clinical Practice Guidelines. In: Malone PM, Mosdell KW, Kier KL, et al., eds. *Drug Information: A Guide for Pharmacists.* 2nd ed. New York, NY: McGraw-Hill; 2001:56-7.

3. Straus SE, McAlister FA. Evidence-based medicine: a commentary on common criticisms. *CMAJ.* 2000;163:837-41.

4. Clinicians for the Restoration of Autonomous Practice (CRAP) Writing Group. EBM: unmasking the ugly truth. *BMJ.* 2002;325:1496-8.

5. Cohn JN. Evidence-based medicine: What is the evidence? *J Card Fail.* 2000;6(4):287-9.

6. Horwitz RI. The dark side of evidence-based medicine. *Cleve Clin J Med.* 1996;63:320-3.

7. Charlton BG, Miles A. The rise and fall of EBM. *Q J Med.* 1998;12:371-4.

8. Charlton BG. Restoring the balance: evidence-based medicine put in its place. *J Eval Clin Pract.* 1997;3:87-98.

9. Hampton JR. Evidence-based medicine, practice variations and clinical freedom. *J Eval Clin Pract.* 1997;3:123-31.

10. Swales JD. Evidence-based medicine and hypertension. *J Hypertens.* 1999;17:1511-6.

11. Echt DS, Liebson PR, Mitchell L, et al. Mortality and morbidity in patients receiving encainide, flecainide, or placebo: The Cardiac Arrhythmia Suppression Trial. *NEJM.* 1991;324:781-8.

12. The Cardiac Arrhythmia Suppression Trial II Investigators. Effect of the antiarrhythmic agent moricizine on survival after myocardial infarction. *NEJM.* 1992;327:227-33.

13. Sackett DL, Richardson WS, Rosenberg W, et al. *Evidence-Based Medicine: How to Practice and Teach EBM.* New York, NY: Churchill Livingstone; 1997.

14. Guyatt GH, Keller JL, Jaeschke R. The n-of-1 randomized controlled trial: clinical usefulness. Our three-year experience. *Ann Intern Med.* 1990;112:293-9.

15. Larson EB, Ellsworth AJ, Oas J. Randomized clinical trials in single patients during a 2-year period. *JAMA.* 1993;270:2708-12.

16. Mahon J, Laupacis A, Donner A. Randomised study of n of 1 trials versus standard practice. *BMJ.* 1996;312:1069-74.

17. Devlin J. Critical Appraisal of Meta-analyses. In: Slaughter RL, Edwards DJ. *Evaluating Drug Literature: A Statistical Approach.* New York, NY: McGraw- Hill; 2001:229-48.

18. Malone PM, Mosdell KW, Kier KL, et al. Glossary. In: *Drug Information: A Guide for Pharmacists.* 2nd ed. NewYork, NY: McGraw-Hill; 2001:689.

19. Cochrane Library Web site. Available at: www.cochrane.org/reviews/clibintro.htm Accessed January 2, 2004 and April 13, 2004.

20. Guyatt G, Hayward R, Richardson WS, et al. Moving Evidence to Action. In: Guyatt G, Rennie D, eds. *Users' Guides to the Medical Literature: A Manual for Evidence-Based Clinical Practice.* Chicago, IL: American Medical Association Press; 2002:190-1.

21. Lau J, Ioannidis JPA, Schmid CH. Quantitative synthesis in systematic reviews. *Ann Intern Med.* 1997;127:820-6.

22. Sackett DL. Centre for Evidence-Based Medicine. Systematic Review worksheet. Available at: www.pdptoolkit.co.uk/Files/ebm/cebm/Doing%20ebm/therapy_worksheet.htm. Accessed April 13, 2004.

23. McColl A, Smith H, White P, et al. General practitioner's perceptions of the route to evidence-based medicine: a questionnaire survey. *BMJ*. 1998;316:361-5.

24. AHRQ Web site. Evidence-Based Practice Centers Overview. Available at: www.ahrq.gov/clinic/epc/. Accessed February 28, 2005.

25. Slawson DC, Shaughnessy AF. Teaching information mastery: creating informed consumers of medical information. *J Am Board Fam Pract*. 1999;12:444-9.

26. InfoPOEMS Web site. InfoPOEMS overview and definition of POEM available on home page. Available at: www.infopoems.com/. Accessed February 26, 2005.

27. Centre for Evidence-Based Medicine. What is a CAT? Available at: www.cebm.net/cat_about.asp#refs. Accessed June 23, 2004.

28. Trip Database Web site. About Trip Database. Available at: www.tripdatabase.com/index.cfm?method=application.about. Accessed February 28, 2005.

29. Users' Guides to the Medical Literature Web site. Overview of Users' Guides to Evidence-Based Practice. Available at: www.cche.net/usersguides/main.asp. Accessed February 26, 2005.

30. New Zealand Guidelines Group: Tools for Guideline Development and Evaluation. Available at: www.nzgg.org.nz/tools/htm. Accessed June 23, 2004.

31. ACP Journal Club Web site. About ACP Journal Club. Available at: www.acpjc.org/index.html. Accessed June 23, 2004.

32. Bandolier Web site. About Bandolier. Available at: www.jr2.ox.ac.uk/bandolier/index.html. Accessed February 28, 2005.

33. PedsCCM and IntensiveCare.com: Resources for Practicing Evidence-Based Medicine Web site. Available at: http://pedsccm.wustl.edu/EBJ/EB_Resources.html. Accessed June 23, 2004.

Telehealth 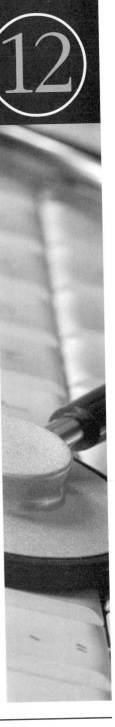 12

Brent I. Fox

Chapter Objectives

After completing this chapter, you should be able to:

- Discuss the history of telehealth.
- Explain key forces driving telehealth's expansion.
- Name three key telehealth disciplines.
- Know how to access telehealth resources.
- List five important goals of successful telehealth initiatives.
- Discuss challenges in adopting telehealth.

i

Telehealth initiatives are growing, with federal funds supporting programs in 46 states. A key force driving telehealth's expansion is advancements in technology that have brought decreased prices and more user-friendly interfaces.

"Telehealth" sounds futuristic, but it's already here—and has been around for decades. The first documented example is from 1920 at Haukeland Hospital in Norway, where radio links were established to provide health care support services to ships at sea. You, too, have engaged in telehealth if you've ever answered a patient's question over the phone or via e-mail, consulted with a colleague over distance regarding patient care, or participated in an online continuing education program. These are some of the more commonly seen examples of telehealth today.

Telehealth uses telecommunication technologies to deliver health care over a distance. Telehealth also provides medical information and education to health care practitioners to help them provide high-quality patient care. "Telehealth" is an umbrella term that encompasses organized initiatives in many disciplines, including "telemedicine" (telehealth activities performed by physicians) "telenursing," and "telepharmacy."

Telehealth initiatives are growing, with federal funds supporting programs in 46 states. A key force driving telehealth's expansion is advancements in technology that have brought decreased prices and more user-friendly interfaces. All the technology in the world is useless, however, if it doesn't address a need—and when it comes to health care, need is a powerful force. Telehealth is a way to reach people in remote parts of the world, as well as people who lack the money or mobility to visit facilities offering the care they need. One catalyst for telehealth is the globalization of the workforce over the past decade and the desire of people working abroad to have the same up-to-date medical practices as at home. Another is recognition by the government, health care providers, and payers that telehealth can be a workable way to give people in rural and underserved areas access to state-of-the-art care.

Telehealth relies on the technologies discussed in Chapter 6 to transfer health care information and services. The specific technology used depends on cost, needs, infrastructure, and other variables. As telehealth programs take root, many obstacles and uncertainties must be addressed. Who will pay for them? How will professionals and patients respond to them? What is the most appropriate approach and technology for each use? How can patients best be trained to use telehealth technology?

Everyday professionals can play a valuable role in finding the answers to these questions and identifying opportunities for telehealth initiatives. As a health care professional, you can help select patients best suited for telehealth technologies based on need, desire, and cognitive functioning; train other professionals and patients in the use of telehealth technologies; and assist with research projects to evaluate telehealth technologies for their impact on the delivery of health care services.

ACTIVITY 12-1

Familiarity with Resources

1. Visit www.clickz.com/stats, click on the "Healthcare" link, and review some of the resources listed to learn more about the status of telehealth and the Internet. This Web site is a part of the Jupiter Web Network and serves as a resource by collecting data gathered from leading research organizations that provide analysis about the World Wide Web.
2. Visit www.ncbi.nlm.nih.gov/entrez/query.fcgi?db=PubMed and search for articles that focus on telehealth, telemedicine, telepharmacy, or telenursing. Determine what articles are available in your area of interest. Select and review several articles to learn about recent advancements in telehealth.
3. If telehealth is a topic in which you have great interest, visit the Web sites listed in Box 12-4 on page 293 and select a print journal or electronic news service to which you can subscribe to keep up with the field.

Definitions

One of the best definitions of telehealth comes from the Office for the Advancement of Telehealth (OAT), established by the U.S. Health Resources and Services Administration as a catalyst for establishing telehealth activities and adopting advanced technologies for health care services. OAT's Web site describes telehealth as "the use of electronic information and telecommunications technologies to support long-distance clinical health care, patient and professional health-related education, public health, and health administration."[1]

Despite what this definition suggests, however, telehealth is not limited to long-distance and can occur within a single building or even a single room. For example, health care professionals or students who log on to a university hospital's server for an online educational program on congestive heart failure are participating in a telehealth learning environment.

The term "e-health," frequently used interchangeably with "telehealth," usually refers to activities over the Internet, whereas

The Office for the Advancement of Telehealth Web site describes telehealth as "the use of electronic information and telecommunications technologies to support long-distance clinical health care, patient and professional health-related education, public health, and health administration.

telehealth—a term that took root before most people had Internet access—encompasses a range of technologies. In this book, the term telehealth refers to both Internet and non-Internet–based information. Box 12-1 lists the goals that should be achieved in successful telehealth initiatives.

BOX 12-1

Goals for Telehealth Initiatives

To be successful and worthwhile, telehealth initiatives should do the following:
- Be based on demonstrated need.
- Ensure patient access to the most appropriate care.
- Ensure equal access to health care.
- Be implemented collaboratively with local providers.
- Be part of an integrated health care service (to ensure information access and dissemination).
- Protect patient privacy and confidentiality.
- Reduce patients' and providers' need to travel.
- Contribute to cost-effective delivery of care.
- Facilitate sharing of expertise among clinicians.
- Provide patient and provider education.

Source: Reference 13.

History of Telehealth

One of the earliest documented telehealth activities took place in the mid-1950s, when the National Institute of Mental Health (NIMH) funded an interactive audio link connecting the Nebraska Psychiatric Institute in Omaha to seven hospitals in teh Nebraska, Iowa, and North and South Dakota. The institute's weekly visiting lecturer series was broadcast to the hospitals, where participants could not only listen, but also ask questions of the lecturer in Omaha.

Then in 1964 microwave technology was used to deliver psychiatric educational programs between the Nebraska Psychiatric Institute and Norfolk State Hospital 112 miles away. These educational programs contained both audio and visual components that could originate at multiple locations within the facilities at each end. Later in the 1960s these facilities received funding to support the use of interactive television to deliver psychiatric consultation and education between specialists and general practitioners. Unlike today's videoconferencing, individuals interacted with content on the TV sceen and used telephones to speak with each other.[2-6]

The National Aeronautics and Space Administration (NASA) became a telehealth pioneer in the early 1960s when it began remote physiological monitoring of astronauts both in space shuttles and in space suits. Other early initiatives are described in Box 12-2.

ACTIVITY 12-2

Learning NASA's Role

The National Aeronautics and Space Administration (NASA) is a leader in telehealth funding, initiatives, and research because putting humans in space requires novel methods for delivering patient care. Visit Google.com and do a search to learn about current NASA telehealth activities. Begin your search with the terms "+nasa" and "+telemedicine" (without the quotation marks). Also try replacing "+telemedicine" with "+telehealth."

BOX 12-2

Important Early Telehealth Initiatives

The following examples, which predate widespread Internet use, describe early examples of point-to-point, non-Internet–based telecommunication for health care delivery. Although not explicitly stated in each example, several driving forces led to these initiatives. What common themes do you see? For a summary of key forces driving telehealth, refer to Box 12-3 on page 285.

Massachusetts General Hospital/Logan International Airport Medical Station. Established in 1967, this medical station provided occupational health care to airport employees and medical attention to travelers passing through Logan International Airport in Boston. A bidirectional audiovisual microwave channel connected physicians at Massachusetts General Hospital with nurses at the airport medical station, allowing the physicians to remotely evaluate nurses' diagnostic and treatment decisions. The nurses performed all hands-on activities at the airport except for the 4 peak passenger hours each day when a physician was present.

Alaska ATS-6 Satellite Biomedical Demonstration. Because of Alaska's remoteness, rural population, and inability of its small communities to support health care providers, it has served as a testing ground for many telehealth initiatives. One of the first, in 1971,

continued on page 282

BOX 12-2 *continued*

used a satellite launched in 1966 in an exploratory field trial to evaluate the reliability of satellite-based communications between the Alaska Native Medical Center in Anchorage and 26 villages scattered across the state. Primarily intended to explore the use of satellite video consultations in improving rural health care, the trial used asynchronous black-and-white television transmission as well as two-way audio to share expertise, knowledge, and advice between health aides in the villages and clinicians at the Alaska Native Medical Center. The project evaluators concluded that health aides could use the system effectively for almost any medical problem except urgent situations.

Space Technology Applied to Rural Papago Advanced Health Care (STARPAHC). One of the first telehealth initiatives, in the early 1970s, took place at the Papago (now Tohono O'Odham) Indian Reservation in Arizona. NASA and Lockheed conceived and engineered it and the Papago people, Indian Health Service, and Department of Health, Education and Welfare put it into effect. Using microwave transmission, a health care van staffed by two Indian paramedics and outfitted with medical instruments was linked with Public Health Service hospitals. It traveled throughout the reservation, providing care to those in need, using the microwave channel and audio transmission to allow those in the field to seek advice and guidance from experts at the Public Health Service Hospital and another hospital.

Memorial University of Newfoundland (MUN). MUN has been involved with telehealth since 1977 as a participant in the Canadian Space Program, when it began developing an interactive conferencing network to deliver educational programs and transmit medical data to institutions across Newfoundland and Labrador via the joint Canadian/U.S. Hermes satellite. The programs were broadcast to hospitals, colleges and universities, high schools, and town halls. MUN has also been part of international teleconferencing initiatives over the past 3 decades, demonstrating consistently that videoconferencing can be effective without expensive equipment.

The North-West Telemedicine Project. This Australian initiative, which began in 1984, used a communications satellite to connect the Mount Isa Base Hospital and the Royal Flying Doctors Service with five remote towns in Queensland. Each site used conference-style telephones, fax machines, and freeze-frame transceivers for transmitting images to improve the health care of residents in these remote locations. By combining these various forms of transmitting information over distance, clinicians in the remote towns were able to discuss patient cases and share information with clinicians in other facilities. Evaluation of the program revealed that it reduced the numbers of patients and providers flying to these locations for routine care and that fewer patients had to leave their towns to receive emergency medical care.

continued on page 283

NASA SpaceBridge to Armenia/Ufa. The first international telehealth program, the NASA SpaceBridge was set up in 1989 in response to a massive earthquake in the Soviet Republic of Armenia. A satellite network provided medical consultation via one-way video, voice, and fax between a medical center in Armenia and four medical centers in the United States. During its 3 months of operation, the SpaceBridge allowed professionals in the United States to help 209 patients during 34 clinical sessions. In all, 422 professionals (247 Armenian/Russian and 175 American) participated in the sessions. One-quarter of the patient consultations resulted in altered diagnoses. That summer the program was extended to Ufa, Russia, to facilitate care to burn victims after a gas explosion.
Source: References 4-7.

Driving Forces Behind Telehealth

The telehealth initiative involving the Nebraska Psychiatric Institute and Norfolk State Hospital, described on page 280, exemplifies a key force behind telehealth: the need to share expertise among professionals. Although the project's ultimate goal was to ensure that patients received appropriate psychiatric care, it called on general practitioners and psychiatric specialists to share knowledge. Today's general practitioners are equipped to handle many clinical scenarios, but sometimes an expert's special training is required. Telehealth offers a convenient way to reach experts when they are not available on site.

NASA, recognizing that health care providers cannot routinely be sent into space with astronauts, has been a telehealth leader, pioneering remote monitoring to track astronauts' health in space. NASA's experience has produced many lessons useful to the care of patients here on Earth, as described in the STARPAHC example in Box 12-2.

With its vast resources, NASA is at one end of the telehealth spectrum, but at the other end are underserved patients in rural and outlying areas who historically have had limited access to quality health care. Financial constraints usually make it difficult for remote locations, such as the Alaskan Bush or the Australian Outback, to support health care providers. Through telehealth initiatives, however, locals trained in rudimentary health care skills can provide basic health care services with the assistance of qualified professionals. For example, health aides in remote Alaskan villages are able to dispense prescription medications using remote dispensing stations connected to the Alaska Native Medical Center. Clinicians

Telehealth offers a convenient way to reach experts when they are not available on site.

Remote monitoring allows patients to stay home, monitor their health conditions, and have the information transmitted to the appropriate health care provider.

in remote Australian villages can consult with medical specialists (such as psychiatrists) using telehealth connectivity.

Telehealth proves a useful way to combat the shortages of pharmacists, physicians, and nurses that have been reported for the past several years. The growing elderly population is also boosting the need for telehealth. The entire health care system, regardless of location, is facing higher demands for care as the number of people over age 50 (the "baby boomers") increases—a group that tends to have more concurrent health issues and take more prescription medications than younger patients. One area of telehealth growth is remote monitoring, which allows patients to stay home, monitor their health conditions, and have the information transmitted to the appropriate health care provider. For example, technicians at cardiology offices can monitor a patient's pacemaker functioning via a portable box in which the patient places the telephone handset while holding a magnet to his or her chest.

As advances in medicine extend people's life expectancy, the general focus of health care is shifting from managing acute conditions to providing chronic, long-term care. Five chronic diseases—heart disease, cancer, stroke, chronic obstructive pulmonary disease, and diabetes—account for more than two-thirds of deaths in the United States, and the associated costs of care account for 75% of the nation's total health care expenditures.[8] These diseases typically require strict monitoring of patients' therapeutic response and adherence to treatment, much of which can be handled by outpatient methods. The Well@Home device from Patient Care Technologies (www.ptct.com), for example, allows stable, chronically ill patients to record and transmit blood pressure, pulse, oxygen saturation, temperature, electrocardiogram, and respiratory rate information to their health care providers. Telehealth initiatives allow virtually constant monitoring of patients to identify problems before they occur, decreasing emergency room visits and their associated costs.

Health maintenance organizations (HMOs), preferred provider organizations (PPOs), and other third-party payers, which focus on the bottom line by negotiating contracts and developing payment systems, sometimes promote telehealth approaches as a way of keeping costs down. Telehealth initiatives can lower costs in many ways:

1. Saving time.
2. Using information for multiple purposes instead of requiring a clinician to repeatedly present information that could be recorded and delivered when needed.

3. Allowing patients to leave the hospital sooner by sharing expertise among clinicians who may not be physically located together.
4. Allowing patients to be monitored at home remotely, instead of staying in the hospital or coming in for appointments.

In the 1990s, large drops in the cost of home computing technology and the emergence of the Internet in people's everyday lives propelled telehealth forward. At the same time, consumers became increasingly interested in being involved in their own care. Many people today, especially baby boomers, feel empowered to ask questions of their health care providers, learn important signs and symptoms of their conditions, and look into alternative treatments. Nearly 75% of the U.S. population has Internet access at home, with women making up a larger portion of regular Internet users than men. Many other countries have similar rates of use, including the United Kingdom and Canada.[9] Among adults who use the Internet at home, 39% have high-speed connections—a number that increases to 55% when broadband access at work is included.[10]

Recent data suggest that 20% of Americans obtain health care information online "often" and another 30% use the Internet "sometimes" to access health information, mostly to learn more about specific topics.[11] Although data indicate that health-related Internet use has plateaued, at least temporarily, consumer use of the Internet for health care information remains important.[12]

> Many people today, especially baby boomers, feel empowered to ask questions of their health care providers, learn important signs and symptoms of their conditions, and look into alternative treatments.

BOX 12-3

Forces Driving the Growth of Telehealth

- The need for generalists and specialists to share clinical expertise.
- The limited access of patients in remote locations to health care clinicians.
- The aging of the population, which is creating a larger pool of patients needing care. At the same time, the number of physicians, nurses, and pharmacists is not keeping pace with the demand.
- Shifting focus away from acute care to managing chronic conditions.
- Pressures to reduce the cost of care.
- Decreasing price of consumer computing technology.
- Increasing availability of Internet connectivity.
- Desire among consumers to be more involved in their care.

Telemedicine

Some of the first telemedicine activities were undertaken so that physicians could share expertise despite geographic obstacles. Early on, telemedicine also allowed physicians to send radiology images via store-and-forward video, which allowed electronic storage of the images for subsequent sending when desired. Today, radiologists routinely use telecommunication channels to remotely view X-rays, CT scans, or MRIs from nearly anywhere in the world.[3,13,14]

Faraway Services

One of the most publicized examples of telemedicine occurred in 1999 at the South Pole, when a physician on a 41-person research team at the Amundsen-Scott Station found a lump in her breast at the beginning of the Antarctic winter season—8 months during which the weather does not allow air travel in or out. She was forced to use the tools and resources available to perform a biopsy on herself.[15]

The only physician on the research team, she had to rely on the help of nonmedical personnel, including a maintenance specialist who used the Internet to learn how to make pathology slides and a computer expert who used a camera and an old microscope connected to a computer to send the biopsy results back to the United States via satellite. The biopsy indicated breast cancer that needed immediate treatment, so the doctor used chemotherapy agents at the station as well as agents later airdropped to see her through until she could be airlifted back to the United States for treatment.[16]

In July 2002, a bidirectional voice and video link between the Amundsen-Scott Station and physicians in Massachusetts was used to perform remote knee surgery—the first telesurgery in the station's 50-year history. Before the actual surgery, physicians in the United States explored treatment options using transmitted digital X-rays of the patient's knee and a live video of the knee examination. Of the various treatment options the physicians suggested, the patient decided on tendon repair because it offered the best chance to restore maximum knee mobility. An orthopedic surgeon and an anesthesiologist in Massachusetts communicated with the physician at the South Pole using the telemedicine connection. They then guided the physician in administering anesthesia and suturing the damaged tendon.[17]

These two examples, though fascinating, do not represent usual and customary telemedicine activities. Typically telemedicine is used to share patient information between physicians, as in a store-and-forward consulting program that Blue Cross recently implemented in rural California. In this program, primary care physicians in rural areas create electronic medical records for their patients, which include both patient data and images. Each record can be securely sent via e-mail to specialists participating in the telemedicine program, who review the record, make a recommendation, and securely send the information back to the primary physician—thus saving time and eliminating the need for an appointment with the patient, primary care provider, and specialist. In this arrangement, the primary care physician is reimbursed for a standard office visit and the specialist is reimbursed for a second opinion.[18]

> Typically telemedicine is used to share patient information between physicians, as in a store-and-forward consulting program that Blue Cross recently implemented in rural California.

Urban Care

In Orange, California, videoconference equipment is being used to give rape victims specialized medical attention that minimizes additional stress placed on them once they enter the health care system. The telemedicine initiative connects providers at St. Joseph Hospital with those at the University of California Davis Medical Center for second opinions and help in gathering evidence. Before the telemedicine program's launch, victims often were sent to Davis after being examined at St. Joseph.[19]

Videoconferencing can also be used to deliver health care in busy urban areas, as in South Central Los Angeles, where residents—including those with high-risk conditions—must wait months to receive specialized care, or they do not receive care at all because they lack insurance, efficient transportation, and child care while they travel several hours to reach a clinician. They may even have to travel through gang territory to reach a health care provider. There are 1.5 million people living in this inner city area, many of whom wait to see a doctor until their condition has progressed so far they must go to the emergency room. The result is high medical bills and patients who are much sicker than they should be. Located at the King/Drew Medical Center, the program connects clinicians throughout the inner city with specialists who diagnose patients, provide consultation, review objective information, and even perform videoconferences with patients. Unlike rural telemedicine programs that often provide care to small groups of people, programs such as the one in Los Angeles can affect millions of people in a small geographic area.[20]

One distinct area of telemedicine activity expanding in use is telepsychiatry—delivery of psychiatric care over distance using telecommunication technologies. Experts believe it will expand psychiatrists' opportunities to care for patients by allowing them to be in two places at one time, virtually. As with any health care provider, the ideal situation would allow psychiatrists to see patients in person, but in situations where face-to-face assessment isn't possible, telepsychiatry may be the next best alternative. Several states, including Oklahoma, Arizona, Montana, and North Carolina, have already implemented telepsychiatry programs with varying levels of complexity. Generally, the programs focus on evaluation, treatment, and education when the psychiatrist is unable to physically be with the patient. Countries with widely dispersed populations, such as Australia, Sweden, Norway, and Canada, have developed telepsychiatry programs as well.[21]

In 1998, federal funds supported telemedicine programs in 46 states. From 1993 to 1998, the number of telemedicine programs in the United States grew 1500% and telemedicine consultations increased from 1750 to 58,080.[22] The common theme among telemedicine programs is to "bring care to patients instead of patients to care"—which is reminiscent of the beginnings of health care in the United States, when physicians made house calls and patients were so widely dispersed it was difficult to get to them all. Today, population growth and a shortage of providers—especially in rural areas—strain physicians' capacity. Telemedicine may be the answer to overcoming these limitations.

The Internet helps pharmacists connect with patients and providers, process prescriptions, and streamline workflow.

Telepharmacy

Pharmacists are often surprised to learn that many things they do daily fall under the telehealth label—such as answering a patient's question on the telephone or calling another health care professional regarding a patient's care. In the 1990s, pharmacy's use of videoconferences to communicate with patients and colleagues lagged behind physicians,[3] but today pharmacists are ramping up their connectivity via the Internet and other channels.

Central Processing

The Internet helps pharmacists connect with patients and providers, process prescriptions, and streamline workflow. In an approach called "central processing," for example, pharmacists in one location securely transmit prescriptions over the Internet to a central location off site, often known as a call center. These call centers are staffed by people (including pharmacists) specially trained to handle tasks that pharmacists would normally perform when they dispense medications, including drug use review (DUR), third-party adjudication, and prescription clarification/verification with the prescriber. After the call center processes the prescription in terms of payment and clinical checks, it sends it back to the originating pharmacy where, meanwhile, the pharmacist has been dispensing the medication and counseling the patient about how to use it properly.[23]

Another telepharmacy operation, "central fill," is closely related to central processing in that a single location handles dispensing activities for patients who do not directly interact with the facility. Central fill operations vary considerably depending on their business model, but most usually focus on refill prescriptions and handle large volumes. Central fill operations use sophisticated automated dispensing machines to handle large volumes of prescriptions. Mail-order pharmacies typically use central fill to dispense and package medications before they are shipped to the patient. Many chain pharmacies have also become involved in central fill approaches to meet increasing prescription demands.[23]

Remote Dispensing

Telepharmacy can be helpful for delivering prescription medications to underserved locations that are too remote, small, or poor to support a pharmacy. In Anchorage, Alaska, for example, the Alaska Native Medical Center implemented a remote dispensing program in December 2003, In this program, which started with nine rural communities and is expected to expand to dozens more, dispensing cabinets placed in clinics in remote villages contain packaged medications—including antibiotics and even, in some cases, narcotics. After a nurse practitioner or other health worker diagnoses a patient he or she faxes this information to the medical center in Anchorage, where a pharmacist reviews the diagnosis and prescription order, checks for potential drug interactions, adds the prescription information to the patient's profile, and transmits the prescription order electronically to the village, where two labels with bar codes are printed out on a standard desktop computer. The health care clinician scans the first bar code to make sure the prescription is for the correct patient and scans the second to initiate release of the medication. The appropriate prescription bottle then falls to the collection area in the bottom of the cabinet. A final scan of the bar code on the bottle ensures that it matches the

Telepharmacy can be helpful for delivering prescription medications to underserved locations that are too remote, small, or poor to support a pharmacy.

FIGURE 12-1

The PickPoint™ remote dispensing cabinet used by the Alaska Native Medical Center to remotely dispense prescription medications to patients located in outlying communities.

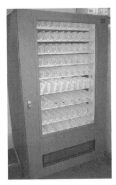

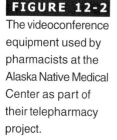

FIGURE 12-2

The videoconference equipment used by pharmacists at the Alaska Native Medical Center as part of their telepharmacy project.

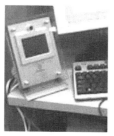

prescription order. Figure 12-1 on page 289 shows a PickPoint remote dispensing cabinet used by the Alaska Native Medical Center program.

Before switching to dispensing cabinets, the medical center used large containers with little security, but now, thanks to secure dispensing cabinets and bar codes, it can better track inventory, prevent medication shortages, prevent theft, and avoid wasting medication due to overstocking. The Veterans Administration has similar programs for remotely dispensing medications, which, like the Alaska program, are being evaluated for cost-effectiveness, safety, accuracy, and timeliness.

In telepharmacy initiatives around the country, pharmacists remotely oversee the dispensing of packaged medications—often using cabinets similar to those in Alaska—and they concurrently counsel patients over the telephone, via videoconference equipment, or by store-and-forward videos. Figure 12-2 shows a videoconference camera and display screen that pharmacists use to counsel patients as part of the Alaska Native Medical Center program.

ACTIVITY 12-3

Web-Based Telepharmacy for Patients

Develop a better understanding of services available through retail pharmacies' Internet sites by creating an online profile at one of the well-known pharmacies below or another of your choosing.

■ CVS Pharmacy: www.cvs.com
■ Duane Reade Drug Store: www.duanereade.com
■ Longs Drugs: www.longs.com
■ Rite Aid Pharmacy: www.drugstore.com
■ Walgreens Pharmacy: www.walgreens.com

In addition, do the following:
■ Explore health and medication information available on the site.
■ Note which services require additional fees or personal information for access.
■ Identify household items such as toothpaste, contact lens solution, and toilet paper that you need, compare the price with what you normally pay, and buy these items from the online pharmacy.
■ Evaluate your experience overall, including ease of use, availability and accuracy of health and medication information, and information required to create your online profile.

Telenursing

Because nurses are so highly involved in direct, hands-on patient care, it may seem that their role in telehealth would be limited, but telenursing is crucial—allowing patients to be monitored in their homes even when a nurse can't be there physically. Thanks to videoconferencing technology, nurses can assess wounds or monitor a patient's gait remotely in nonemergency situations.

Telenursing also allows nurses in different locations to consult about patient care or train student nurses. Using video and audio capabilities, a nurse in North Carolina might talk a nurse in Texas through a complete patient assessment, for example, helping him or her to assess a patient's mental status.[24] Nurses are increasingly acting as triage specialists at call centers to help patients get the appropriate level of care with no unnecessary delays.

Telenursing initiatives are designed to enhance care and decrease costs by keeping people out of hospitals, shortening hospital stays, and reducing home health care visits. Routine monitoring that spots problems before they become serious is a key way to keep people out of the hospital. Patients can perform daily health checks at home using products such as well@home from Patient Care Technologies (see Figure 12-3) and send the information electronically to nurses who review and analyze it. Well@home can record patients' weight, blood glucose, blood pressure, blood oxygenation, and an electrocardiogram. Patients can also record medication adherence information, all of which is presented to the nurse electronically in flow sheet form, as shown in Figure 12-4. Patients can use the touch screen to get answers to questions about medications and treatments, and the device can prompt them to perform daily activities (such as measuring oxygen saturation) that would otherwise be handled by a home health nurse and send medication adherence data to the patient's health care providers, as shown in Figure 12-5.

> *Telenursing initiatives are designed to enhance care and decrease costs by keeping people out of hospitals, shortening hospital stays, and reducing home health care visits.*

The well@home™ health check device from Patient Care Technologies.

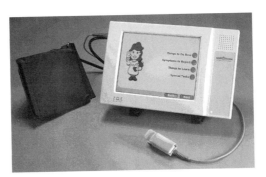

Used with permission of Patient Care Technologies, Inc.

FIGURE 12-4

The well@home™ flow sheet.

Patient Care Technologies, Inc.®

Patty Patient: Female, 75

Flowsheet for Patty Patient

Previous / Next

	8/21 Fri	8/22 Sat	8/23 Sun	8/24 Mon	8/25 Tue	Yesterday	Today
ECG Qod	✓			✓			✓
Blood Glucose TID	110 145 78	289 192 60	274 110 69	199 165 78	301 131 78	275 121 62	279 113 63
Blood pressure BID	129/74 141/86	189/96 130/79	129/74 124/71	140/89 135/81	131/75 141/90	136/76 126/73	128/80 133/76
Pulse Ox BID (%Spo2/bpm)	97/71 99/72	87/74 95/82	? 96/77	97/69 99/71	98/74 100/72	? 99/79	99/113 97/74
I & O Qd (Input/output in mL)	3000/3500	5200/3700	5400/3900	4800/3300	4600/3600	4900/3800	5100/3700
Avandia 4mg tablet BID	✓ ✓	✓ ✗	✓ ✓	✓ ✓	✓ ✗	✓ ?	✓ ✓
Norvasc 5mg tablet TID	✓ ✓ ✗	? ✓ ✓	✓ ✓ ✓	✓ ✓ ✓	✓ ✓ ?	✗ ✓ ✓	✓ ? ✓
Lasix 40mg tablet Qd	✓	?	✓	✗	✓	✓	✓
Lotensin 10mg tablet QID	✓ ✗ ✓ ✓	✓ ✓ ✓ ?	✓ ✗ ✗ ✓	✓ ? ✓ ✗	? ✓ ✓ ✓	✓ ✓ ✗ ✓	✓ ✓ ? ✓
Ambien 5mg tablet Qd	✓	✓	✓	✗	✓	✓	?
Dyspnea Qd		Moderate +					Severe -
Chest pain Qd							
Cough Qd							
Fatigue Qd							

✓ Scheduled item was performed
✗ Non-compliance
? Item scheduled to be done, but compliance not reported
+/-/= Symptom reported better(+)/worse(-)/same(=) (mouse-over for details)

Alerts ▾ go

Used with permission of Patient Care Technologies, Inc.

FIGURE 12-5

Adherence monitoring using the well@home™ device.

Patient CareWare by PtCT - PTCT In-House

PtChart-TRAD   Tricia Friends   AR

Tools
Show Detail
Return
On-Line Doc
Options
Fact History

Med - Glucophage on 12/24/2003 at 2:37pm by pt@hm
Dose compli   Yes
amt taken   500mg Glucophage

Dose compliance

Patient Care Technologies®

Used with permission of Patient Care Technologies, Inc.

At first, some providers may react negatively toward such devices out of fear that they will replace humans and minimize the importance of trained professionals. When used in appropriate situations, however, telenursing devices offer substantial benefits, such as[25,26]:

■ Allowing homebound patients to have their clinical status monitored even if they can't afford home nursing visits.

■ Freeing home health nurses to focus on patients with more serious conditions.

■ Allowing patients more control over their lives by performing these activities at their discretion instead of on an appointment basis.

ACTIVITY 12-4

Getting Involved in Telehealth Planning

Inquire within your facility about current or planned telehealth initiatives. Explore any opportunities for you to be involved in the process, such as identifying and recruiting patients, assessing and selecting equipment, or evaluating the overall project. In accordance with your area of involvement, record your impressions of implementing or evaluating a telehealth initiative and share them with your colleagues.

ACTIVITY 12-5

Web-Based Telehealth in Your Practice

Examine your current practice or, if you are a student, envision the type of practice you expect to have and identify opportunities for telehealth to help you reach patients or colleagues more efficiently. Develop a practical strategy (information, online scheduling, e-mail, video consultations, etc.) for improving your delivery of care using a Web-based telehealth approach. After developing a strategy, visit Web sites such as www.buildwebsite4u.com, www.homestead.com, and www.learnthenet.com/english/section/webpubl.html for help with Web site development, the next step in your progression to telehealth.

BOX 12-4

Online Telehealth Resources

The following organizations offer telehealth resources and have Web sites with a wealth of information and tools.

- American Telemedicine Association: www.atmeda.org/
- Association of Telehealth Service Providers: www.atsp.org
- California Telemedicine and eHealth Center: www.cttconline.org/
- Canadian Society of Telehealth: www.cst-sct.org/
- Health Informatics World Wide Telemedicine: www.hiww.org/TEL.html
- International Society for Telemedicine: www.isft.org/
- Journal of Telemedicine and Telecare: www.uq.edu.au
- Office for the Advancement of Telehealth: telehealth.hrsa.gov/
- Telemedicine Information Exchange: tie.telemed.org/
- Telemedicine Today: www.telemedtoday.com/
- Texas Tech University Health Sciences Center: www.ttuhsc.edu/telemedicine/
- U.S. Department of Veterans Affairs: www.va.gov/occ/THinVA.asp

Internet, EHR, and Other Telehealth Initiatives

Millions of Americans use the Internet to learn about health issues affecting them or their family, often bringing printouts of information to their health care appointments. The Internet lets professionals read primary literature articles online before the print journal lands in their mailbox, and it allows quick access to articles that may be decades old—but still important. As described in Chapter 10, the Internet also helps professionals find concise clinical guidelines, free of charge.

Patients can take part in online communities to share experiences and learn about resources, such as support groups. Health systems and care providers are beginning to use the Internet to reach out to local patients as well as those across the country.

Some pharmacies have developed extensive Internet offerings that let patients request refills online, get health and medication information, purchase durable medical equipment and other goods, create an online record of their medications—including over-the-counter and herbal products—and record other pertinent health information, such as blood pressure readings. The pharmacies benefit because it gives them access to current information about patients' health and helps establish loyalty from patients—who have invested time and effort into creating their profile.

The electronic health record (EHR), slowly becoming a reality in the United States, is expected to enhance the efficiency and safety of health care delivery by giving providers immediate access to complete, up-to-date information about patients' medical history. Much remains to be determined about EHRs, including standards and protocols; regulatory issues, such as transferring information across state lines; practical matters, such as which professionals will be allowed to read the record or make changes to it; and what patients' role will be in maintaining the record. Fortunately, the Department of Health and Human Services has taken the lead in developing a national strategy to develop and implement the EHR.

As an example of innovations in telehealth today, take a look at Medicine Online (www.medicineonline.com), an auction site similar to eBay. Potential patients create an online post for a desired procedure; doctors respond with their credentials and complete price, after which patients follow up for a free consultation with selected doctors. Then the patient and doctor work out a mutually satisfactory agreement, and after the procedure is completed, the patient pays a fee to Medicine Online.

Although Medicine Online's unorthodox approach may raise eyebrows—understandably so—the site is only for elective procedures such as cosmetic surgery, cosmetic dentistry, LASIK surgery, and podiatric surgery. Given that most people find such providers by asking for names from family and friends, Medicine Online offers potential improvements such as broader pool of providers to choose from, the providers' credentials, the "out the door" price, detailed information about the practice, and patient references. However, patients have to rely on Medicine Online and the providers using it to supply accurate information. Only time will tell if this novel approach to selecting a health care provider will be successful.

ACTIVITY 12-6

Assessing Electronic Health Records

Visit www.informatics-review.com/thoughts/PHR_Site_Comparison.htm, which gives an extensive listing of companies and Web sites that offer electronic health records (also called personal health records). Compare at least three of these records for:

- Functionality
- Accessibility
- Security
- Portability (the ability to run on multiple operating systems)
- Extensibility (the ability to incorporate new functions)
- Cost
- Other desirable features

Challenges in Adopting Telehealth

As telehealth grows in popularity, it will affect professionals from many disciplines and change the way health care is delivered. Access to care will improve for the underserved, clinicians will have increased access to information and specialists, patients will be able to stay at home for routine monitoring, and costs may decrease.

Turf Issues; Buy-In

Although the lines between telepharmacy, telenursing, and telemedicine may get blurred, it is helpful to define telehealth initiatives in terms of the primary professional involved so that patients know who is ultimately responsible for their care plan and practitioners understand their specific roles. Some practitioners resist telehealth because they fear it will minimize their role or affect their autonomy. Telehealth initiatives are more likely to be accepted on the grassroots level when they are openly endorsed by a respected colleague or leader.

End users must be involved in telehealth initiatives from their inception, since no one is more qualified to evaluate a proposed change than the person who will use it daily. The perfect fit in theory does not always translate to the best solution in practice. Health care providers from all disciplines—regardless of their technical knowledge—should define, test, and evaluate the desired functionalities.

Funding

Financial issues can be a barrier in telehealth initiatives that connect providers with patients (or other providers) across large distances because they often require considerable time and resources to study the problem, propose a solution, develop the technology, train users, and evaluate the initiative. At each step along the way, new issues can come up that raise the project's cost.

To overcome financial barriers to telehealth, you must demonstrate (perhaps through a pilot project) that money spent now will save money in the future, especially for third-party payers.

Key funding resources already available for telehealth include agencies of the U.S. government, which you can explore online at http://tie.telemed.org/funding, a site sponsored by the Telemedicine Information Exchange (TIE), a clearinghouse developed with funding from the National Library of Medicine. Nongovernmental funding can come from third-party payers, foundations, telecommunication companies, and other private sources.

Demonstrating Effectiveness

Because telehealth can involve new, exciting technologies, it may be tempting for practitioners, patients, and administrators to focus on the technology instead of outcomes, but telehealth initiatives must demonstrate clinical effectiveness.

Any telehealth project that does not include a research component on clinical effectiveness is missing an important opportunity to contribute to the telehealth knowledge base. Critically evaluating a telehealth project provides key information about the project at hand and serves as a resource for future projects. For example, estimates from the Los Angeles example on page 287 indicate that patient waiting times were reduced from months to days, and even hours in some circumstances.

Reimbursement

Historically, reimbursement has been lacking for telehealth services that do not include interactive audio and video components. Diagnostic and consultative services using teleradiology are the exception, generally being covered by third-party payers even though patients and physicians do not interact directly. Recent changes suggest that the reimbursement barrier may be shrinking: for example, a managed care plan in New York announced that it will reimburse primary care physicians for online consultations with patients in nonurgent situations.[27]

Regulatory Issues

Regulatory issues related to telehealth are complex. For example, can a professional licensed in Montana legally use telehealth channels to care for patients in California? Such questions are currently being answered state by state, but a potential long-range solution is a federal license to deliver care through telehealth channels.

The Health Insurance Portability and Accountability Act's (HIPAA) privacy and security standards affect telehealth. Any telehealth initiative must comply with HIPAA to ensure that patient information is accessible only to approved entities and that patient information is secure from unauthorized activities (i.e., manipulation).

Technology Issues

The fast pace at which technology is advancing—weighing less, doing more, and decreasing in cost—leads to problems when standards are not set concurrently for interoperability between systems. If telehealth systems end up operating as islands, what good are they? Any telehealth initiative must focus on how information will be shared among appropriate people.

Any telehealth initiative must comply with the Health Insurance Portability and Accountability Act to ensure that patient information is accessible only to approved entities and that patient information is secure from unauthorized activities.

Simple lack of technology can be a huge issue. Patients in remote areas may not have a telephone, let alone high-speed connections for interactive video.

Rapid advancements can lead to rapid obsolescence. It's not unusual for a personal computer purchased in January to be replaced by a cheaper, more powerful computer in June—sometimes resulting in incompatibilities and wide variations in the technology used in telehealth initiatives. Because telehealth is multidisciplinary, months or years can pass from a project's inception to implementation. Those selecting technology for telehealth must be diligent in their research, recognize that "something better" is always around the corner that they may have to pass up, and be able to identify when a change in technology is necessary.

Simple lack of technology can be a huge issue. Patients in remote areas may not have a telephone, let alone high-speed connections for interactive video. Although satellite communication can reach far corners of the earth, its cost can be prohibitive and its reliability depends on the weather.

Access to technical support can be a problem, too, especially in remote locations. Telehealth professionals practicing at a tertiary care facility in a major city can expect to have technical support personnel nearby, but in rural, far-off places, what happens if something breaks down? Steps that can be taken to decrease the need for technical support are listed in Box 12-5.

ACTIVITY 12-7

Overcoming Telehealth Barriers

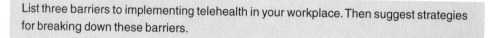

List three barriers to implementing telehealth in your workplace. Then suggest strategies for breaking down these barriers.

Telehealth is an exciting and promising opportunity to positively impact health care on many levels. Underserved patients can receive appropriate care, providers and patients can access vast amounts of information, and health care costs can be reduced. Telehealth may help alleviate clinician shortages across the health care system as well. Challenges exist on several fronts, but the extensive growth in new programs suggests that telehealth can meet a critical need.

BOX 12-5

Ensuring Effective Implementation

1. Interview current users of the technology to get details about its use in the real world, including how to avoid pitfalls. One of the best ways to understand the capabilities of a technology is to see it in use. If you are considering implementing a telehealth technology, contact the Department of Veterans Affairs, a telehealth leader.

2. If possible, thoroughly test the telehealth technology before it is installed. Although it would be nice to test how the technology performs in all conceivable scenarios, it's more feasible to test scenarios most likely to occur and those perceived as most challenging. For example, test a remote monitoring device (like well@home) with a group of patients who are likely to understand the device's components and functions. Results may be less accurate if the device is given to a patient with dementia who cannot operate it.

3. Train users carefully, including clinical use of the technology and general troubleshooting steps. New technology can be intimidating for new users. For example, electronic prescription vendors often provide unlimited Internet-based training for prescribers to alleviate apprehension.

References

1. Office for the Advancement of Telehealth. So what is telehealth? Available at: http://telehealth.hrsa.gov/welcome.htm. Accessed May 5, 2004.

2. Leiner BM, Cerf VG, Clark DD, et al. A brief history of the Internet. Internet Society. Available at: www.isoc.org/internet/history/brief.shtml. Accessed January 13, 2004.

3. Angaran DM. Telemedicine and telepharmacy: Current status and future implications. *Am J Health Syst Pharm.* 1999;56(14):1405-26.

4. Brown N. Telemedicine 101: A brief history of telemedicine. Telemedicine Information Exchange. 1995. Available at: http://tie.telemed.org/telemed101/understand/tm_history.asp. Accessed May 5, 2004.

5. Klein JA. Introduction to telemedicine. iTeleHealth. 2000. Available at: www.itelehealth.com/telemed1.asp. Accessed May 5, 2004.

6. Perednia DA, Allen A. Telemedicine technology and clinical applications. *JAMA.* 1995;273(6):483-8.

7. Scott JC. Telemedicine in disaster applications. 1996. Available at: www.uku.fi/english/organizations/helina-l/msglog/1996/0019/html. Accessed May 5, 2004.

8. National Center for Chronic Disease Prevention and Health Promotion. The burden of chronic diseases and their risk factors: National and state perspectives 2002. Available at: www.cdc.gov/nccdphp/burdenbook2002/01_tables.htm. Accessed May 8, 2004.

9. ClickZ Stats Staff. Population explosion! ClickZ Stats. Available at: www.clickz.com/stats/web-worldwide/article.php/151151. Accessed May 10, 2004.

10. Greenspan R. The broadband tipping point. ClickZ Stats. Available at: www.clickz.com/stats/sectors/broadband/article.php/3342131. Accessed May 8, 2004.

11. Greenspan R. Net attracts health-seeking surfers. ClickZ Stats. Available at: www.clickz.com/stats/sectors/healthcare/article.php/3339561. Accessed May 10, 2004.

12. Greenspan R. Senior surfing surges. ClickZ Stats. Available at: www.clickz.com/stats/sectors/demographics/article.php/3111871. Accessed May 10, 2004.

13. Felkey BG, Fox BI. Telehealth for pharmacy care. In: Mueller BA, Bertch KE, Dunsworth TS, et al. eds. *Pharmacotherapy Self-Assessment Program*. Vol. 2. 4th ed. Kansas City, MO: American College of Clinical Pharmacy; 2001:117-41.

14. Brown N. What is telemedicine? Telemedicine coming of age. Telemedicine Research Center. 2002. Available at: http://trc.telemed.org/telemedicine/primer.asp. Accessed May 11, 2004.

15. Nielsen J. Ice bound: Part III of III. 2001. Available at: www.jrcwebexchange.com/Shared/images/icebound/icebound3.html. Accessed May 11, 2004.

16. ABC News. Survival at the South Pole. 2001. Available at: www.abcnews.go.com/sections/primetime/2020/PRIMETIME_nielsen_feature.html. Accessed May 11, 2004.

17. National Science Foundation. Telemedicine link with South Pole allows remote knee surgery. 2002. Available at: www.nsf.gov/od/lpa/news/02/pr0261.htm. Accessed May 12, 2004.

18. Association of Telehealth Service Providers. Blue Cross of California launches store and forward telemedicine site at Sablan Medical Corporation. 2004. Available at: www.atsp.org/news/spo.asp?contentID=1240&FullStory. Accessed May 12, 2004.

19. Association of Telehealth Service Providers. California hospital uses telemedicine to perform sexual assault examinations. 2004. Available at: www.atsp.org/news/spo.asp?contentID=1610&FullStory. Accessed May 13, 2004.

20. Association of Telehealth Service Providers. Los Angeles telemedicine program fills urban healthcare need. 2004. Available at: www.atsp.org/news/spo.asp?contentID=1599&FullStory. Accessed May 13, 2004.

21. Association of Telehealth Service Providers. Telemedicine advances could expand psychiatric care. 2004. Available at: www.atsp.org/news/spo.asp?contentID=1574&FullStory. Accessed May 13, 2004.

22. National Conference of State Legislatures. Telemedicine. 2004. Available at: www.ncsl.org/programs/health/telemed.htm. Accessed May 13, 2004.

23. Felkey BG, Fox BI. Using the Internet to enhance pharmacy-based patient care services. *J Am Pharm Assoc.* 2001;41(4):529-38.

24. International Council of Nurses. Telenursing. 2004. Available at: www.icn.ch/matters_telenursing_print.htm. Accessed May 14, 2004.

25. Stumbo SD. Medical house calls. The News-Review. 2004. Available at: www.newsreview.info/apps/pbcs.dll/article?AID=/20040401/NEWS/104010015. Accessed May 20, 2004.

26. Association of Telehealth Service Providers. Telemedicine advances could expand psychiatric care. 2004. Available at: www.atsp.org/news/spo.asp?contentID=1629&FullStory. Accessed May 20, 2004.

27. Health Data Management. Payer to reimburse online consults. 2004. Available at: www.healthdatamanagement.com/html/PortalStory.cfm?type=vend&DID=11571 Accessed May 21, 2004.

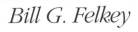

E-Commerce 13

Bill G. Felkey

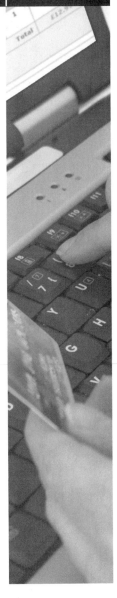

Chapter Objectives

After completing this chapter, you should be able to:

■ Name four types of e-commerce commonly in use.
■ Describe e-commerce approaches and formats that have been found to be workable.
■ Discuss ways that e-commerce is being applied in health care.
■ Explain the basics of establishing an e-commerce Web site.
■ Provide an overview of what to look for in a hosting service.
■ Discuss ways to create and market an e-commerce site that brings consumers back repeatedly.

A 2003 U.S. Department of Commerce report detailed a larger increase in sales through e-commerce than through normal retail channels.

With the advent of the Internet, a powerful new way of conducting business has emerged: electronic commerce or "e-commerce." Doing business over the Internet is becoming a significant commercial channel in many parts of life, including health care.

Among advantages of e-commerce is that it allows companies to analyze transactions and predict individual consumer behavior. As a result, sellers can present goods, services, and information targeted to each person. E-commerce can also provide consumers with 24-hour-a-day, 7-day-a-week access to services and organizations, including health care. And because e-commerce transactions occur via automated methods, they decrease the need for personnel involvement.

"E-commerce is poised to explode in the U.S., reaching $370 billion by 2004," Forrester Research predicted at the end of 1999.[1] This was a little optimistic—other statistics suggest that e-commerce for all types of businesses may not yet have attained quite this level—but there's no question that e-commerce is expanding and is changing consumer habits. Already, 32% of online consumers shop on the Web for health products ranging from vitamins to motorized scooters. Forrester Research predicted that 8% of all retail health sales—$22 billion dollars—would be transacted on the Internet by 2004.

Many traditional businesses now produce activities geared for e-commerce. A 2003 U.S. Department of Commerce report detailed a larger increase in sales through e-commerce than through normal retail channels. In 2001, online sales grew 22% while retail sales grew only 3%. Also, the report pointed out that "while business-to-consumer activity is the focus of much public attention, 93% of e-commerce is business-to-business,"[2] suggesting that e-commerce is an effective way for businesses to purchase the goods and services needed for everyday operations.

Sears, like many large retailers, still produces traditional paper catalogs and flyers, but also has a Web site where customers can compare prices, look for sales, get complete specifications on products, or search by name or category for specific items. Some companies—such as airlines—offer discounts on fares or frequent flier miles as an incentive for ordering online. E-commerce helps these businesses reach more consumers and satisfy their needs. Invoicing, delivery arrangements, and other transactions that used to take place by phone or on paper also take place via Web and e-mail.

BOX 13-1

E-Commerce Types and Terminology

The two primary types of e-commerce are:

■ Business to consumer (B2C)—retail sales on the Internet, such as Amazon.com

■ Business to business (B2B)—wholesale networks such as McKesson

Secondary types of e-commerce include:

■ Government interacting with businesses or consumers (G2B/G2C)

■ Consumers doing business with other consumers (C2C), as on eBay

With the advent of e-commerce, terminology has emerged to describe different entities. For example, businesses and practices with a physical presence in the community are known as "brick and mortar" operations. Those with both a physical presence and e-commerce access are called "brick and click" businesses. Companies that operate entirely as e-commerce entities are known as "pure play" businesses.

Amazon.com, the popular online source of books and merchandise, is a great example of a pure play business—you can't walk into an Amazon store. Barnes & Noble, on the other hand, is a brick and click competitor. Most brick and clicks get the bulk of their revenue from retail outlets, but the e-commerce channel is an important complement.

Although Dell Computers started as a pure play business, its products have gained such name recognition that they are now sold in retail outlets. Gateway computers was a pure play competitor to Dell until they determined that retail outlets could help showcase their product line. Different permutations will emerge as e-commerce evolves.

Electronic storefronts for large retailers, electronic malls, banking industries, personnel placement businesses, travel services, and real estate are also earning tremendous revenues in e-commerce.

Just like any business, health care organizations can use their Web sites to give consumers additional access, flexibility, and value. And just like in any business, health care e-commerce needs to be profitable. An article in the *Journal of Healthcare Information Management*[3] noted that electronic claims submission, a widespread e-commerce activity in health care today, decreases claims processing costs by 50% to 75% (see Table 13-1).

Health care organizations can use their Web sites to give consumers additional access, flexibility, and value.

TABLE 13-1

Documented Ways E-Commerce Adds Efficiency in Health Care

Organization	Efficiency
Physician practices and hospitals	35%-50% decrease in accounts receivable days
	35%-60% decrease in billing and transaction costs
Payers, independent practice associations (IPA), and medical groups	50%-75% decrease in claims processing costs
	60%-80% percent of claims received process without human intervention
Physician practices	Referral/authorization turnaround times in 1-2 days
	Decreased costs by $7,000 at a single-physician practice
IPA and medical groups	50% decrease in use-review cost
	Decreased customer service phone volumes

Source: Journal of Healthcare Information Management, vol. 14, no. 2, Summer 2000.

E-Commerce Categories

E-commerce operations can take many forms, but the most commonly used are listed below. Before investing in any of these options, organizations should carefully consider their appropriateness. Ask yourself, Does this method of doing business fit the image we want to project? Is it consistent with the position we seek in the marketplace? Will the e-commerce model we've chosen significantly undercut revenues produced by our traditional channels?

- **Virtual storefront.** This model opens up an opportunity to conduct transactions over the Internet that would traditionally have taken place by consumers walking into the business or calling on the telephone. Blockbuster.com and CVS.com, for example, offer goods and services online in a way that reproduces the experience of walking through their doorways

- **Auction.** eBay, one of the most successful e-commerce businesses, has over 2 million regular visitors to its auction site, annual revenues of more than $20 billion, and more than 19 million products offered for sale. People can find merchandise ranging from vintage Tasmanian Devil dolls to bed-and-breakfast accommodations in Sicily. In like fashion, hospitals are listing their old equipment for resale on sites such as Usedequip.com.

- **Reverse auction.** When consumers turn the tables on retailers and get businesses to bid for *their* business, it is called a reverse auction. Web sites such as lendingtree.com let banks bid to provide loans to consumers. Medicineonline.com allows surgeons and Internet pharmacies to bid for patients' out-of-pocket dollars for procedures and supplies.

- **Aggregator.** Intisoft.com is an example of an aggregator, which specializes in collecting and sharing information. If a large health system needs assistance in sharing information with employees, partners, suppliers, and customers collaboratively, it might enlist an aggregator to collect and distribute these data. Shopper.com, an aggregator for technology products, displays over 100,000 technology products on behalf of online retailers, who constantly rework their pricing to be displayed in the site's top positions. Shopper.com does not sell any of these products directly.

- **Content provider.** Any health care entity that creates and publishes information for patients or practitioners would be classified as a content provider. The Mayo Clinic (mayo.com) is one example. Some content providers, such as yourhealthinformation.com, produce consumer health information for hospitals and health care providers to display on their Web sites.

- **Online service provider.** Nearly every medical specialty has a second opinion service where patients with serious medical problems can get a second viewpoint from an expert. Gynecology, for example, has gynsecondopinion.com, which provides questions, answers, and advice from the book *A Gynecologist's Second Opinion* by William Parker, MD, Clinical Professor at the UCLA School of Medicine. Other online providers triage patients, helping them understand when and where to receive care; provide psychological counseling; or help people select diets and make lifestyle changes. At these sites people can interact with health care professionals outside their community and tap knowledge in faraway cities and academic centers.

- **Digital product delivery.** Anything that can be delivered digitally—movies, photography, music, software, and even advanced academic degrees—falls into this category. Packaging and shipping can be completely eliminated when you buy a media download and transfer funds digitally. At MP3.com, for example, you can experience music without ever handling a CD. These businesses usually have a global perspective and target industries where challenges exist in the flow of raw

> Other online providers triage patients, helping them understand when and where to receive care, provide psychological counseling, or help people select diets and make lifestyle changes.

materials, replacement parts, or delivery. FineGround (www.fineground.com), recently acquired by Cisco Systems, provides digital products to the health care industry.

■ **Information broker.** These companies offer access to information in key topic categories, such as Quote.com, a free information broker for the stock market. The health care industry may use an information broker such as Sterling Commerce to retrieve information on regulatory affairs or research and development projects. The Baptist Leadership Institute of the Baptist Health System in Pensacola, Florida (www.baptistleadershipinstitute.com), offers information to help other health care systems improve organizational management and operations.

Applications of E-Commerce in Health Care

Here's an overview of functions that can be placed on a Web page or in a kiosk at your facility or around your community. Just as automatic teller machines (ATMs) give you access to your banking needs, your e-commerce Web site or kiosk can serve your patient's health care needs. Some of the following applications are appropriate only inside your facility while others are beneficial from any location.

Wayfinding (how to get to where you need to go) is a self-service function that supports your internal business processes. It may include self-service scheduling, consumer information—everything from product instruction manuals to presurgery informed consent documents—or gift store access. If your site makes it convenient for people to send flowers to sick loved ones, it's not only a service to them, but an opportunity for revenues.

Support group enrollment can be featured online, and people can enroll in self-care management classes or be recruited into clinical trials using your e-commerce site. The site can give patients suggestions for associated equipment rentals such as oxygen tanks, wheelchairs, and crutches, and it can handle material transactions such as video rentals or self-help book sales.

Clinic-based e-commerce sites can promote key services, facilitate patient registration procedures, and provide access to insurance options so patients are processed faster when they arrive for appointments. Offering interactive health risk screening is not only a way to engage patients in their own health but also great for informing clinics about other problems patients may need to have addressed. Sites can also sell online weight loss programs, smoking cessation, and other services to help patients achieve goals.

A recent CNN news broadcast featured a story about seven day care centers using virtual doctor visits from one of their locations in Rochester, New York. When children develop symptoms, instead of calling parents away from their jobs, the centers contact a local pediatrician who remotely assesses the child and makes recommendations for medical interventions. In the story, a 2-year-old girl having ear problems was prescribed antibiotics after a telemedicine-trained day care staffer worked over the Internet with the pediatrician. When the child's mother picked her up after work, everything had already been taking care of. The program, launched in 2001, has been so successful it is expanding to five more day care centers and seven public schools.

RelayHealth (www.relayhealth.com), which provides secure online health care communication between patients and health care professionals, offers a platform for Web-based office visits that is being used by providers in several states. The American Medical Association has even created a new procedure code for online medical evaluation—intended to supplement, not replace, face-to-face visits.

My own experience supports the value of "virtual visits." I saw my physician 6 months ago for my annual checkup, and as I write this, allergy season in my hometown is reaching its peak. Having used Allegra successfully in the past to relieve my symptoms, I go online and complete a Web page form that tells my doctor all the symptoms I'm experiencing. It costs me an additional $5 in my copay, but allows me to head to work instead of to the doctor's office. Between exam room visits, my doctor reads my Web information and decides that sending a prescription electronically to my pharmacist is appropriate. When I'm ready to leave work, I check online and discover that my pharmacy has e-mailed to say my prescription is ready for pickup. Experts generally agree that this type of e-commerce transaction would be appropriate for roughly 20% of clinic office visits currently made.

Many health organizations have difficulty wrapping their arms around e-commerce because they think selling retail items is beneath them. But consider this scenario. A patient who suffers from migraines is searching the Internet for information that will bring relief. She finds a health system Web site that recommends vitamin B2, 400 mg, once a day, based on a peer-reviewed reference. What do you suppose she wants to do next? Buy it, of course. And

RelayHealth (www.relayhealth.com), which provides secure online health care communication between patients and health care professionals, offers a platform for Web-based office visits that is being used by providers in several states.

if she can't order it somewhere on that site, she's going elsewhere. Once she forms a business relationship with another health care entity on the Internet, that may be where her loyalty remains.

Using a fulfillment service for e-commerce is a good idea. Fulfillment services take orders generated by a health care organization's patrons and send out products in a timely manner. Although it is possible to do your own fulfillment, this task requires the proper personnel, facilities, and inventory to provide excellent customer service.

BOX 13-2

Benefits of E-Commerce in Health Care

Benefits of adding an e-commerce component include:

1. **Wider visibility.** Health care organizations can expand their market share nationally and internationally. When people from other parts of the world search for services that your Web site highlights, they may become your customers or patients. The Mayo Clinic, for example, known for treating patients with rare diseases, is familiar internationally thanks to its Web site. A well-designed Web site also enhances your presence with locals and lets them know about services they may not be aware of otherwise, such as specialized clinics or wellness seminars.

2. **Cost savings.** Reduced paper and postage account for some of the savings you get from electronic transactions, but efficiency and speed are also key aspects. E-commerce streamlines many business processes, thus decreasing the cost of doing business.

3. **Creating loyalty in constituencies.** When consumers invest their time and energy to establish a Web-based connection to your organization and they have a good experience, they tend to return—both in person and on the Internet. Conveying the sense that you truly care about the well-being of patients brings them back. Good service is getting harder to find—so if you excel in this area, people will remember you.

4. **Taking work out of systems.** Managing transactions without using personnel and delegating tasks to your Web site frees customer service personnel for tasks with the potential to create new revenues. Delta Air Lines now charges customers a $5 processing fee if they call a Delta agent and book their tickets over the telephone rather than booking online.

5. **Keeps you in the business you want to be in.** E-commerce lets you outsource tasks that fall outside your core business. When you call for help with your printer problem, the person you talk to is probably sitting in East India. Burger King now outsources much of its drive-through order-taking. If your health system offers a triage service, does the nurse who answers the telephone have to be in your community?

Nuts and Bolts of E-Commerce

Like other computer-based functions, e-commerce involves inputs, processing, and outputs. In health care e-commerce, consumers handle most of the inputs—requests, orders, questions—while the organizations are responsible for the processing and the outputs—supplying the necessary goods and services.

E-Commerce Web Sites

Two fundamental steps when you are creating an e-commerce Web site are registering a domain name for the business and securing a Web hosting service. Of course you also need to have the proper business infrastructure for providing goods and services electronically—and you must develop the actual Web site and e-commerce pages.

Registering a Domain Name

All the Web sites listed below sell domain names. Commercial ventures usually use the ".com" ending of the domain name. If you don't already own a domain name, you can search for available domain names by completing the on-screen form.

Domain registration sites have become a commodity item on the Internet. Competitors look at each other's sites daily and try to outdo the "deal of the day," so check each to determine the best bargain. Here's a sampling:

- Register.com
- NetworkSolutions.com
- GoDaddy.com
- MyDomain.com
- EasySpace.com

Hosting Services

Web hosting companies are businesses that provide server space, file maintenance, and other Web services. A server is the computer that stores and "serves up" your Web site. One server can hold many Web sites, and each site can be made up of many Web pages. (Each Web page is essentially a separate document on a Web site, identified by a unique URL.)

Web hosts suitable for e-commerce sites should offer credit card processing features and shopping cart functionality. Onboard calculators can determine shipping costs, generate package labeling, and provide automated links to let consumers

i

Two fundamental steps when you are creating an e-commerce Web site are registering a domain name for the business and securing a Web hosting service.

track their orders. Real-time credit card processing can save substantial time when orders are being fulfilled during times of high sales volume and is a great option for businesses that don't have any other way of processing credit cards offline. Box 13-3 provides tips for choosing a hosting service for your e-commerce operation.

BOX 13-3

Tips for Choosing an E-Commerce Hosting Service

1. Match the capabilities of the host's server to the needs of your business. For example, some hosts sell as little as 5 megabytes of space, but a business may require several gigabytes. Hosting services charge differentially by the amount of space used. Some restrict the number of pages they host for a given fee, while others allow unlimited Web pages. You can estimate your likely storage requirement by taking a sample of the kind of information you want to offer your Web visitors and then look at the properties of the folder on your computer that holds the Web site data offline (the online and offline measures will be the same) and add a "cushion" to give yourself room to grow. Should your space needs change, most hosting services offer ways to instantly expand your space for additional fees. Be sure that your space requirements will not exceed the upper limit of the hosting service you choose.

2. Check the amount of data transfer. Data transfer is a traffic-related measure. If you are offering an educational film online that is 1 gigabyte in size, you need at least 1 gigabyte of space to store it. If 1000 patients decide to download that film in a month, you use 1 terrabyte of data transfer. Some hosting services grant unlimited data transfer for traffic between the site and visitors. Others charge on a per-megabyte basis for data uploads and downloads.

3. Know what kind of support you'll get. Customer service is crucial in this kind of business, so you may want to select a vendor that gives "24/7" support. When you depend on the Internet for even a portion of your business, your support for keeping it running needs to be reliable. Some health care information technology support people carry pagers that alert them when systems malfunction.

4. Check out compatibility issues. Are the hosting service's features compatible with the software and languages used to develop your site? Among these are Microsoft FrontPage extensions, scripts such as CGI, and programming and markup languages such as Java and UNIX. For example, the popular Microsoft

continued on page 311

BOX 13-3 *continued*

FrontPage Web development application uses a set of extensions that will not get full functionality unless they are supported on the server running your Web site. The best course is to select the hosting service after you determine how your Web site will be developed and maintained.

5. Learn about their promotion services. Many hosting services will help you optimize your position on search engines and hyperlink with associated Web sites (see Box 13-6 on page 316). Anything you can do to increase traffic to your site usually results in a greater revenue stream. These services can be expensive, so try to get a performance metric as part of your negotiated price. Be aware that a computer program can be set up to "hit" your site automatically, so examining how visitors actually use your site can help you assess whether the traffic is bona fide.

6. Learn the capabilities for streaming media support. Running multimedia material such as narrated video from your Web site may require that your Web hosting company have additional licenses and software. Ask for a list of these capabilities and match this list with your media formats. Also, make sure that operating the streaming media products will not exceed your data transfer limits.

7. Inquire about database support. Usually, information from your Web site will be collected by a database program such as Microsoft Access or Microsoft Excel. A connection called open database connectivity (ODBC) will download forms filled out on your Web site into an industry-standard database program. Most health care Web sites need this kind of support, so be sure it is available on your hosting service.

8. Assess whether the number of e-mail accounts meets your needs. Having your own e-mail address—something like yourname@Dailyhospital.com—is one of the advantages of creating a Web site. A standard Web-hosting service will supply anywhere from 5 to 300 e-mail accounts as part of your Web site account.

9. Find out if the hosting service offers Web development support. The person or team who develops your Web site can be internal—part of your organization— or you can outsource it to a Web development company. Some Web-hosting services do Web site development as well. Pricing may be on a per hour basis, fixed-price contract, or a combination of both. Make sure that you understand the pricing structure and have a good sense of what developing the site is likely to cost given its features and size. Have an exit strategy in place if you find you've entered into a Web development agreement with a company that proves to be unresponsive to your needs.

E-Commerce Payment Systems

E-commerce payments can be handled in many ways:

- **Electronic checks.** These secure transactions require authorization of an electronic funds transfer directly from a consumer's bank account. Just as with a debit card, consumers can only spend up to the limit of funds in their account. The advantage of this approach to the e-commerce site is usually lower transaction fees and lower levels of repudiation.

- **Credit cards.** Using credit cards is routine today for e-commerce transactions. To achieve security, the site can require the purchaser to supply the three- or four-digit number printed on the back of the card. This prevents the waiter or store clerk who copies a receipt with someone's name, card number, and expiration date from making an online purchase.

- **Debit cards.** These cards provide the same connection to the consumer's bank account as with electronic checks. If the transaction is taking place at a kiosk, a personal identification number (PIN) may be requested, but these are usually not part of transactions over the Web because consumers are reluctant to give this information online.

- **Electronic cash.** Also called cybercash, in this type of money transfer a consumer's money is held in escrow (for a small fee) by a company that does not release the funds to sellers until the buyer is satisfied with the e-commerce transaction. Many years ago this approach was touted as the future of money, but given all the other methods for funds transfer within the normal banking system, it never gained much traction.

Anytime money is being transferred, it's critical to have in place proper systems for authentication, encryption, and verification of the purchaser. Thankfully, secure protocols are commonly in place in consumer browsers so that these transactions are reasonably well protected.

Online sales and payment systems are now routine. Any health care organization that wants to receive money electronically simply decides which type of payment it prefers, incorporates the proper features into its Web site, and pays a small percentage of the transaction as a processing fee.

E-Commerce Sites That Enhance Business

Nearly anyone can develop simple Web sites. Common word processors such as Microsoft Word and Microsoft Publisher provide wizards for novice users. Web page development software such as Dreamweaver and Microsoft FrontPage have a larger learning curve but are more powerful. Your Web site must reflect the same level of quality and sophistication as your business or health care practice. Some people's very first impression of your organization will come from your Web site, so this is no place to cut corners. Take time for the due diligence necessary to create a professional-looking Web site that is highly functional and supports the vision and mission of your organization.

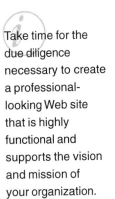

Take time for the due diligence necessary to create a professional-looking Web site that is highly functional and supports the vision and mission of your organization.

Professional developers charge between $80 and $110 per hour to create pages. The adage, "You get what you pay for," may apply to Web site development. You want someone knowledgeable and experienced who understands not only how to make the site look good, but also how to structure it—known as information architecture—so it is highly functional.

Although there are many companies and individuals to choose from, keep in mind that using someone local may have advantages. He or she may already have a feel for your organization and will be able to take part in regular sit-down meetings. That said, your designer can live in another state, time zone, or country and do a terrific job for your organization. For each Web site developer you consider, look at previous designs and test some sites' functionality. Make sure the Web developer is not using a standard template that makes your site look like all others on the Internet. Your Web site's look should be consistent with your printed brochure's color scheme, font selection, inclusion of logo, etc.

E-Commerce Advertising

Advertising your e-commerce capability should piggyback onto your normal operations. When you send out mailings, include a line suggesting a visit to your Web site. Put signs in waiting areas, add announcements about your site on printed brochures, list your Web address on receipts, and announce your Web address on giveaway objects such as ballpoint pens.

BOX 13-4

'Must Haves' in a Professional E-Commerce Web Site

- Attractive design, overall visual appeal.
- Solid architecture so site is constructed for ease of use.
- High-quality content: written well and arranged properly for online readability.
- Links all work properly.
- Everything kept up to date.
- Engaging material—it keeps people coming back.
- Interactive features that capture the attention of passive visitors.
- Integration features—the Web site "talks" to your office systems.

BOX 13-5

A Successful Marketplace for Online Patrons

An ideal marketplace where online consumers feel satisfied doing business must:

- **Recognize returning users.** The best sites make it easier to do business with them the second time around. Think of establishing a relationship with the consumer that allows you to offer those things in which they seem to be interested. Save any information the consumer is comfortable having you store such as credit card number, addresses, and shipping preferences.
- **Support complicated negotiations.** Make it easy for consumers to stay online and not have to pick up a telephone to talk with one of your employees. Most consumers who have a preference for working on your Web site will want to be able to take the transaction to its conclusion online. Allowing a flexible policy on returned goods will facilitate their peace of mind.
- **Support complex product configuration** (e.g., multiple component requirements). Plastic surgeons take a digital picture of their patients and manipulate the image to show how they will look after a procedure. Automobile manufacturers allow people to build a virtual Corvette and see how it will look when it arrives from the factory. For durable medical equipment, it should be possible for prospective buyers to see how products will appear with various options and add-ons installed.
- **Match requests for products and services automatically.** Services such as extended warranties or installation can be tied to product sales. Try to anticipate when a related item might benefit someone buying a certain product so you can call their

continued on page 315

BOX 13-5 *continued*

attention to it. Some Web sites even share how other consumers have bundled goods and services during previous transactions.

- **Compute and apply prenegotiated multilevel discounts.** Consumers appreciate any business that tries to protect their pocketbooks. When someone notes that he or she is a member of AARP, your Web site should retain this information and apply appropriate discounts for future transactions without placing additional burdens on consumers to reenter the information.

- **Support arrangements for ancillary services.** Make it possible for consumers to select additional services such as installation, when available, or special/expedited delivery during the purchase sequence online rather than forcing them to take additional steps for these options after the initial transaction.

- **Execute services in a timely manner.** Consumers appreciate acknowledgment of their order, updates on progress, projections on when to expect delivery, and confirmation that your records show the transaction has been completed. Don't contract with a fulfillment agency that does not maintain inventory of your most popular products. In the same way that the person who answers your telephone can make or break the first impression your customers form, timely and well-executed fulfillment is a powerful boost for repeat business.

Mass media advertising—newspapers, radio, television, and on the Internet—can be expensive, but may be worth it if the potential return on investment is high. Make sure your Web site URL is included in any standard advertising or public relations work your organization does. Regularly remind your constituencies of this valuable connection to your organization.

For example, the Web site of a physical therapy facility could provide exercises helpful to people with low back pain. The site could also allow patients to schedule appointments and buy products such as exercise bands, floor mats, dumbbells, and topical rubs—items that reinforce the facility's procedures and recommendations.

Make sure your Web site URL is included in any standard advertising or public relations work your organization does.

Viral Marketing

When a Web site contains something so interesting that lots of people go to it, download it, and send it to friends and family, it's known as "viral marketing." In viral marketing, people share a resource that contains your Web site address. When it's something of key interest, both your resource and contact information

Web Site Optimization: Search Engine Positioning

When consumers seek content using search engines, they pay the most attention to the first 10 to 20 "hits." Thus, for businesses to have the greatest likelihood of purchasers choosing their products or services, they need to appear near the top of search results—and they can pay for this type of placement. An entire business has emerged on the Internet for improving placement strategy, known as "Web site optimization." Prices start at about $1000 to improve a business's positioning on search results. Search engines such as Google also allow businesses to pay for placement so they come up first—often in a banner at the top or along the side. On Google, these placements are called "sponsored links."

can quickly spread globally—which in today's jargon is called "going viral."

For example, if your site has an excellent video clip that details how to handle patients with diabetes who come down with the flu, the clip might spread quickly. By offering the clip and other information on the topic, you might cut down on phone calls from patients asking how to manage their blood sugar during their illness and decrease after-hours interruptions. Anything that builds traffic on your Web site had potential for increasing e-commerce revenues.

Customer Relationship Management

In viral marketing, people share a resource, such as a video clip or article, that includes your Web site address and thus gives you visibility.

Customer relationship management (CRM)—an approach in which businesses target individual preferences as they learn specifics about each customer—is changing the nature of e-commerce. Based on how a customer interacts with the Web site, the company can examine that customer's characteristics, buying decisions, and interests, and use these data to engage him or her further. For example, if a patient looks up information about asthma on a Web site, a CRM software application can pick up clues and infer that she or someone close to her has this condition. In future visits, or even the current visit, the site displays targeted information on asthma-related goods and services. It's sort of like a salesperson at Nordstrom saying, "And we have this nice shirt and fabulous tie to match that suit."

The site might invite patients to sign up for regular e-mail notices of asthma-related products and services. To respect a consumer's privacy, "opt out" links are usually included in correspondence and notifications. Some organizations have consumers fill out profiles as part of their registration process before they can access certain parts of the site, which gives them key marketing information.

Specific tips for good customer relations mangement:

1. Analyze how visitors use a Web site to be sure it is relevant to their needs. Programs are available to help with this task. For example, Webtrends (www.webtrends.com) creates an activity log for every click a visitor makes on a Web site. You purchase software from them or one of their competitors to watch your site's traffic and give you a report to help you modify your layout and links. Some hosting services offer this analysis as part of their service package.

2. Make sure links are arranged according to Web site visitors' interests, which increases traffic and exposure to your offerings. What seems logical or practical to you—including the names you give links on your site—may not be useful to your audience.

3 Consider hiring a consultant to help you maximize CRM opportunities on your Web site. Do site visits to assess the consultant's work and ask for references to assure that other customers were satisfied.

ACTIVITY 13-1

Promoting Your Site

This chapter lists several ideas for letting consumers know about your site and driving traffic to it. What other approaches can you come up with? To generate ideas, conduct some searches to learn ways that other health care entities similar to yours are marketing their sites.

BOX 13-7

Brave New World of Medical E-Commerce

When health care practitioners first visit the auction site Medicine Online (www.medicineonline.com), they are usually shocked. It allows consumers to pick a surgical or dental procedure and then gives providers 1 week to bid by offering the patient a flat fee to carry out the service. Providers supply their medical education, credentials, practice history, and philosophy for the patient to review. They also provide references from patients, statistics on typical outcomes, disclosure on financing availability, and information on their surgical facilities, offices, and language capability. Consumers in the transaction are not obligated to take the low bidder nor do they pay a fee to use the site.

Let's say that John, age 48, wants to investigate LASIK surgery. Like most people, he asks for recommendations from friends, family, and coworkers who had the procedure and are satisfied with the results. He calls a few of them and finds that LASIK surgery might cost him $3500 per eye. On the Medicine Online site, however, the same procedure may cost as little as $499.99 per eye.

Of course when it comes to health, people don't necessarily want the low bidder. But if Medicine Online's experience is a good gauge, many patients don't think higher cost always means better results and they negotiate heavily for any procedure that must be paid for out-of-pocket, from dental whitening to cosmetic surgery. There are not large numbers of these sites being constructed on the Internet, but the ones that exist are an indication that when patients are paying, they view health care as a commodity and scrutinize options carefully.

Medicine Online also offers a reverse auction process for prescription drugs, medical supplies, equipment, dietary supplements, and over-the-counter medications. Patients list their requirements and check back in three days to see how Internet pharmacies have bid for their business. The pharmacies bidding for this business must contact the patient's physician for prescription orders before they can dispense your medication. Veterinary medicines and vision care products are burgeoning online, allowing consumers to buy heartworm pills or contact lenses at very competitive prices.

Ways that E-Commerce is Changing

In presentations to health care professionals I always ask how many have purchased something online—and I always get about 90% raising their hands. With very few exceptions they indicate it was a positive experience. When we try something and it works, in our minds it illuminates the light bulb of opportunity.

Certain products work better online. At holiday time, gift items that are shipped directly to recipients are popular, allowing you to avoid the hassle of packaging and shipping. Anything that produces a large transaction total is more likely to be profitable. I heard one expert say, "Kmart doesn't sell bags of dirt on the Internet." Finding the right product mix is important in your e-commerce business.

There may be opportunities related to conditions that carry a stigma or that people find embarrassing to talk about, such as sexually transmitted diseases or erectile dysfunction. It can be more comfortable to go online for information, goods, and services for certain problems than to interact with another person, even an anonymous supplier on the telephone.

Several factors are impacting e-commerce and making it a very dynamic environment. Try to imagine how each factor will have a positive or negative effect on any e-commerce venture you are considering.

- **Technological changes.** Hardware is going to weigh less and do more, and any consumer can potentially check pricing and product features from anywhere in the world 24/7. Shopping software will assist consumers throughout any purchasing process.
- **A global market.** Certain products, such as exercise equipment, are designed in the United States and a few weeks later, an Asian manufacture introduces a knockoff at half the cost. Restrictions and extra costs you face in your market do not exist in Italy—and even with shipping costs your price is undercut. This is a market in which it can be cost-effective to ship beef from Argentina to Texas rather than buying beef for Texas in Texas.
- **Evolving societal factors.** When e-commerce was first introduced, consumers were very tentative about using it. Now it's routine for many people—and its use is becoming more prevalent among the elderly, a large percentage of the health care market.

There may be opportunities related to conditions that carry a stigma or are embarrassing, allowing people to go online for information, goods, and services rather than interact with another person, even an anonymous supplier on the telephone.

■ **Cost of labor.** Geographic boundaries disappear on the Internet. Some companies cut expenses by locating their order processing and fulfillment in countries where the labor force receives only a fraction of U.S. wages. When businesses stay entirely on U.S. turf, they still have the option of selecting inexpensive real estate if they are pure play and don't rely on local traffic for their revenue. Amazon.com, for example, located in Seattle, doesn't have an expensive building on desirable real estate. As long as the U.S. Postal Service and parcel delivery such as FedEx and UPS are available, you can situate order fulfillment facilities in large empty warehouses in depressed real estate markets.

■ **Around-the-clock availability.** Because the Internet makes it easy for consumers to buy anytime, day or night, they are no longer held back by holidays, weekends, darkness, or bad weather.

■ **Better payment mechanisms.** The banking industry has quickly adapted its product lines to support e-commerce. Easier transactions globally are being negotiated to handle problems with international banking regulations.

■ **Instant delivery.** As soon as you buy items that can be delivered electronically, such as software programs or video rentals, you receive them. Anything digital that is not an object you can hold in your hand has the potential to be delivered via the Internet.

■ **Online troubleshooting and feedback.** E-commerce purchases can be done entirely online including troubleshooting when there is a problem. E-commerce sites can post feedback from customers on product performance and the business's reliability—information previously available only in publications like *Consumer Reports*. For example, the Web site pdaphonehome.com has more than 5000 members commenting on a single PDA smart phone.

All these factors, and many more, will shape e-commerce over the coming years. Like any other industry, e-commerce will mature and evolve to a higher level of sophistication as society changes, new technologies emerge, and the business environment adapts.

BOX 13-8

Critical Success Factors

Undertaking an e-commerce initiative requires that you consider several factors. Do you have the following?

1. **A committed executive team.** Unless executives in an organization truly understand the benefits of adding an e-commerce channel, it is probably not a good idea.
2. **A knowledgeable project team.** Many organizations do not have the expertise internally to launch and maintain a successful e-commerce venture. Make sure the necessary personnel are in place before getting started. Conduct site visits with organizations operating successful e-commerce operations and learn from their experience.
3. **The appropriate information system.** Ideally, e-commerce should be integrated into the practice management software. Integrating e-commerce efforts with banking and fulfillment centers can be equally important. To round out the e-commerce information technology suite, have the proper telephone equipment integrated with computers and software for your support personnel. If you employ a customer relations management (CRM) strategy, support personnel have the tools to document troubleshooting, resolve quickly future problems that are similar, and work more efficiently overall.
4. **Integration to vendor partners**, such as banking and product fulfillment. Outsourcing to specialists is often more cost-effective than taking patient care staff, or even shipping and receiving personnel, out of their normal roles.
5. **The right look and feel.** Your e-commerce venture should represent the image and personality you want to project to your public.
6. **Scalability.** You must be able to ramp up your capacity or cut it back in the event of wild success—more hits and sales than you'd expected—or disappointing failure. Planning for scalability allows you to build your infrastructure according to anticipated business and then adjust accordingly.
7. **Customer relationship management**, CRM, mentioned on page 316, allows an organization to do something called micromarketing—where you focus a campaign at a single individual. The transactions of each new Web site visitor go into a database and return visits are monitored so that each time the person logs on to the site, he is greeted personally and receives suggestions and material relevant to his interests.

As with anything, careful planning from conception through implementation will help ensure that your e-commerce efforts are rewarded. Evaluate your processes from time to time to determine whether reengineering is necessary.[4]

ACTIVITY 13-2

Your Site's Targets ✓

1. Identify the demographics of consumers who would connect to your practice's Web site for e-commerce. For information, start with your local Chamber of Commerce and expand into U.S. Census Bureau data. For more sophisticated assistance, consider hiring a marketing firm to determine the level of computer use in your community.
2. List transactions that consumers could perform on your Web site that would take work out of your system.
3. List products you could market through your Web site that are in line with your practice's focus. Pick three and perform a price comparison through such sites as shopper.com, mySimon.com, pricewatch.com, and buy.com. What kind of pricing would be appropriate for an Internet market? Remember, Internet pricing is usually lower than retail pricing in walk-in outlets.

References

1. Boehm E. Sizing Healthcare Ecommerce. December 1999. Available at: www.forrester.com/ER/Research/Report/Summary/0,1338,8667,00.html. Accessed July 7, 2004.

2. Measuring the electronic economy. US Census Bureau E-Stats Report. Available at: www.census.gov/Press-Release/www/2003/cb03-50.html. Accessed July 7, 2004.

3. Arbietman D, Lirov E, Lirov R, et al. E-Commerce for healthcare supply procurement. *J Healthc Inf Manag.* 2001;15:1.

4. Healy JL, DeLuca JM. Electronic commerce: beyond the euphoria. *J Healthc Inf Manag.* 2000;14 (2):97-111. Available at: www.himss.org/asp/ContentRedirector.asp?ContentID=832. Accessed July 7, 2004.

Patient and Professional Education ⑭

Margaret R. Thrower

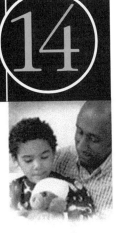

Chapter Objectives

After completing this chapter, you should be able to:

■ Discuss the relationship between information and quality of care.
■ Define "information therapy."
■ Instruct patients where to find self-care information on the Internet to empower them and involve them in their health care.
■ Find high-quality sources of patient education.
■ Find high-quality sources of professional education.

▷ **Health To**
Start here with ove
diseases and welln

▷ **Drug Info**
About your prescri
medicines

▷ **Medical E**
Includes pictures a

▷ **Dictionar**
Spellings and defir

▷ **News**
Health News from

▷ **Directorie**
Find doctors, denti

▷ **Other Res**
Local libraries, hea
sites and more

Many Web sites promote a "patient-centered" approach that helps consumers be informed, active participants in their health care.

The Internet can be a great learning tool for both patients and health care providers, accommodating all types of learners: those who learn by reading, seeing, listening, or doing. The Internet can teach many things—allowing health care providers to complete continuing education on pain management or cancer therapy, for example, and making it easy for patients to learn about diabetes, menopause, and other conditions affecting them or their families. Many Web sites promote a "patient-centered" approach that helps consumers be informed, active participants in their health care.

Thanks to the unlimited amount of information it hosts, the Internet offers vast resources for professional and patient education. It also helps health care providers research clinical questions and stay abreast of the most current information on diseases and therapies. This chapter talks about where to find instant information—current facts and learning tools at the moment you and your patients need them.

Information Technology: Crucial in Health Care

The use of information technology is key to improving quality in the U.S. health care system, according to a report released in 2001 by the Institute of Medicine: *Crossing the Quality Chasm*. The report argues that our disjointed, inefficient health care industry has difficulty providing consistent, safe, high-quality care to all Americans and emphasizes that part of the solution is better use of multidisciplinary teams, evidence-based practice, and technological advances such as e-mail, computerized prescription order entry, and computerized reminders. The report also identifies 10 rules to incorporate in a redesign of the health care system.[1-3]

1. Care is based on continuous healing relationships. Patients should receive care in many forms, whenever they need it, not just during face-to-face visits. For the health care system to be responsive 24 hours a day, there must be access by way of the Internet, telephone, and other means in addition to office visits.
2. Customization of care is based on patient needs and values. The system of care should be designed to meet the most common types of needs but have the capacity to respond to individual patients' choices and preferences.

3. The patient is the source of control. Patients should have the information they need, as well as the opportunity, to control health care decisions that affect them. The health system should be able to accommodate differences in patient preferences and encourage shared decision making.
4. Knowledge is shared freely. Patients should have unfettered access to their own medical information and to clinical knowledge. Clinicians and patients should communicate effectively and share information.
5. Evidence-based decisions are made. Patients should receive care based on the best available scientific knowledge. Care should not vary illogically from clinician to clinician or place to place.
6. Safety is a system property. Patients should be safe from injury caused by the care system. Reducing risk and ensuring safety requires greater attention to systems that help prevent and mitigate errors.
7. Transparency is necessary. The health care system should make available to patients and their families information that allows informed decisions when they select a health plan, hospital, or clinical practice or when they choose among alternative treatments—including information on the system's performance related to safety, evidence-based practice, and patient satisfaction.
8. Needs are anticipated. The system should anticipate patient needs, rather than reacting to events.
9. Waste is decreased continuously. The health system should not waste resources or patient time.
10. Cooperation among clinicians is a priority. Clinicians and institutions should actively collaborate and communicate to ensure an appropriate exchange of information and coordination of care.[1-3]

> Healthwise defines information therapy as "the prescription of evidence-based medical information to a specific patient, caregiver, or consumer at just the right time to help the person make a specific health decision or behavior change."

A concept known as "information therapy" can help bridge the quality chasm in health care, according to Healthwise Inc., (www.healthwise.org), an organization that develops evidence-based medical information to meet the needs of patients, caregivers, and consumers. Healthwise defines information therapy as "the prescription of evidence-based medical information to a specific patient, caregiver, or consumer at just the right time to help the person make a specific health decision or behavior change."[3] In other words, information therapy is patient education based on clear evidence and delivered at the most useful moment.

Information therapy helps patients ask useful questions of health care providers, form realistic expectations, manage their conditions more effectively, actively participate in treatment, and make better decisions.

Gwinn and Seidman of the Center of Information Therapy, a Healthwise division, wrote in a white paper that ways to address health care quality include encouraging self-care of acute illness and ongoing self-management of chronic conditions, sharing decision making between patient and provider, and improving patient knowledge, self-care skills, clinical quality, patient experience with care, and cost-effectiveness.[3]

Consumers today have access to millions of health care Web sites and more than 12 million bibliographic citations[4] linked to articles and abstracts. Research has shown that patients benefit from information therapy in the following ways[3]:

■ Improves their ability to ask health care providers useful questions regarding their conditions and understand the answers.
■ Helps them have more realistic expectations about outcomes.
■ Raises their confidence about managing their conditions effectively.
■ Equips them to actively participate in the treatment and decision-making processes.

Therefore, it's important that you help patients find the most useful information so they can take better care of themselves.

The Internet for Teaching and Learning

The Illinois Online Network (ION), made up of almost 50 community colleges and the University of Illinois, promotes the use of

---

BOX 14-1

How the Internet Accommodates Learning Styles

1. Visual/verbal learners benefit greatly from the Internet because they perform best when information is presented in writing or using visual aids such as PowerPoint.
2. Visual/nonverbal learners grasp material most readily when it is presented in pictures or designs, which are abundant on the Internet.
3. Auditory/verbal learners do best when they hear information in lectures or group discussions; therefore they benefit from online information that uses streaming audio and conferencing.
4. Tactile/kinesthetic learners learn by doing "hands-on" activities, which the Internet provides by way of simulations and three-dimensional graphics.

---

information technology to improve instruction and has identified ways that online learning can accommodate learners' different ways of processing information (outlined in Box 14-1). Online training, with its infinite possibilities, has expanded greatly in the past five years and continues to evolve as technology advances.[5]

Special Populations and Languages

The Internet is a great learning tool for people who are deaf or hard of hearing. Because it's a highly visual medium, the Internet is not so useful for people with eyesight problems, despite some Web sites' efforts to use larger fonts, better contrast, and text-only pages that will work with screen readers—software programs that read the contents of the screen aloud to the user—and magnification software—which can magnify text, menus, and icons on the computer screen.

In one study performed in 2002 by the Pew Internet and American Life Project, which studies Internet use, 63% of American adults were online—but only 38% of adults with disabilities were online.[6]

Language differences are no longer a significant problem on the Internet because so many translation functions are available, such as tools through Google.com that can translate words and even Web pages from one language to another. Figure 14-1 shows where the Language Tools link is on the Google home page.

> Online training, with its infinite possibilities, has expanded greatly in the past five years and continues to evolve as technology advances.

FIGURE 14-1

The Language Tools link on the Google home page.

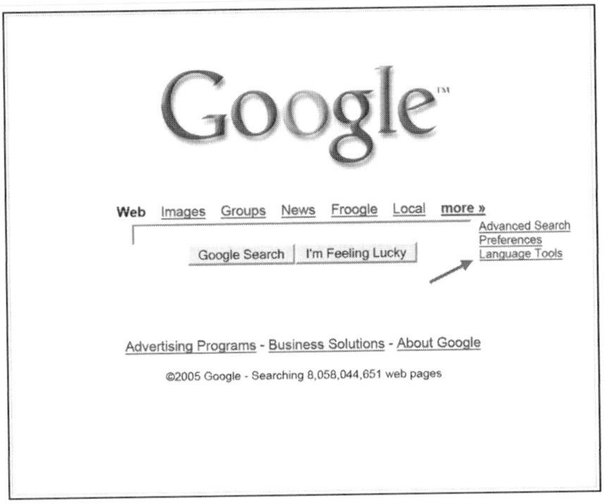

Consumer Use of Patient Education

In 2002, as many as 110 million American adults used the Internet to find health information.[7,8] Many people do not properly interpret the information they find, however, according to a 2003 study in Australia[9]—a problem that the authors concluded could lead to anxiety and poor compliance with therapy.[9] A key problem is that the Internet lacks the quality control and standardization of other forms of published information.

In the Australian study, made up of 46 people in six focus groups, many participants were largely unaware of how they found and evaluated Internet-based information on medicines. All participants used a search engine to find information on medicines. Opinions varied on which sites were credible sources: some participants thought that information given by the pharmaceutical company was "official." Others preferred sites that they deemed as "impartial," such as governments, organizations, and educational institutions. The authors reported that while most participants were skeptical of trusting information on the Internet, they viewed it as an important source of medication information and did not pay conscious attention to how they selected information. The authors recommend that health care professionals teach consumers how to find and interpret Internet-based information on medicines.

Web-based information can be potentially dangerous, according to a 2004 study in the *American Journal of Emergency Medicine,*[10] especially in emergency medical situations. The study compared 20 of the most popular consumer Web sites with four generally accepted as "gold standards" for medical information, which they believed would contain complete, accurate information on emergency medicine. They used checklists to assess four topics—suspected myocardial infarction, stroke, febrile children, and influenza. In addition, they noted whether the Web site has a certification emblem such as Health On the Net (HONcode) indicating compliance with certain standards. They found no correlation between certification emblems and completeness of information—and even identified some information on these sites as potentially dangerous. Overall, they concluded that Web sites are not good sources for patients seeking guidance in an emergency, further evidence that patients must be taught how to evaluate Internet information.

Selecting Patient Education Sources

Using the information in this chapter, you can play an effective role in helping patients select and assess medical information. Emphasize that information alone does not replace medical advice from a provider and that they need to carefully evaluate all information. Some reliable sources of patient information on the Internet are discussed below.

Medline Plus: www.medlineplus.com

Medline Plus, the consumer version of Medline (discussed in Chapter 9), contains comprehensive, consumer-oriented information about health and medications. A service of the National Library of Medicine and National Institutes of Health, one of its unique features is that it uses specific selection guidelines to determine which materials and links to include.[11] Under "cough," for example, you find the topic "Chronic Cough: Causes and Cures;" if you click on it, a page pops up from the site of the American Academy of Family Physicians that has been evaluated with the Medline Plus selection guidelines. Criteria that Medline Plus follows include:

- The content is high quality, authoritative, and accurate.
- The Web site is from an organization that is well established, respected and dependable and it publishes a list of advisory board members or consultants.
- The information provided is appropriate to the audience level, well organized, and easy to use.
- The information is from primary resources (i.e., textual material, abstracts, Web pages).
- The Web page's primary purpose is educational, not commercial, and most content is available at no charge.
- The Web page and links are well maintained and the site is consistently available.
- The source for the content of the Web page and the entity responsible for maintaining the Web site (webmaster, organization, creator of the content) are clear.
- The information is current.
- You do not need to register to view the information on the site.
- The site offers unique information on the topic with little redundancy and overlap between resources.
- The site contains special features, such as graphics, diagrams, and glossaries.
- The content is accessible to people with disabilities.

Medline Plus, the consumer version of Medline contains comprehensive, consumer-oriented information about health and medications.

In addition to providing access to Medline, Medline Plus links to ClinicalTrials.gov, the database of research studies from the National Institutes of Health, and contains a medical dictionary by Merriam-Webster and a drug information database compiled by the United States Pharmacopeia and the American Society of Health-System Pharmacists. The site also covers 650 health topics and offers a health encyclopedia by Adam.com, a well-known provider of health information, with 4000 articles on diseases, diagnostic tests, symptoms, injuries, and surgeries. You can also use Medline Plus to find doctors, dentists, hospitals, libraries, health organizations, and other resources.[12] See Figure 14-2 for an image from Medline Plus.

FIGURE 14-2

The Medline Plus Web site home page.

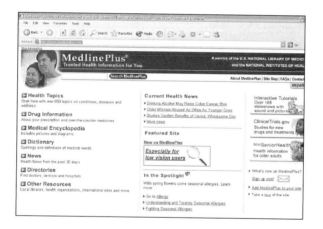

DrugDigest: www.drugdigest.org

This evidence-based, consumer-oriented Web site is a great place to refer patients because its writers are all residency-trained pharmacists affiliated with a leading pharmacy school. The site's special features include medication administration videos demonstrating such techniques as inhaler use; insulin mixing, administration, and injecting; eye and ear drop administration; and use of rectal suppositories. The site also compares different classes of drugs and has a side effects checker that compares the incidence of side effects of different drugs in the same class.[13] See Figure 14-3 for a picture of DrugDigest's Web site.

FIGURE 14-3

The Drug Digest Web site home page.

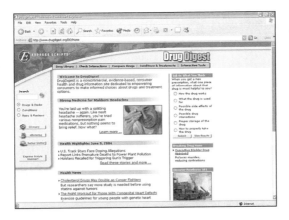

WebMD Health: www.WebMD.com

WebMD Health, sponsored by the WebMD Health Corp., is a popular consumer-oriented Web site with more than 20 million visitors every month. One special feature is that this site hosts a message board where patients can interact with others who have similar conditions and with medical experts as well. The site encourages patients to become active players in their own health care by providing valuable health and medication information and tools to empower patients. See Figure 14-4 for a picture of the WebMD Web site. Other features of WebMD include services for health care professionals and the health care field.[14]

FIGURE 14-4

The WebMD Web site home page.

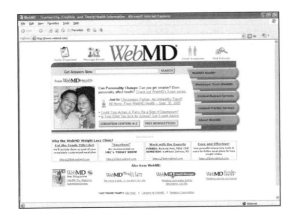

Kartoo presents results on a visual map you can save and use for future searches.

Dr. Koop: www.DrKoop.com

Broadcasts of television segments on important topics such as chronic pain and other health issues are a great feature of this site, which is a leading source of free health and medication information for consumers.[15] Topics of the broadcasts change; recent ones included chronic pain, erectile dysfunction, and diabetes. The site offers lively, comprehensive information on a huge number of subjects as well as an interactive medical dictionary with 3D animation that lets patients visualize health conditions and hear short explanations. In the "health tools" section, people can take quizzes to learn if they need more sleep or determine whether their symptoms are consistent with a cold or the flu, for example.

Kartoo: www.kartoo.com

Kartoo is a different kind of search engine; it's a metacrawler that summarizes the results of various search engines. Useful for both patients and health care professionals, Kartoo presents results on a visual map you can save and use for future searches. A difference from other search engines, such as Google, is that Kartoo groups the results into a sort of topical "family" rather than listing every site in a linear format.[16] Figures 14-5 and 14-6 show examples of the Kartoo Web site, allowing you to see how it differs from others.

FIGURE 14-5

Kartoo Web site showing a search for the keyword "diabetes."

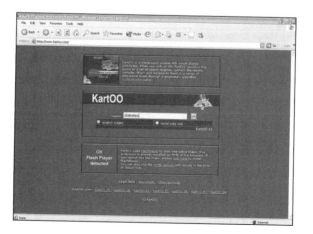

FIGURE 14-6

Kartoo Web site showing search results for the keyword "diabetes."

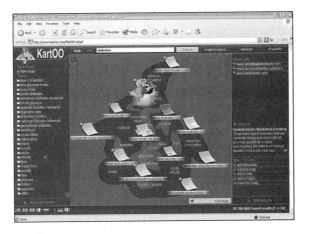

WorldDoc: www.worlddoc.com

This site takes a markedly different approach to health care information by providing decision support for consumers. Created by a team of physicians, the site advertises that it helps patients answer the question, "What might I have and what should I do?" Its mission is to "shape the future of global medicine by empowering patients, physicians, and payers to make better health care choices."[17] People can subscribe to the service for $99.95 for 1 year or $9.95 per month. The site, which includes text, images, and sound, uses its "personal evaluation system" (PES) to answer patients' questions. You click on the image of a body to show where the symptom arises, answer a few questions, and the PES guides you to the most likely diagnosis. It was developed as a form of education to help patients make good decisions and is not intended to replace face-to-face medical advice.

WorldDoc helps patients answer the question, "What might I have and what should I do?"

Services on WorldDoc include a medical library so patients can read about conditions, symptoms, diagnoses, and treatment options, including self care, and an educational database called Health Helps with details on preventing illnesses and complications. Smoking cessation, managing chronic disease, and weight loss are a few of the topics in the database. The pharmacy section provides information on medications, what they are used for, how to take them properly, and drug interactions. In the "Ask the Doctor" section you get information on 50 of the most commonly asked questions in 15 topic areas.

Companies can subscribe to WorldDoc and give their employees free access to information. WorldDoc maintains that its service benefits everyone: patients, payers, and providers of health care services. Benefits for patients include detecting diseases early and learning how to take care of themselves. Benefits for payers include reduced health care costs, healthier, more productive employees, and satisfied health plan beneficiaries. Health care providers benefit because they can improve efficiency, effectiveness, patient communications, profitability, and market share. The Web site offers a free demonstration of its services.[17] See Figure 14-7 for a picture of this Web site.

FIGURE 14-7

The WorldDoc Web site home page.

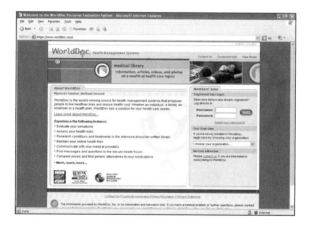

Healthwise: www.healthwise.org

Healthwise.org is an online health information provider with a simple mission: "To help people make better health decisions."[18] It aims to help people think more like partners in their health care and less like patients—assisting them in making informed decisions and learning self-care approaches. Launched in 1975, Healthwise also offers a self-care handbook explaining common diseases, such as sinusitis, with information on symptoms, prevention, self care, and when to call a health professional. To find healthwise.org content, go to www.WebMD.com and look for the Health Guide A-Z. Many health plans and hospitals also license information from Healthwise, which is identified by the Healthwise logo.[18] See Figure 14-8 for a picture of the Healthwise home page.

> Healthwise.org is an online health information provider with a simple mission: "To help people make better health decisions."

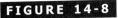

FIGURE 14-8

Healthwise Web site home page.

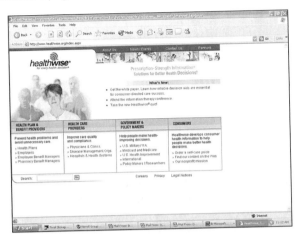

Continuing Education for Professional Education

Internet-based educational tools for health care professionals make learning easier and more accessible than ever. In addition to gaining valuable continuing education (CE) credit, you can apply much of the information you learn directly in caring for patients and teaching them about their conditions.

Many states now mandate that a specific number of the continuing education hours you earn each year must be obtained "live" and in person.

FindThatCE: www.findthatce.com

Many states now mandate that a specific number of the continuing education hours you earn each year must be obtained "live" and in person. Findthatce.com is particularly helpful in identifying live programs. One of the main topics in the directory on the home page is "Live CE," which leads you to a page where you can search by state, date, and type of location (such as cruise or resort). If you create a personal profile, the site will send you e-mail notices of live CE coming up in your area for whichever discipline you choose: medical, nursing, dental, or pharmacy. The site also lets you search for topic-specific CE in the geographic area of your choice.[19]

Power-Pak: www.powerpak.com

Power-Pak CE is a source of free CE for pharmacists, pharmacy technicians, nurses, physicians, and physician assistants.[20] You can read, complete, and submit the CE online and receive a

A portal for health care professionals, MedConnect links you with news and information in the areas of medicine, family practice, pharmacy, and managed care.

grade immediately. If you get a score of 70% or higher a certificate of completion appears on screen for you to print. Clicking on Exam History shows you a record of all the exams you have taken through the site.

The Center for Health Care Education: www.chce.net

Primarily a resource for physicians, this site lets you know about both live and online CE programs, some of which are suitable for other disciplines. For example, a recent live CE listing was the Art of Active Listening Workshop, targeted to health plan administrators, providers, nurses, pharmacists, and clinical staff. For online CE, listings give the title, target audience (such as primary care, cardiologists, or emergency medicine) and a link to the site hosting the assessment activity, such as MedScape.com or Neurocasereviews.com. The site also has information about CE in a variety of formats, including symposia, conferences (audio and video), grand rounds, teleconferences, digital media (CD-ROMs and DVDs), monographs, journal supplements, and slide kits.[21]

Health Communication Research Institute, Inc.: www.hcri.com

This site offers CE and online courses for a nominal fee for physicians, nurses, and other health care professionals. The HCRI Learning/Research Center is designed to provide quick access to information, course enrollment, and other services, including participation in research.[22]

MedConnect: www.medconnect.com

A portal for health care professionals, MedConnect links you with news and information in the areas of medicine, family practice, pharmacy, and managed care. It also provides free CE and a weekly updated list that includes coverage of primary care meetings and conventions throughout the United States and Canada.[23]

ContinuingEducation.com: www.continuingeducation.com

These low-cost online CE programs are targeted toward seven disciplines: physicians, pharmacists, pharmacy technicians, nurses, medical assistants, massage therapists, and engineers.[24]

CECity.com: www.cecity.com/elearning.htm

At this site, you click on your profession to see a catalog of activities. The search engine lets you select from a wide range of topics—everything from allergies to women's health. Many of the programs are free, but some require a fee.[25]

MediCom: www.medicaled.com

MediCom Worldwide is a medical communications company specializing in continuing education for physicians, pharmacists, and nurses. It offers both online courses and teleconferences, many for free.[26]

Ways for Professionals to Keep Up

Systematic ways to keep up with new information are critical for busy health care professionals. E-mail lists, newsletters that summarize biomedical literature, and easily scannable tables of contents are tools that work well and are available electronically. Here's an overview of some of the most useful resources.

The Medical Letter: www.medicalletter.com

Published since 1959, *The Medical Letter*—for physicians, pharmacists, educators, and students—is a highly respected, peer-reviewed monthly resource that evaluates new medications and reviews old ones when new information emerges on their safety and efficacy. Generally the newsletter covers two or three new medications and related topics per issue. Supported entirely by subscription, the newsletter accepts no advertising, in keeping with its goal of providing unbiased, reliable, timely information. If a new drug offers genuine advantages over older drugs, *The Medical Letter* says so, and is equally candid if a drug offers no advantage, has limited effectiveness, or is too toxic or too expensive to justify its use.[27] It is available in paper and online versions as well as for download to handheld personal digital assistants (PDAs). The Web site also offers continuing education.

Treatment Guidelines from The Medical Letter: www.medicalletter.com

From the same publisher as *The Medical Letter* and with the same standards for quality, unbiased information without the pharmaceutical industry's influence, this monthly newsletter

337

provides review articles of drug classes for treating common disorders. A valuable feature is that it recommends first-choice and alternative medications and compares effectiveness, cost, and safety. Here's a sampling of topics covered in past issues: drugs for use in cardiovascular intensive care units, diabetes, asthma, postmenopausal osteoporosis, rheumatoid arthritis, hypertension, cancer, heart failure, epilepsy, tobacco dependence, weight loss, and HIV infection. Online access is available and advantageous because you can search all past issues. The newsletter is also available for download to handheld PDAs.[28]

Prescriber's Letter: www.prescribersletter.com

The Prescriber's Letter, published by the Therapeutic Research Center, is a monthly newsletter that helps prescribers keep up to date on new developments in drug therapy. Subscribers receive issues in the mail and have online access to past issues. A link can be sent via e-mail, where you can read the whole publication online after logging on with your subscriber password. *The Prescriber's Letter* also lets you get CE credit for reading the content and answering questions. The concise newsletter, written in a conversational yet professional tone, gives information and advice about new developments in drug therapy and includes "Detail-Documents" with comprehensive information supplementing the newsletter, which are available online or by fax.[29]

Pharmacist's Letter: www.pharmacistsletter.com

Also published by the Therapeutic Research Center, *The Pharmacist's Letter* is similar to *The Prescriber's Letter* except it's tailored to provide valuable information for pharmacists. It offers concise, clear information on new developments in drug therapy and recommendations for the practice of pharmacy. "Detail-Documents" available 24 hours a day via online access or fax provide more comprehensive information.[30]

For subscribers, the Web site includes many useful tools such as comparison charts, patient handouts on important topics, a "truth vs. rumors" section that dispels rumors floating around in the world of pharmacy, and a section allowing colleagues to interact online. Pharmacists can also subscribe to a service that provides CE credit after they read the content and take a quiz.

E-mail Delivery of Tables of Contents

Receiving tables of contents by e-mail is a useful tool for browsing journals to find articles pertinent to your practice. Although it's tempting to subscribe to the maximum number of tables of contents published, cluttering your inbox with more than you can review is a nuisance. A better way is to subscribe to tables of contents for journals in your specialty area. Generally, you can browse titles linked to abstracts (summaries of clinical trials and review articles) and determine if you want to read the abstract or if the material is important enough to get a copy of the entire article.

It can also be useful to subscribe to the tables of contents for popular journals such as *The New England Journal of Medicine* or *The Journal of the American Medical Association* (*JAMA*), which are often cited in newspapers or on the evening news, prompting patients to ask questions. Because e-mailed tables of contents usually arrive before the journals are distributed, you can familiarize yourself with recent studies before the general public hears about them.

Webinars and Webcasts

The Foundation for Retrovirology and Human Health (www.retroconference.org) has been a leader in Web broadcasting since 1997, when it sponsored the first seminar on the Web, or "webinar." Webinars let attendees participate by receiving and sharing information and asking questions. Webcasts, a similar approach, generally allow participants only to receive information rather than interact in real-time. You can typically view webcasts anytime, night or day, and get access to audio and slides from past conferences that were presented live. Webinars are frequently used by pharmaceutical companies, technology companies, and health plans as an efficient means for disseminating their message to a widely scattered audience.[31]

PowerPoint Presentations

Any search engine, such as Google, offers unlimited access to PowerPoint presentations, many put together by health care professionals for patient and professional education. While information must be evaluated for quality and currency, it provides a good starting point for many educational endeavors. A couple of good places to start are reputable organizations and universities.

Webinars let attendees participate by receiving and sharing information and asking questions. Webcasts, a similar approach, generally allow participants only to receive information.

ACTIVITY 14-1

Finding Educational Material ✓

1. Find and bookmark at least five high-quality patient education sites you can refer patients to so they can learn more about their condition or medications.
2. Locate a PowerPoint presentation using a search engine such as Google or Kartoo on a topic that you currently manage in your practice.

References

1. Berwick DM. A user's manual for the IOM's 'Quality Chasm' report. Patients' experiences should be the fundamental source of the definition of "quality." *Health Aff.* 2002;21:80-90.

2. Institute of Medicine. *Crossing the Quality Chasm: A New Health System for the Twenty-first Century.* Washington DC: National Academy Press; 2001.

3. Gwinn BR, Seidman J. The IX Evidence Base: Using Information Therapy to Cross the Quality Chasm. Center for Information Therapy. Available at www.healthwise.org. Accessed May 24, 2004.

4. Forkner-Dunn J. Internet-based patient self-care: the next generation of health care delivery. *J Med Internet Res.* 2003;5:c8.

5. Illinois Online Network Web site. Learning Styles and the Online Environment. Available at: www.ion.illinois.edu/IONresources/instructionalDesign/learningStyles.asp. Accessed May 3, 2004.

6. Pew Internet and American Life Websites. Report: The Ever-Shifting Internet Population: A new look at Internet access and the digital divide, Part 7: Americans with Disabilities: A Special Analysis. Available at: www.pewinternet.org/reports/toc.asp?Report=88 Accessed May 6, 2004.

7. Fox S, Rainie L. Vital decisions. How Internet users decide what information to trust when they or their loved ones are sick. Pew Internet and American Life Project, 2002. Available at: www.pewinternet.org/reports/toc.asp?Report=59. Accessed May 6, 2004.

8. Harris Interactive, Cyberchondriacs update. Available at: www.harrisinteractive.com/harris_poll/index.asp?PID=299. Accessed May 6, 2004.

9. Peterson G, Aslani P, Williams KA. How do consumers search for and appraise information on medicines on the Internet? A qualitative study using focus groups. *J Med Internet Res.* 2003;4:e33. Available at: www.jmir.org/2003/4/e33/. Accessed April 3, 2005.

10. Zun LS, Blume DN, Lester J, et al. Accuracy of emergency medical information on the web. *Am J Emerg Med.* 2004;22(2):94-7.

11. MedlinePlus Selection Guidelines. Medline Plus Website Available at: www.nlm.nih.gov/medlineplus/criteria.html. Accessed April 21, 2004.

12. Medline Plus Web site. Available at: www.medlineplus.com/ Accessed April 21, 2004.

13. Drug Digest Web site. Available at: www.drugdigest.org. Accessed May 21, 2004.

14. WebMD Web site. Available at: www.WebMD.com. Accessed June 11, 2004.

15. Dr. Koop Web site. Available at: www.DrKoop.com. Accessed June 11, 2004.

16. Kartoo.com Web site. Available at: www.kartoo.com. Accessed April 15, 2004.

17. World Doc Web site. Available at: www.worlddoc.com. Accessed May 24, 2004.

18. Heathwise.org Web site. Available at: www.healthwise.org. Accessed May 24, 2004.

19. FindThatCE.com Web site. Available at: www.findthatCE.com. Accessed April 23, 2004.

20. Powerpak Web site. Available at: www.powerpak.com/. Accessed April 23, 2004.

21. The Center for Health Care Education, LLC Web site. Available at: www.chce.net/html/intro.html. Accessed April 23, 2004.

22. The Health Communication Research Institute Inc. Web site. Available at: www.hcri.com/index.html. Accessed April 23, 2004.

23. MedConnect Web site. Available at: www.medconnect.com/cme/login.asp?url=/index.asp. Accessed April 23, 2004.

24. ContinuingEducation.com Web site. Available at: www.continuingeducation.com/pharmacy/index.html. Accessed April 23, 2004.

25. CE City Web site. Available at: www.cecity.com/elearning.htm. Accessed April 6, 2005.

26. MediCom Web site. Available at: http://medicaled.com. Accessed April 23, 2004.

27. The Medical Letter on Drugs and Therapeutics Website. Available at: www.the medicalletter.com. Accessed April 22, 2004.

28. The Medical Letter Treatment Guidelines. Available at: www.themedicalletter.com. Accessed April 5, 2005.

29. The Prescriber's Letter Web site. Available at: www.prescribersletter.com. Accessed April 5, 2005.

30. The Pharmacist's Letter Web site. Available at: www.pharmacistsletter.com. Accessed April 5, 2005.

31. The Foundation for Retrovirology and Human Health Web site. Available at: www.retroconference.org. Accessed July 6, 2004.

Privacy, Security, HIPAA, and Related Matters

15

*Bradford N. Barker**

Chapter Objectives

After completing this chapter, you should be able to:

- Define the main types of privacy.
- Discuss the changing legal system's philosophy on medical information privacy.
- Identify privacy issues arising from computerization.
- Discuss the importance of confidentiality in dealing with patient information and give examples of ways in which security can be breached in a health care environment.
- Determine the impact of new technologies on ensuring medical information privacy and confidentiality.
- Summarize key provisions of HIPAA.

*Bradford N. Barker, guest author of this chapter, is an informatics research associate at Auburn University.

"The makers of the Constitution conferred the most comprehensive of rights and the right most valued by all civilized men—the right to be let alone."[1] This statement by Supreme Court Justice Louis D. Brandeis in 1928 reflects the current predominant view in America, that our culture was founded on principles of freedom and individual rights. However, the right to privacy is not explicitly stated in the Constitution or the Bill of Rights. Privacy wasn't developed as a legal concern until 1890, when Louis Brandeis and Samuel Warren published their article "The Right to Privacy" in the *Harvard Law Review*. Brandeis later argued in the Supreme Court case Olmstead v. United States that wiretaps should be illegal without a warrant, using the fourth amendment as the basis of a right to privacy.

In the late 1950s the Supreme Court's majority opinions regarding privacy started to change, and some amendments to the Constitution were reinterpreted as providing privacy protection. In the 1960s and 1970s, the Supreme Court defined the concept of privacy to include personal decisions concerning reproduction, sex, and marriage.

Interestingly, today's high-tech society clashes in many ways with "the right to be let alone." Scott McNealy, chief executive officer of Sun Microsystems, put it bluntly when he said in 1999: "You have zero privacy anyway. Get over it."[2]

Privacy and security go hand in hand. The right to privacy is recognized today in all U.S. states and by the federal government, either by statute or by common law, although the level of privacy protection varies widely by state. Generally, federal laws provide a "minimum" legal standard, and stricter state laws take priority. In health care, once the appropriate level of privacy protection has been identified by the health care organization, ensuring that level of privacy falls in the realm of security.

Although most people agree that privacy is to be respected, their definitions of privacy vary and few see eye-to-eye on what efforts are reasonable for maintaining a person's privacy. Courts interpret laws relating to privacy and confidentiality of medical records and information in several ways. The Heath Insurance Portability & Accountability Act (HIPAA) of 1996 attempts to provide a standard for both the courts' and the health care industry's interpretation of privacy. Changes are still taking place, so what constitutes "privacy" constantly changes—especially since any state law stricter than federal HIPAA law takes precedence.

Types of Privacy

In the realm of informatics, privacy has to do with collecting, storing, and disseminating information. Anita Allen, professor of law at the University of Pennsylvania and a noted legal theorist, defines privacy as: "modes by which people, personal information, certain personal property, and personal decision-making can be made less accessible to others."[3] Theoretically, there are at least three types of privacy:[4]

- **Physical privacy**, which restricts the ability of others to experience a person through one or more of the five senses. For example, we have the right to seek to be "left alone," to not answer telephones unless we choose to, etc.
- **Informational privacy**, which is the right to determine when, and to what extent, information about a person can be communicated to others. Informational privacy is at issue in cases about access to medical records, employer access to e-mail, online anonymity, data encryption, and executive privilege. Confidentiality and secrecy are informational privacy concerns. Concerns about informational privacy go by many names, including secrecy, confidentiality, anonymity, security, data protection, and fair information practices.
- **Decisional privacy**, which excludes others from decisions or restricts the dissemination of facts related to decisions made by a person and his or her group of intimates, such as health care decisions or marital decisions.

For both health care professionals and patients, privacy means being free from unauthorized intrusion and protecting personally identifiable information, including name, birth date, Social Security number, and financial data. Thus, privacy in health care organizations involves policies that determine what information is gathered and stored, how the information is used, and how patients are informed and involved in this process.

Organizations that fail to address privacy issues can suffer substantial financial loss and significantly damage the trust of their patients. For example, if personal information is stolen—such as records indicating that a patient has a sexually transmitted disease or terminal cancer—it's a problem of both privacy and inadequate security, not to mention a situation that would make any patient angry.

For both health care professionals and patients, privacy means being free from unauthorized intrusion and protecting personally identifiable information, including name, birth date, Social Security number, and financial data.

BOX 15-1

Privacy of Prescription Records

According to a report in the *Wall Street Journal* on April 11, 2001, a lawsuit over the privacy of prescription records at a former family-owned pharmacy could complicate the way pharmacies acquire competitors.

The suit challenges the common but little-known practice of "file buying," in which chains purchase patients' prescription files from pharmacies they acquire and add them to their own. The lawsuit, brought by an AIDS patient in state court in New York, contends that CVS Corp. illegally obtained his prescription records when it bought and later closed a family-owned pharmacy he patronized and then logged his medical information into its giant database without his consent.

The plaintiff said only a few people know he has AIDS, and he had been dealing with the same pharmacist for years, with whom he felt comfortable. He was shocked to be stopped at the front door in August 1999 by three CVS employees who reported that the pharmacy had been sold. When he replied that his medical records were inside, he was barred from entering and directed to a CVS store around the corner, he said.

The case has broken legal ground. A state court judge ruled that both the former pharmacy in midtown Manhattan and CVS could be sued for damages on grounds that they breached a duty of confidentiality to the plaintiff, who was allowed to file the suit anonymously. The ruling is the first to establish that pharmacy customers have a right to expect that their pharmacy records, like their medical records, will remain confidential. "Because pharmacists have a certain amount of discretion, and an obligation to collect otherwise confidential medical information, the court must find that customers can reasonably expect that the information will remain confidential," New York state Judge Charles Edward Ramos wrote in his opinion.

Source: Reference 5.

In health care, privacy issues relate to these basic questions.

For the organization:

- What kind of surveillance can we use that will not infringe on privacy (such as video cameras strategically placed so they do not capture views of patients)?
- Where should information be electronically stored?
- How should we control access to information?

For the patient and the employee:

■ What do I have to reveal?
■ What can I keep to myself?
■ Do I have the right to access my own personal information?

HIPAA is one step toward clarifying each group's rights and responsibilities.

Based on past court decisions in many countries, the following two tenets have emerged about privacy:[6]

■ The right of privacy is not absolute. Privacy must be balanced against the needs of society.
■ The public's right to know is superior to the individual's right of privacy.

Sometimes it is difficult to balance these tenets to determine and enforce privacy regulations. Courts in different areas of the country prior to HIPAA's enactment have concluded that health care workers may disclose medical information without liability under a number of different circumstances:

■ When information is already available to others. For example, medical information in an employee's records has been exempted from confidentiality protection with respect to the patient's employer.
■ To protect patients' interests. The states may obtain medical records to determine whether a patient needs to be committed.

BOX 15-2

Top 10 Tips for Good Corporate Security

Any good security program has a positive balance of four key data components: confidentiality, integrity, availability, and accountability. Achieving this balance typically involves a combination of technology, people, and process, as well as an understanding of internal communication and politics. Consider the following:

1. Understand what assets are critical to the business. How can you protect something when you don't know what you're protecting? It is nearly impossible to expect that companies will provide the highest levels of security around every piece of data they

continued on page 348

BOX 15-2 *continued*

hold, and in most cases they should not. If we determine that 10% of the organization's data is critical, we can focus priorities and funding around these assets first, then move on to less critical data.

2. Know what regulatory drivers you are subject to. All too often, we see security departments deploying technologies without knowing why or what they are protecting. Will this new security control meet all the requirements of your specific information technology (IT) governance issues? If it doesn't, then why invest in it?

3. Know what new technology initiatives may negatively impact your risk position. Traditional firewall and intrusion detection system (IDS) technologies won't stop someone from stealing confidential information in your e-commerce applications. As we push content to the edge and transform the way we do business, we must address security upfront, before these new initiatives take place.

4. Understand where your security program stands today (controls, skills, policies, etc.) and use a gap analysis to uncover strengths and weaknesses. Do the security controls you have in place today support the business objective, or do they fall short? Providing a report card-formatted gap analysis of your security controls and processes allows you to better understand which areas you need to address first. If you identify something that is grossly deficient, it does little good to shore up the other areas and leave a gaping hole in one.

5. Design a security program that fosters collaboration. In developing a good overall security program, different business groups, IT, and management must work together, and current skill sets, capabilities, processes, and policies must be assessed. Many companies struggle with this area due to internal politics, culture, organizational structure, and lack of direction. Consider forming a security council that incorporates members from security, business continuity, disaster recovery, business, human resources, etc.

6. Invest in effective incident detection, monitoring, and response capabilities. Many organizations purchase intrusion detection technology in order to meet compliance, but have not built the strategies around it to make it an effective tool. They collect gigabytes of data, yet aren't able to detect, prevent, and learn from the incidents. Using the technology to stop intrusions requires having a response program in place.

continued on page 349

BOX 15-2 *continued*

7. Provide periodic vulnerability assessments and regularly test the effectiveness of your security controls. How do you know what you don't know? Most organizations today have firewalls and other security controls, but rarely test them. Although daily testing is not possible for most companies, consider implementing monthly tests by your internal team and annual or biannual tests by an outside firm to check both the controls and the overall vulnerabilities of the environment, including servers, storage, and laptops.

8. Provide accountability and audit capabilities. How do you really know who has seen your corporate financials, and can you prove it? Today, having security controls and policies in place is not enough. There are too many regulatory requirements, with more to come, each calling for proof of who has seen what data and when. Eventually, you may even need to provide accountability of your data trails from beginning to end as a business or consumer requirement.

9. Document everything and provide feedback to management and team members showing the effectiveness of your security program. How will you ever receive funding or buy-in if you don't share your results? Keep a record of everything you are doing to put security in place and document why you're not doing certain things. Some organizations can be exempt from installing expensive security controls for financial reasons, but then they need to extensively document why. Some regulations require organizations to notify affected parties when personal information has been stolen. The Sarbanes-Oxley Act requires that financial data be accurate and timely; a possible security breach could harm the validity of that information be it in real-time format or recovered data from backups. Get management involved so they can buy-in to the process and provide continued financial support. Management may not care that you were infected by the latest worm, but they will care if you make them aware of how that worm will affect their ability to meet regulatory compliance.

10. Invest in security awareness training. The best way to develop an effective security environment is to be proactive about combating social engineering, which is the practice of tricking people into revealing confidential information. Human nature, especially in America, is to help other people and to trust. Why do you think we all have "help desks?" How is your help desk helping or hurting you now? What have you done to verify that they are not being too helpful?

Source: Reference 7. Adapted with permission from Line56 magazine.

BOX 15-3

Protect Your PC

What You Should Do:

■ Purchase and install a firewall, if you do not have Windows XP Service Pack 2 or greater. The same people who sell antivirus software usually sell firewall software as well (McAfee, Norton, etc.).

■ Make sure the operating system has the latest patches. For the Microsoft operating system, go to http://windowsupdate.microsoft.com and follow the on-screen instructions. After the patches are uploaded, reboot the computer, go back to the same site, and rescan. Continue this until the tool can no longer find any patches to apply.

■ Set up antivirus software to scan the hard drives at least once a week. Make sure the virus checker has the latest update (most update automatically, usually by purchasing a subscription).
   Note: Microsoft currently provides a "security wizard" to walk people through the above three processes, which you can access at www.microsoft.com/athome/security/protect/default.mspx.

■ Install antispyware software on the PC. Microsoft offers a free beta version at www.microsoft.com/athome/security/spyware/software/default.mspx .

■ Use a password entry program like RoboForm or Login King as a way around phishing and pharming. If a site has been phished, RoboForm will not fill in the fake form. If pharmed, the falsified Web site must have the exact underlying address and code for RoboForm to function.

■ Keep browser security settings at as high a level as possible to protect yourself against infections. (In Internet Explorer, choose "Tools, Internet Options, Security." Click on Default Level and set the setting to Medium.)

■ Check the license agreement of any program you install to confirm it does not come bundled with other programs. License agreements are supposed to explain if the software you are downloading will cause advertisements or other downloads. Always carefully read what you agree to before you download software.

What You Shouldn't Do (or at least do carefully):

■ Download or exchange files from sources you don't trust. Viruses and other Internet security threats can look like valid files or photos. Set up the software on your PC to always scan files with a virus scanner before opening them.

■ Click on popup ads. Regardless of how you feel about them, you should never click on them. Popup ads can secretly download software onto your computer.

■ Open e-mail attachments. Viruses can be sent out as e-mail attachments to infect your computer if you open them. Again, set up the software on your PC to always scan files with a virus scanner before opening them. Don't download files from unknown sources.

continued on page 351

BOX 15-3 *continued*

- Instant messaging. Everything said here applies to instant messaging as well. Infections look like valid files or photos, so always be careful accepting file transfers, even from sources you trust.
- Music downloads. Web sites that advertise free music downloads usually provide a hefty dose of spyware, as well. Some sites will download spyware onto your PC just by visiting the site without manually starting a download.
- Adult-related Web sites. Many of these sites make a profit by forcing viewers to download spyware and adware to access their site. You may not be able to view these sites if you are using a secure browser or have your security settings too high.
- Use Person-To-Person sharing programs like Kazaa or Limewire. If you share files using peer-to-peer networks, you will share viruses, popups, spyware, etc.

Source: References 8-11.

Security Issues

Before the electronic age, most health care information security needs were limited to corporate accounting and medical records—needs that could be met by a shredder. Now an organization's information usually permeates its infrastructure, including business partners' and employees' home computers. As electronic information expands, all information technology components are potential security risks. Examples of potential risks:

- Discarded hospital computers given away to schools, which have had their hard disks reformatted but not wiped clean of information.
- Buildings formerly rented by a hospital that still contain direct, unsecured connections to the hospital's intranet.
- Unsecured wireless access points or a personal router with wide-open wireless connection on the corporate network.
- A laptop computer accidentally left on a plane, which contains 5 years' worth of an entire hospital's patient data and lab reports.
- A 12-year-old using an Internet workstation in a school library to hack into a hospital's medical records.

> An organization's information usually permeates its infrastructure, including business partners' and employees' home computers.

Most health care organizations have thousands of potential risk points like these, and the risks will become greater as the means for capturing and transporting data become cheaper and more prevalent. The growing use of cell phones containing digital cameras demonstrates the speedy onset of new security issues. Anyone can quickly take a picture of a computer screen,

351

Some health systems restrict access to data by giving authorized users electronic name badges with a short-range radio frequency or infrared identification signal.

for example. As these devices pervade our lives, how will hospitals handle the need to protect patients' identities? Will tinted windows or a lack of external windows become the norm? Will visitors be allowed in patient wards at all?

Data Access

Traditionally, the method for dealing with data security is compartmentalization, which used to be accomplished physically. Locked filing cabinets, keys, and number-punch door locks were sufficient to secure most areas, keeping out everyone except authorized employees. Now, electronic tools are used to restrict who can view material, using login IDs or passwords.

In health care systems, physical security issues can be a major challenge. For example, nurses can pull up a patient's chart at the nursing station, get what they need, and walk away, leaving the patient's information on the screen. Although screen savers with password protection (which come on after a predetermined time of no activity, requiring you to type in your password to get back to the data) are security aids, they can be annoying and detract from patient care. Some health systems restrict access to data by giving authorized users electronic name badges with a short-range radio frequency or infrared identification signal. When no one with the correct security rights is in range, the computer screen goes blank.

To help protect data and keep different data elements separate, most organizations have an intranet that is connected to an external network, usually through the Internet. The intranet allows data to be transferred with minimal risk because its connection to the Internet is protected by one or more layers of firewalls. Firewalls usually consist of a set of security-related programs, which protect a network from unauthorized users from other networks. These can either run on individual computers (which is the way they're primarily used at home) or are installed in a separate computer, usually for a business. Firewalls can determine whether to forward messages between the PC or internal network and the internet. A firewall is usually installed in the electronic "no man's land" between networks, so that no incoming request can reach the organization's protected network resources directly. Firewalls also screen messages to make sure they come from previously identified computers. Mobile users can get remote access to private networks that have firewalls by using secure logon procedures and authentication certificates (this is called virtual private networking, or VPN).

Computer Crimes

Computer crimes are increasing exponentially. Examples of the types of crimes taking place include:

- Unauthorized network access, such as using wireless computers to find and access wireless networks without the owner's permission or knowledge. This is known as "wardriving."[12]
- Unauthorized computer use, such as infecting a computer with a virus that allows it to be controlled by others to retransmit spam e-mail or store files remotely. This is known as "turning a computer into a zombie."[13]
- Theft or inappropriate use of data.
- Theft of computer equipment or programs.
- Malicious damage or sabotage, including causing destruction via computer viruses or worms.
- Computer crimes occur in several different ways: by employees misusing privileged information, by hackers breaking in through an institution's network or Web site, or by hackers masquerading as trusted individuals, also known as identity theft. The methods range from passively viewing protected data to modifying data. The more sophisticated crimes involve installing such malicious programs as:
- Viruses—software programs capable of reproducing themselves, which infect files and programs: executables, documents, or the boot sectors on floppy and hard disks. Viruses are spread through sharing infected files or disks.[14] A form of electronic vandalism, viruses don't target only desktop or laptop computers—they have now been found on personal digital assistants (PDAs), cell phones, ATMs, and high-end cars.
- Spyware that secretly tracks computer users' activities, keystrokes, login names, passwords, and Internet usage.
- Worms that automatically copy themselves and distribute the copies to other computer systems via e-mail attachments or direct connections. Worms don't necessarily infect other executables; instead they proactively spread themselves over a network (which can including mass e-mailing). A specialized type of worm or virus is a Trojan Horse, which does something malicious while running as an innocent program.

Worms and viruses are now globally distributed via the Internet. A virus or worm runs on a personal computer like any other program, but usually masks its use of the operating system's

> A virus or worm runs on a personal computer like any other program, but usually masks its use of the operating system's resources so that the operating system is unaware that the virus or worm is there.

Phishing is a form of identity theft in which a scammer uses an authentic-looking e-mail to trick recipients into giving out sensitive personal information.

resources so that the operating system is unaware that the virus or worm is there.

Programs to protect against viruses, such as Norton Antivirus, Symantec Security, and McAfee VirusScan are constantly updated by the manufacturer as new virus threats emerge. Whether a virus on your computer can be detected depends on the virus's speed in spreading over the Internet (formerly measured in months, now in days or even hours[15]) versus the ability of these companies to recognize the threat and provide an update to their software. Most virus programs now have software built into the virus checker that keeps the virus protection software automatically updated.

Viruses are starting to be introduced that are more subtle than the ones that first emerged years ago. Like the common cold virus, these viruses "rewrite" themselves every time they propagate, making each strain harder to detect. Viruses can be automatically programmed to tell a computer to access a targeted Web site continuously, which your computer does in a way that masks this interaction from you. When hundreds or thousands of computers are infected with such a virus they can disable even a very large Web site—what is know as a "denial of service" or DOS attack, now one of the most prevalent uses of viruses. Incorporating the code for a DOS attack into a worm or virus is relatively easy. During the time the Web site is being bombarded by requests from the infected computers, the system is unavailable, which could result in lost revenue or inability to access a patient's records.

Identity theft as a computer crime has risen significantly in the past several years. Individuals will probably not know if their personal information has been compromised unless a company informs them.[16]

Phishing is a form of identity theft in which a scammer uses an authentic-looking e-mail to trick recipients into giving out sensitive personal information, such as a credit card, bank account, or Social Security numbers. Usually, the Internet addresses are off by only one character from the address they want to mimic. Recipients may receive a note from a bank asking them to go to its site (link provided, of course) to reenter personal information. Initially, the facts requested might tip off the person (a bank wouldn't really need a mother's maiden name) or there are misspellings in the phony e-mail, but scammers have gotten much more savvy (see Box 15-4).

Pharming is much more dangerous than phishing in that no action has to be performed to hand over personal information to identity thieves. Rather than sending e-mail requests, pharmers attack the servers on the Internet that direct network traffic (referred to as the DNS servers) and tell them to redirect the Web request somewhere else. As far as the browser is concerned, it is connected to the right site with the exact same look and feel.

BOX 15-4

Can You Spot Differences in These Web Addresses?

Original:
http://locator.regions.com/servlet/Locator/
SearchResults.jsp?zipCode=36832&state=&city=&branchSw=1&atmSw=0

False Address #1:
http://locator.regions.com/serv1et/Locator/
SearchResults.jsp?zipCode=36832&state=&city=&branchSw=1&atmSw=0

False Address #2:
http://locator.regions.com/servlet/Locator/
SearchResults.jsp?zipCode=36832&state=&city=&branchSw=1&atmSw=O

False Address #3:
http://locator.regions.com/servlet/Locator/
SearchResults.jsp?zipCode=36832&state=&city=&branchSw=1&AtmSw=0

Answers:
#1 – The 1 in "serv1et" is a number, not a character.
#2 – The last character is an "O", not a zero.
#3 – the A in "AtmSw" is capitalized (capitalization matters in a Web address).

Security Administration

Security systems are only as good as their ability to adapt to a changing environment. The best security system in the world is nonfunctional if it allows an employee who was fired yesterday access to the company's information today. Yet many health care systems don't tie together the databases between their personnel files and the security systems. A person who has been terminated from the corporation will very likely have their

BOX 15-5

Recommended Steps If Your Identity's Stolen

If you think your identity has been stolen, here's what the Federal Trade Commission (FTC) says to do now:

1. Contact the fraud departments of any one of the three major credit bureaus to place a fraud alert on your credit file. The fraud alert requests creditors to contact you before opening new accounts or making changes to your existing accounts. As soon as the credit bureau confirms your fraud alert, the other two credit bureaus will be automatically notified to place fraud alerts. Once the alert is placed, you may order a free copy of your credit report from all three major credit bureaus.
2. Close the accounts that you know or believe have been tampered with or opened fraudulently. Use the ID Theft Affidavit when disputing new unauthorized accounts.
3. File a police report. Get a copy of the report to submit to your creditors and others that may require proof of the crime.
4. File your complaint with the FTC. The FTC maintains a database of identity theft cases used by law enforcement agencies for investigations.

Source: Reference 17.

status changed in the personnel database (the one that determines whether they get a paycheck), but not necessarily get their name taken out of the security database (the database that determines which doors can be automatically entered by keycard or number pad) or the databases that determine whether a person can login to a particular system (they may be taken out of the main computer system, but not taken out of a specialized, nonconnected system such as the blood bank or pharmacy system).

Questions to ask in any health care environment include these:

- How long does it take new employees to gain access to the network and the applications needed to do their jobs?
- When employees are transferred or promoted, how long does it take before they have the rights to the applications they need? Are they still allowed access to applications that aren't in their new position's responsibility?
- How often are manual audits performed to ensure that the people who have rights are the ones who should have rights?

The results of these audits, especially for computer systems that have an automated connection to the personnel computer (and therefore are rarely checked manually), can be highly informative. As an example, if a person is automatically assigned a set of access rights based on job description when he is initially entered into a computer system, what happens if he is subsequently relocated to another department doing another job? Are his rights automatically updated?

In addition, protection against viruses and other potential threats is only as good as the latest software update on the organization's firewall and servers as well as on the individual PC's antivirus software. These updates include the software in the network components (known as firmware), as well as software in the PCs themselves. Many viruses exploit security holes in software that have not been patched by users, even though the software manufacturers have made a patch available.

Other Security Risks

Any information technology concern that could lead to data being transferred to a person who has no business seeing the data is a security concern. Sometimes, this can be as simple as making sure that none of the terminals at the nursing stations are in a position to be viewed by unauthorized personnel such as visitors or patients. Another recognized concern is the need to secure wireless local area networks throughout a hospital. A less-recognized threat (and a more complex and problematic issue) is whether USB flash drives should be allowed to store and transport patient information. Compact USB flash memory drives are small enough—about the size of a pack of gum—to slip easily into a pocket, on a lanyard around a neck, or on a keychain. They are relatively inexpensive, readily available, will work on most computers today, and are able to store and transport incredibly large amounts of computer data.[18]

Advance planning is critical to ensure that procedures or technologies with security concerns do not become security breaches. With forethought and planning, health care providers can have access to the information they need to care for patients and unauthorized users can be barred. Waiting until there's a fire, flood, power outage, or computer system failure is not the best time to inquire about how to safeguard your data and make your system secure.

> *Waiting until there's a fire, flood, power outage, or computer system failure is not the best time to inquire about how to safeguard your data and make your system secure.*

To decrease the administrative cost associated with health care, HIPAA standardized transactions between third-party payers and health care facilities and provided strict policies for the privacy and security of patient information.

Any computer operation that involves transmitting data off site should be reviewed for possible security concerns, including how these data will be restored during a crisis. Whatever security measures are used should not delay data restoration because such delays can disrupt computer operations, which can have far-reaching consequences for the organization, including long waiting periods for the data to be available again and exorbitant systemwide costs.

Health Insurance Portability & Accountability Act

The Health Insurance Portability & Accountability Act (HIPAA) of 1996 was originated to protect health insurance coverage for workers and their families when they change or lose their jobs. When it was proposed, there was little federal regulation relating to secure and private communication between health care providers and third-party payers. HIPAA's scope grew as it passed through committees in the House and Senate—affecting other programs, including the Internal Revenue Code, Social Security, and the Public Health Service Act.

To decrease the administrative cost associated with health care, HIPAA standardized transactions between third-party payers and health care facilities and provided strict policies for the privacy and security of patient information. In 2003, an average of 26 cents of each health care dollar was spent on administrative overhead, including enrolling people in a health plan, paying health insurance premiums, checking eligibility, obtaining authorization to refer a patient to a specialist, and processing claims.

BOX 15-6

Key Abbreviations Related to HIPAA

There are several abbreviations HIPAA uses:

CMS: Centers for Medicare and Medicaid Services
EDI: electronic data interchange.
EIN: employer identification number
PHI: protected health information
TPO: to carry out treatment, payment, or health care operations

HIPAA called upon the U.S. Department of Health and Human Services (HHS) to publish new rules to do the following:

■ Standardize electronic patient health, administrative, and financial data.
■ Establish unique health identifiers for individuals, employers, health plans, and health care providers.
■ Set security standards protecting the confidentiality and integrity of "individually identifiable health information," past, present, and future.

Health care organizations—including all health care providers, health plans, public health authorities, health care clearinghouses, and self-insured employers—as well as life insurers, information systems vendors, various service organizations, and universities, are affected by HIPAA. Violating HIPAA regulations can result in severe civil and criminal penalties, such as:

■ Fines up to $25,000 for multiple violations of the same standard in a calendar year.
■ Fines up to $250,000, imprisonment up to 10 years, or both for knowing misuse of individually identifiable health information.

BOX 15-7

How HIPAA Affects Health Care Organizations

To comply with HIPAA's requirements, organizations must assess their privacy practices, information security systems and procedures, and use of electronic transactions, develop an action plan, and set up a technical and management infrastructure to implement the plan. The plan must include the following:

■ Developing new policies, processes, and procedures to ensure privacy, security, and patients' rights.
■ Building business associate agreements with business partners to support HIPAA objectives.
■ Developing a secure technical and physical information infrastructure.
■ Updating information systems to safeguard protected health information (PHI) and enable use of standard claims and related transactions.
■ Training all workforce members.
■ Developing and maintaining an internal privacy and security management and enforcement infrastructure, including providing a privacy officer and a security officer.

The Rules Under HIPAA

HIPAA's administrative simplification provision has four parts, each of which has generated a variety of rules promulgated by HHS. The four parts are:

- Electronic Transaction Standards
- Security Rule
- Privacy Rule
- Unique Identifiers Standards

Electronic Transaction Standards

This area includes health claims, health plan eligibility, enrollment and unenrollment, payments for care and health plan premiums, claim status, first injury reports, coordination of benefits, and related transactions. In the past, health providers and plans have used many different electronic formats to transact such business; implementing a national standard is intended to bring about one format, thereby improving transactions' efficiency nationwide.

Providers using nonelectronic transactions are not required to adopt the standards for use with commercial health care payers. However, electronic transactions are required by Medicare, and all Medicare providers must adopt the standards for these transactions or contract with a clearinghouse to provide translation services.

Health organizations also must adopt standard code sets to be used in all health transactions. For example, coding systems that describe diseases, injuries, and other health problems as well as their causes, symptoms, and actions taken must become uniform. All parties to any transaction will have to use and accept the same coding to reduce errors and duplication of effort. Fortunately, the code sets proposed as HIPAA standards are already used by many health plans, clearinghouses, and providers, which should ease the transition.

Security Rule

The final security rule, published February 20, 2003, provides for a uniform level of protection of all health information that is housed or transmitted electronically and pertains to an individual. The security rule requires covered entities to ensure the confidentiality, integrity, and availability of all electronic protected health information (ePHI) that the covered entity creates, receives, maintains, or transmits. It also requires entities to protect against any reasonably anticipated threats or hazards to the security or integrity of ePHI, protect against any reasonably anticipated uses or disclosures of such information that are not permitted or required by the privacy rule, and ensure compliance by their workforces. Required safeguards include applying appropriate policies and procedures, safeguarding physical access to ePHI, and ensuring that technical security measures are in place to protect networks, computers, and other electronic devices.

The security rule does not require specific technologies to be used. Covered entities may elect solutions appropriate to their operations, as long as the selected solutions are supported by a thorough security assessment and risk analysis.

Privacy Rule

The privacy rule is intended to protect the privacy of all individually identifiable health information in the hands of covered entities, regardless of whether the information is or has been in electronic form. It creates national standards to protect individuals' medical records and other personal health information. It gives patients more control over their health information, sets boundaries on the use and release of health records, and establishes safeguards that health care providers and others must achieve to protect the privacy of health information. Violators are held accountable and civil and criminal penalties can be imposed if patients' privacy rights are violated. The rule strikes a balance when public responsibility requires disclosure of some forms of data—for example, to protect public health.

For patients, the privacy rule means that they can make informed choices about how personal health information may be used when they seek care or reimbursement for care and to find out how their information may be used. It generally limits release of information to the minimum reasonably needed for the purpose of each disclosure and it gives patients the right to examine and obtain a copy of their own health records and request corrections.

Before HIPAA, there was little in the way of standardized legislation dealing with the PHI that moves across doctors' offices, hospitals, or insurers. Patient information held by a health plan was not protected from lenders, who could deny the patient's application for a home mortgage or a credit card, or from employers, who could use it for personnel reasons. The privacy rule establishes a federal floor of safeguards to protect the confidentiality of medical information. State laws with stronger privacy protections apply over and above the federal privacy standards.

The privacy rule creates national standards to protect individuals' medical records and other personal health information. It gives patients more control over their health information, sets boundaries on the use and release of health records, and establishes safeguards that health care providers and others must achieve.

Unique Identifiers Standards

In the past, health care organizations used multiple identification formats when conducting business with each other—a confusing, error-prone, and costly approach. It is expected that these problems will be reduced by using standard identifiers—the numbers used to identify health care providers, health plans, employers, and patients. Over time, this is intended to simplify administrative processes, such as referrals and billing; improve accuracy of data; and reduce costs.[19]

There are two standards planned: one to identify employers and the other to identify the health care provider and third-party payer. The employer identifier standard, published in 2002, adopts an employer's tax ID number or employer identification number (EIN) as the standard for electronic transactions.

General Provisions

Patient consent is required before a covered health care provider that has a direct treatment relationship with the patient may use or disclose PHI to carry out treatment, payment, or health care operations (TPO), with the following exceptions:

- Uses and disclosures for TPO may be permitted without prior consent in an emergency, when a provider is required by law to treat the person, or when there are substantial communication barriers.
- Health care providers that have indirect treatment relationships with patients (such as laboratories that only interact with physicians and not with patients), health plans, and health care clearinghouses may use and disclose PHI for purposes of TPO without obtaining a patient's consent. The rule permits such entities to obtain consent, if they choose.
- If a patient refuses to consent to the use or disclosure of his or her PHI to carry out TPO, the health care provider may refuse to treat that patient.
- A patient's written consent need only be obtained by a provider one time.
- The consent document may be brief and may be written in general terms. It must be written in plain language; inform the individual that information may be used and disclosed for TPO; state the patient's rights to review the provider's privacy notice, to request restrictions, and to revoke consent; and be dated and signed by the individual (or his or her representative).

BOX 15-8

Individual Rights Related to HIPAA

- An individual may revoke consent in writing.
- An individual may request restrictions on uses or disclosures of health information for TPO. The covered entity need not agree to the restriction requested, but is bound by any restriction to which it agrees.
- An individual must be given a notice of the covered entity's privacy practices and may review that notice before signing a consent form.

Administrative Issues

A covered entity must retain the signed consent form for 6 years from the date it was last in effect. The privacy rule does not dictate how these consents forms are to be retained by the covered entity.

- Certain integrated covered entities may obtain one joint consent for multiple entities.
- If a covered entity obtains consent and also receives an authorization to disclose PHI for TPO, the covered entity may disclose information only in accordance with the more restrictive document, unless the covered entity resolves the conflict with the individual.
- Transition provisions allow providers to rely on consents received before April 14, 2003 (the compliance date of the privacy rule for most covered entities), for uses and disclosures of health information obtained before that date.

> The privacy rule does not dictate how consent forms are to be retained by the covered entity.

Security

The final HIPAA security regulations were released in February 2003 and apply to ePHI, with enforcement beginning April 2005. The final rule requires that covered entities:

- Determine appropriate security measures through risk analysis.
- Adjust security practices as circumstances change.
- Revisit the security needs associated with "appropriate administrative, technical, and physical safeguards" for protected information implemented under the privacy regulations.

i Vulnerabilities of ePHI must be identified and the effects of potential threats calculated as if they actually occurred.

Risk Analysis

According to the final rule, risk analysis is a thorough assessment of potential risks to the confidentiality, availability, and integrity of ePHI. Vulnerabilities of ePHI must be identified and the effects of potential threats calculated as if they actually occurred. If potential threats create an unacceptable risk, safeguards are to be implemented. The rule doesn't require a certain risk-analysis approach, but two approaches are well accepted, each with its strengths and weaknesses:

■ Quantitative analysis, a tedious process not often followed in its purest form, which involves measuring and assigning objective numeric value to assets, potential threat impacts, safeguard effectiveness, safeguard costs, uncertainty, and probability. A quantitative approach provides a more workable cost/benefit analysis but requires extensive study for asset valuation and threat probability.

■ Qualitative analysis, sometimes imprecise but helpful in prioritizing risks, which involves ascribing relative rank to threats and vulnerability of assets according to seriousness, then matching potential level of threat to potential asset loss to select the appropriate safeguard. A qualitative approach is relatively simple but depends largely on subjective information.

When conducting risk analysis, basic steps include conducting a complete inventory to identify assets needing protection. The following list is a good starting point for identifying where ePHI is received, stored, and transmitted and who has access to it:

■ **Hardware**—computers, radiology storage devices, medical equipment, front-end processors, workstations, modems.
■ **Information networks**—servers, communication lines, internal and external connectivity, remote access.
■ **Applications**—database and application software, operating systems, utilities, compilers, encryption tools, procedure libraries.
■ **Physical facilities**—heating, ventilation, and cooling systems; furniture; supplies; machinery; fire control systems; storage.
■ **Other assets**—records and data, policies and procedures, customer confidence.

Here is an overview of risk-analysis activities:

1. **Determine the value of every asset.** For example, use financial statements to value physical assets. With ePHI, one method is to consider the cost of creation and protection, attributable revenues, competitive advantages provided, and value to third parties. Initial creation and valuation of an asset inventory can be tedious, but it will be helpful, for example, in contingency and risk-insurance planning.

2. **Identify vulnerabilities and threats for each asset.** A vulnerability is a software, hardware, or organizational weakness that may allow unauthorized access. A threat is any potential danger to the information system that exploits that vulnerability. For example, software code that permits system access without a password is a vulnerability. Someone accessing the system to steal or destroy stored information is a threat. Some vulnerabilities can pose more than one threat, so risk analysis must be thorough.

3. **Evaluate the severity of each threat** for every asset in the inventory. For quantitative analysis, first determine the exposure factor (EF)—the percentage of loss a threat would likely cause the asset and the ePHI connected with it. For example, if a fire in the computer server room could be expected to destroy half the servers, the fire threat is 50%.

4. **Using the EF, determine the single-loss expectancy** (SLE)—the effect of a single occurrence of the threat for each asset and its ePHI. If the EF is 50% and the servers and their ePHI are worth $3 million, the SLE from a fire is $1.5 million. The SLE is used in cost/benefit analysis for selecting safeguards. For qualitative analysis, rate the effect on a scale, such as 0 for none and 5 for severe. In the fire example, effect might be valued at 3 if the organization could function after losing half its servers. If the servers contain all the information needed to function, the rating is 5.

5. **Determine the probability of a threat.** For quantitative analysis, establish the annualized rate of occurrence (ARO). In the example, fire-occurrence averages compiled by local insurance companies could be used. If statistics show there's a server room fire once every 5 years, the ARO would be one-fifth, or 20%. For qualitative analysis, based on the consensus of management and the risk-analysis team, the probability of a fire might be given a 1.

A vulnerability is a software, hardware, or organizational weakness that may allow unauthorized access. A threat is any potential danger to the information system that exploits that vulnerability.

6. **Calculate the annual expected loss or total risk level** for a threat. For quantitative analysis, the amount lost or paid out if the threat occurs is determined by multiplying the SLE by the ARO. The organization experiencing the fire could expect to lose $300,000 annually ($1.5 million ´ 20%). For qualitative analysis, determine total risk by multiplying the threat's effect by its probability. Since a 5-point scale was used for each in the example, total risk is measured on a 25-point scale. Effect (5) ´ probability (1) = total risk of 5, a relatively low score on a 25-point scale.

7. **Identify safeguards for each vulnerability**—those currently used and those addressable or required by HIPAA (e.g., a fire suppression unit in the server room). For quantitative analysis, measure the cost of purchasing, installing, and maintaining each safeguard against the cost of a threat occurrence. With a fire costing $300,000, a $50,000 fire suppression unit is well worth the price. For qualitative analysis, the cost of each safe guard is important even though exact expense calculations aren't required. For example, spending $200,000 to counter a low-probability risk makes little sense.

Transferring or Accepting Risk

When eliminating or mitigating risk to an acceptable level is impossible, one option is to transfer it, which is usually accomplished by buying insurance. More insurance companies are beginning to offer cyber insurance, but policies seldom cover fines and cannot restore good will lost during a security incident. Another option is to accept a technical risk that, though potentially very harmful, is unlikely to occur (for example, a hurricane in Oklahoma) after full disclosure of this intention to legal, risk management, and executive personnel and the board of directors. But even with transfer or acceptance of risk, the security regulations require some form of risk analysis.

The Gramm-Leach-Bliley Act

HIPAA isn't the only major legislation recently enacted to deal with privacy. While HIPAA deals primarily with clinical data privacy, the Gramm-Leach-Bliley Financial Modernization Act of 1999 (GLB) deals with the privacy of financial information. Enacted by Congress to remove barriers between financial institutions and modernize financial services regulations, GLB applies to banks, credit unions, securities firms, and insurance companies.

Why does a health care provider need to know about a bill that applies to financial institutions? Because, just as HIPAA holds hospitals responsible for information they send to third-party payers, the same third-party payers have a parallel responsibility under GLB when they share information with a health care provider. For health insurers, GLB is administered at the state level. Under GLB, each state's insurance commissioner adopts privacy legislation and implements regulations conforming to GLB requirements. Multistate health insurers have to comply with the maximum GLB privacy requirement of the states they serve.

GLB uses the phrase "nonpublic personal information" (NPI) to mean the same as PHI. Health insurers can only share nonpublic personal information with nonaffiliated companies under the provisions of the act. These are GLB's main health information requirements:

> Third-party payers have a parallel responsibility under GLB when they share information with a health care provider.

- Financial service companies must notify consumers and allow them to opt out of sharing their PHI with unaffiliated third parties for non-insurance–related reasons.
- Financial service companies that handle PHI must provide customers with descriptions of their privacy policies and give them the opportunity to opt out.
- Financial service companies must protect and audit the information in electronic format.

Both HIPAA and GLB rules apply to health insurers. Therefore, health insurers have to comply with HIPAA even if an NPI disclosure or an opt-out notice is permissible with GLB. This can be a nightmare situation for a hospital that provides insurance to its own employees.

What's a health care provider to do? Since HIPAA is the more comprehensive of the two laws, complying with HIPAA privacy statutes should result in GLB compliance, as a general rule. There are differences, however:

- HIPAA requires an initial privacy notice where GLB requires an annual notice.
- HIPAA requires a patient's authorization for a health care provider to share PHI for a reason outside of TPO. GLB places

the burden on the consumer to choose not to permit a disclosure. It is unclear whether an insurer needs to obtain both an authorization and an opt-out form for information that is both PHI and NPI.

Other Confidentiality Issues

In health care, some confidentiality issues occur are that either unique or occur often enough to deserve merit.

The Physician-Client Privilege

At one time, a physician (and by relation, other health care professionals) could assume that any health care-related information communicated between the patient and the physician could be treated as confidential, even in a court of law. However, the legal statute for this privilege is not federal and varies widely between states. Many states use a system accepted by the Canadian Supreme Court, called the Wigmore test, to determine whether physician-patient confidentiality exists. Communication is privileged under these circumstances:[20]

- The communications must originate in confidence with the understanding that they will not be disclosed.
- This element of confidentiality must be essential to the full and satisfactory maintenance of the relationship between the parties.
- The relationship must be one that, in the opinion of the community, ought to be assiduously fostered.
- The injury that would result from the disclosure of the communication must be greater than the benefit that would be gained by the correct disposal of litigation.

One interesting legal interpretation of the physician-client privilege in some court cases is that it can be waived if the physician asks a patient to sign a "limited confidentiality consent statement," which includes a clause recognizing that "… as a result of legal action, the physician may be required to divulge information obtained in the course of this research to a court or other legal body."

Identity Theft

According to the Federal Bureau of Investigation, an average robbery involves $3000; an average white-collar crime involves

$23,000; but an average computer crime involves about $600,000.[21] A significant portion of these crimes occur through identity theft.

A large percentage of identity thefts are committed by insiders, notably at health care and financial institutions. The FTC received about 117,000 complaints about identity theft in 2001 and nearly 300,000 in 2002.

Recently, new federal laws have been proposed to deal with this problem. For example, the 2004 Identity Theft Penalty Enhancement Act aims to punish identity theft by increasing criminal penalties and creating a new crime of "aggravated ID theft," defined as using a stolen identity to commit certain other crimes. Conviction for aggravated ID theft will require a mandatory sentence enhancement of 2 years, and aggravated ID theft committed for the purpose of terrorism will have an additional mandatory 5-year penalty. The bill also directs the U.S. Sentencing Commission to revise guidelines for punishing individuals who abuse positions of trust to commit insider identity theft.[22] Laws will continue to develop to deter employees from ID theft.

> A large percentage of identity thefts are committed by insiders, notably at health care and financial institutions.

Spyware

Currently, spyware is legal under federal law, but several bills making their way through Congress and state legislatures would regulate this and force software makers to notify consumers before installing some kinds of monitoring programs on their PCs.

The issue of spyware, otherwise known as adware or malware, has been building slowly over several years, with many people complaining about popup advertisements triggered by adware or about the potential of software spying on their online actions. Most bills under consideration bar key logging (recording every stroke of computer users' actions on the keyboard and reporting this remotely) and the display of uncloseable advertisements.

State Laws

In terms of HIPAA and GLB, each state's medical privacy laws must be analyzed by affected organizations to determine what steps are important to ensure health information privacy. The effect of the law for each situation depends on many factors and varies widely by state, so it's best to engage legal counsel with experience in this area to assess and help minimize legal liability based on your particular requirements. The information in this chapter is in no way a substitute for legal advice.

ACTIVITY 15-1

Changing Laws ✓

Find any new laws, either federal or state, that have been enacted since this book has been published on information identity theft by employees. For the set of laws you find, answer the following questions:

- Which laws will take a higher precedence?
- Which laws are directly applicable to you?

Ethics is the science that points out standards and ideals of life in harmony with natural law. It helps us to answer the question: "What ought I to do?"

Ethical Issues

Why do you as a health care professional care about ethics in information services? Because if you do what is generally considered to be right in regard to patient privacy, your conduct will be explainable to your peers and defensible in a court of law. Most important, it will allow you to sleep well at night, knowing you've done the best you could in a given situation.

It's essential to make the distinction that we can't, as health care professionals, subscribe to one set of ethics at our facility and another outside our profession: our ethics are who we are. Ethics is the science that points out standards and ideals of life in harmony with natural law. It helps us to answer the question: "What ought I to do?"

Ethics is arguably the most important component of a profession, especially one that deals with people's lives, as the health care professions do. The subject has been defined as "the standards of conduct of a given profession." This "agreement among people to do right and to avoid wrong" is paraphrased in Hippocrates' famous statement "First, do no harm."[23]

What is unethical is not necessarily illegal. Thus, an individual or organization faced with an ethical decision, such as what to tell the family about a patient's condition or whether to share patient-related information with a colleague who can help the patient, is not necessarily breaking the law. Adopting health care

BOX 15-9

Principles of Medical Ethics

Following is a summary of ethical principles adopted by the American Medical Association, which define the essentials of honorable behavior for the physician. Each physician shall:

- Be dedicated to providing competent medical care, with compassion and respect for human dignity and rights.
- Uphold the standards of professionalism, be honest in all professional interactions, and strive to report physicians deficient in character or competence, or engaging in fraud or deception, to appropriate entities.
- Respect the law and also recognize a responsibility to seek changes in those requirements which are contrary to the best interests of the patient.
- Respect the rights of patients, colleagues, and other health professionals and safeguard patient confidences and privacy within the constraints of the law.
- Continue to study, apply, and advance scientific knowledge, maintain a commitment to medical education, make relevant information available to patients, colleagues, and the public, obtain consultation, and use the talents of other health professionals when indicated.
- In providing appropriate patient care, except in emergencies, be free to choose whom to serve, with whom to associate, and the environment in which to provide medical care.
- Recognize a responsibility to participate in activities contributing to the improvement of the community and the betterment of public health.
- While caring for a patient, regard responsibility to the patient as paramount.
- Support access to medical care for all people.

Source: Reference 24.

information technology without taking into consideration patient risk is an unethical decision but it is not (at the time of this writing) illegal. Each profession's code of ethics (see Box 15-9) serves as an important guide. Codes are inspirational—aiding young members of a profession and inspiring its elders—and they help to maintain a high moral tone among those in active practice. Codes of ethics should delineate principles underlying a profession's duties and the practitioners' responsibilities and rights. These principles apply to relationships with administrators, medical and nursing staffs, pharmacy committees, rank-and-file personnel, students, visitors, the health care facility, the general public, the community, and others such as paramedics, the medical record librarian, the social worker, and the dietitian, and others in the health care field.

Codes of ethics should delineate principles underlying a profession's duties and the practitioners' responsibilities and rights.

ACTIVITY 15-2

Codes of Ethics

Obtain a copy of the codes of ethics for your organization. In private, write a description of an unethical situation you either observed or performed. In the description, answer the following questions:

- What was there about the situation that made it unethical?
- Was the action performed, despite the fact it was unethical? Why or why not?
- Could anything have been done to change the situation to make it ethical?

References

1. *Olmstead v United States*, 277 U.S. 438, US Supreme Court (1928).

2. Sprenger P. Sun on privacy: 'get over it'. *Wired*, 1999;26.

3. Allen AL. Privacy Matters. Payment Cards Center Workshop on the Right to Privacy and the Financial Services Industry at University of Pennsylvania; Philadelphia; 2001.

4. University of Nebraska Medical Center. Ethics Glossary. Available at: www.unmc.edu/ethics/words.html. Accessed July 2, 2004.

5. Geyelin M. Do prescription records stay private when pharmacies are sold? *Wall Street Journal.* April 11, 2001.

6. Turban E, Ranier RK, Potter RE. *Introduction to Information Technology.* 2nd ed. Hoboken, NJ: John Wiley & Sons, Inc.; 2003.

7. Smith E. Good IT Security Policy Starts Here. Available at: http://line56.com/articles/default.asp?articleID=5558&TopicID=3. Accessed June 3, 2005.

8. Microsoft. Security At Home - Protect Your PC. Available at: www.microsoft.com/athome/security/protect/default.mspx. Accessed June 3, 2005.

9. Microsoft. Microsoft Windows AntiSpyware (Beta). Available at: www.microsoft.com/athome/security/spyware/software/default.mspx. Accessed June 3, 2005.

10. Williamson B. Feedback - pharm relief. *PC Magazine.* June 7, 2005:24,83.

11. Vamosi, R. Alarm over pharming attacks: identity theft made even easier. Available at: http://reviews.cnet.com/4520-3513_7-5670780-1.html. Accessed February 18, 2005.

12. Anon. Define Wardriving. Available at: http://havenworks.com/vocabulary/a-z/w/war-driving. Accessed July 3, 2004.

13. Anon. Your computer could be a 'spam zombie'. Available at: www.cnn.com/2004/TECH/ptech/02/17/spam.zombies.ap. Accessed July 3, 2004.

14. The Cognitive Science Laboratory at Princeton University. The WordNet lexical database - Virus. Available at: www.cogsci.princeton.edu/cgi-bin/webwn2.1?s=virus. Accessed June 2, 2005.

15. Quainton D. The record shows the net's taking blows - it did it Mytob way. Available at: www.scmagazine.com/news/index.cfm?fuseaction=newsDetails&newsUID=bc5789cf-e448-4a6e-bee9-a5dd291405ed&newsType=Latest%20News&s=n. Accessed June 3, 2005.

16. U.S. Department of Justice. U.S. Announces What Is Believed the Largest Identity Theft Case In American History; Losses are in the millions. Available at: www.usdoj.gov/criminal/cybercrime/cummingsIndict.htm. Accessed June 3, 2005.

17. Federal Trade Commission. Your Natural Resource for ID Theft. Available at: www.consumer.gov/idtheft. Accessed June 2, 2005.

18. USB Flash Drive Alliance. USB Flash Drive FAQ. Available at: www.usbflashdrive.org/usbfd_faq.html#whatis. Accessed June 2, 2005.

19. Workgroup for Electronic Data Interchange. Administrative Simplification under the Health Insurance Portability and Accountability Act. Available at: www.wedi.org/snip/public/articles/details~6.shtml. Accessed June 26, 2004.

20. Lowman J, Pal T. Going the Distance: Lessons for Researchers from Jurisprudence on Privilege. Available at: www.sfu.ca/~palys/Distance.html. Accessed June 29, 2004.

21. Fisher D. Group Fights Online ID Theft. Available at: www.eweek.com/article2/0,1759,1257072,00.asp. Accessed July 1, 2004.

22. Carlson C. Congress Passes ID Theft Bill. Available at: www.eweek.com/article2/0,1759,1618523,00.asp. Accessed July 1, 2004.

23. American Medical Association. Frequently asked questions in ethics. Available at: www.ama-assn.org/ama/pub/category/5105.html#oath_oblig. Accessed June 3, 2005.

24. American Medical Association. Principles of Medical Ethics. Available at: www.ama-assn.org/ama/pub/category/2512.html. Accessed June 3, 2005.

The Future of Health Care Informatics

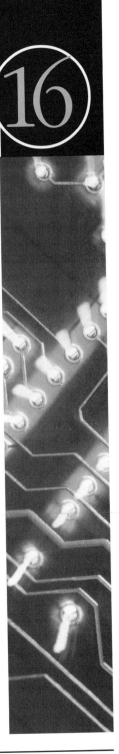

Bill G. Felkey

Chapter Objectives

After completing this chapter, you should be able to:

- Define the term "disruptive technology."
- Identify disruptive technologies that could affect the business side or clinical operations of health care organizations.
- Name several technology-driven trends in health care.
- Describe key wireless innovations that could have an impact on health care.
- Describe the likely components of future "wearable computers."
- Give examples of robotics and artificial intelligence in today's health care practice.
- Discuss important ways to plan ahead for bringing new technology into your organization.

Other industries are already far ahead of health care when it comes to information technology—surprising when we consider that life-and-death consequences hover around health care decisions.

When Yogi Berra quipped that "It's tough to make predictions, especially about the future," he could have been talking about health care informatics. One thing is certain: technology has the capability to fundamentally change the way health care organizations operate.

We are quickly moving to a level of digital information capability where all aspects of workflow, along with empirically derived research, can be electronically integrated into every process within an organization. Other industries are already far ahead of health care when it comes to information technology—surprising when we consider that life-and-death consequences hover around health care decisions.

Although there's no question that health care will use greater levels of technology in the future, by no means do we want to go from "hugging patients"—letting them know their desires are respected—to "hugging technology"—being fascinated with technology at the expense of human contact. When used properly, however, technology can give us more time to spend with patients.

It's Good to Plan Ahead

Because so many wonderful technological capabilities are available right now, we seldom feel the need to look very far into the future. Some organizations do, however, try to plan ahead and get ready for what's coming. The Health Technology Center or "HealthTech" (www.healthtechcenter.org), a nonprofit that does research, education, and technology forecasts for health systems, looks 2 to 5 years into the future to prepare its members for what are known as "disruptive technologies": any new device or information processing breakthrough with a profound effect on technologies that preceded it (such as cell phones replacing traditional landline phones). Any technology in the pipeline has the possibility of being a boon or a threat to existing work processes.

The people at HealthTech recognize that looking ahead can help organizations be more proactive and efficient, preparing them to modify operations if necessary. For example, for United States military, completing a global telecommunications satellite network is an opportunity to provide health care using experts at the National Naval Medical Center in Bethesda, Maryland, rather than deploying top surgeons in range of a scud missile. A threat to surgical centers that perform kidney surgery and lithotripsy would be a new technology that lets family practitioners dissolve kidney stones noninvasively in a typical exam room.

Tracking Technology

The HealthTech Center emphasizes how important it is for organizations to prepare for the potential positive and negative effects of technological innovation. By monitoring trends and identifying strategic and tactical implications of these trends, you can prepare for disruptive technologies, keeping in mind capital investment, workforce issues, facility considerations, and clinical program impact.

Just as we can stay abreast of what's happening with medications from their early development to the point where they enter the market—the medication pipeline—we can track technologies in various stages of research and development. Several technological "push" publications send regular electronic newsletter updates on new products. The Google search engine's "alert" function (www.google.com/alerts), which sends hyperlinks to news on specific topics as soon it becomes available, is a great tool for staying on top of technology.

Match Problems with Solutions

There is never a "perfect technology" for everyone in an organization. It's helpful to have technology-savvy personnel on staff who look for innovative tools that could be beneficial. In my organization, I monitor what's new and use a matching process where I identify problems people are experiencing and refer them to possible solutions.

Organizations need to ask themselves, "Do I want to be a 'first in' adopter? Or do I want to make sure products are fully mature before I investigate them?" I call this my "tool or toy" question. Sometimes you find something interesting and buy it before you really know how it's going to fit into your work. For staff in my organization I investigate, preselect, and precertify technologies to let them know what is ready for incorporation.

Think of technology as part of nearly everything you are doing now or plan to do in the future. Before implementing any plan, ask yourself, "Am I using the Internet appropriately in this process? How can we use technology to make this work better? What will be the ripple effect through our organization after making this change?" Technology can potentially enhance any work process or replace work done by humans and perform it more efficiently and effectively.

Monitor technologies coming down the pipeline and identify how they can enhance or disrupt your operations. Before implementing any plan, ask, "How can we use technology to make this work better?"

Fear of Change and Other Challenges

Most health systems are afraid of making a mistake by purchasing technologies that do not produce a return on investment. Health care organizations tend to avoid being innovators or early adopters of technology. Although a few step out as leaders, many simply react, acquiring technology only because they perceive threats from competitors in their market. Careful

---

BOX 16-1

Technology Trends in Health Care

Through its research, the Health Technology Center has zeroed in on 10 top technology-driven trends in health care expected to unfold in the next decade. Ask yourself how any of these would change the way you practice. You need to be ready when disruptive technology becomes viable in the marketplace. Are you aware of any technologies beyond those mentioned below? How are you preparing to adopt or defend against these and other trends?

1. Health care interventions will occur earlier, causing a shift in treatment patterns to screening, prevention, and minimally invasive therapies—which will be increasingly provided in ambulatory and home care settings.
2. Chronic conditions will be addressed in their early stages via biosynthetic drugs and drug implants.
3. Cancer treatment will advance to the point where acute care is less prevalent than chronic care and prevention.
4. Improved management of cardiac patients will reduce surgical interventions—which will create fiscal challenges for hospitals as surgery revenue drops.
5. Patients and physicians will benefit from real-time data access, thanks to medical informatics platforms and networking technologies with open architecture that allow integration with other tools and devices.
6. Technology will improve productivity throughout the health care workforce.
7. Smaller, high-tech surgical devices will allow more than 80% of current invasive surgeries to be replaced by minimally invasive and noninvasive procedures.
8. The success of end-stage therapies will drive up the demand for long-term care services.
9. Pharmaceutical companies will find markets for blockbuster drugs evaporating as genetic testing and imaging define the nature of disease more precisely.
10. Imaging, genetic testing, and improved drug therapies will converge to dramatically improve outcomes for psychiatric conditions as the relationship between behavioral and organic factors becomes more clear.

Source: Reference 1.

---

research and planning are the best hedge against the capital risks inherent in purchasing new technologies.

Although adopting new technology can be costly, it can be even more expensive not to—especially if patients and providers choose to do business with a competing organization that they perceive as more "cutting edge."

When organizations implement a new technology, many challenges follow. You need to hire technicians or have contractors on call to do maintenance, adjustments, and repairs. You must offer on-site training and continuing education to help existing clinical staff and new hires master the new technology. You may need to develop backup systems that are very different from the old manual systems—and people must be trained to use the backup systems before you're faced with unscheduled downtime. For example, if the electronic medical record (EMR) system goes down, staff may need to know how to use a portable, offline workstation that stores information and later updates the EMR when the system comes back online. Writing notes on paper may no longer be an acceptable backup.

Organizations that are best positioned to take advantage of new technologies promote a "culture of change." When organizations view change as a constant, they have a certain momentum. From a leadership perspective, it is almost always easier to redirect a moving organization than to get a stagnant or "stuck" organization in motion. A good approach is to take advantage of opportunities to pilot-test new technologies and infuse them into the organization while you're waiting for the "perfect" technological solution to emerge.

For example, Ridgeview Medical Center in Waconia, Minnesota, determined that requirements of the Heath Insurance Portability & Accountability Act (HIPAA) prevent sending e-mails containing protected health information to patients. But because they want to communicate with patients by e-mail and know that they will eventually have an EMR in place that displays patient data securely, they figured a solution would be to send e-mails to patients directing them to new information on the secure Web site.

The technology for this may be several years away, however, so Ridgeview identified an approach that works in the interim. Using secure e-mail from ZixCorp (www.zixcorp.com), Ridgeview puts the word "secure" or "confidential" in the subject line to encrypt the protected health information in the body of the e-mail. The person receiving the e-mail gets a link to log in to, which allows her to examine her information after authenticating her identity via password.

Careful research and planning are the best hedge against the capital risks inherent in purchasing new technologies.

Organizations that are best positioned to take advantage of new technologies promote a "culture of change."

Let the World Know About Your Innovations

Americans are particularly interested in new developments in health care technology, so anytime you move forward with something innovative, you should have little trouble getting coverage from local media. Press releases pertaining to health care news are usually picked up by syndicated new services and distributed widely.

Focus on the scientific advances possible with the new technology you've acquired, such as robotic patient movers or virtual colonoscopies, and explain how the technology will help patients recover faster, reduce pain, save money, or do whatever it does to give patients a more positive health care experience.

Technology in Our Future

From a connectivity standpoint, we almost have an end to geographic separation. Imagine a future with a pervasive wireless network that lets you move information to every other person on the planet.

Is any "fun stuff" coming down the pike? In truth, the things discussed in this section are already here, but in their earliest stages. We take for granted technology that is now commonplace. Today's cellular telephones were the stuff of fantasies and Dick Tracy cartoon strips not many years ago. We can go anywhere in the world and use an ATM card to obtain cash. How many years will it be before our medical records follow us during our global travels?

Wireless Keeps Us Connected

We all were very enthusiastic when the first wireless networks came online in the mid-1990s, with people drinking coffee and surfing the Internet in cafés or using wireless kiosks in airports. Health systems and clinics put access points into their buildings and connectivity at reasonable speeds was a reality. Marconi paved the way with his "magic box" radio in the 1890s; little did we know that another revolution in wireless communication would take place in the early 2000s.

Wireless connectivity is beginning to include automobiles, public transportation, and even kitchen appliances. From a connectivity standpoint, we almost have an end to geographic separation. Wireless-friendly cities like Dayton, Ohio, and Philadelphia, Pennsylvania, and even some rural towns, are making it easy for people to go online, sometimes for free.

The paradigm I recommend to every discipline and specialty in health care can be summed up in a slogan coined by Cogon Systems, a clinical software company in Pensacola, Florida: "Always available, strategically connected." Although being connected to all the information and people in our practice is only possible experimentally in target markets, imagine a future with a pervasive wireless network that lets you move information to every other person on the planet.

In the "always available, strategically connected" model, data such as medical results needed for clinical decision making are "pushed" every 30 minutes or when triggered by programmable alerts (based on abnormal lab ranges, etc.). Data can also be pulled any time (by a query initiated by the provider) through the traditional, wireless sync function. This system is a good mix from the standpoint of data availability and battery life—it avoids a constantly open connection, which consumes too much battery power.

Some key wireless innovations are listed below. Each represents an expansion in our ability to be connected and each could potentially have a major impact on health care.

From a connectivity standpoint, we almost have an end to geographic separation.

- The Federal Communications Commission has opened up the frequency for a WiFi variant called WiMax, which is faster and longer range than WiFi. WiMax is a way of networking computing stations or devices together across roughly 30 miles. In this way, a single tower atop a hospital could allow a rural community to be fully connected whenever a health care practitioner or patient requires information transfer.
- Satellite phones, which make calls from even the remotest mountaintop, are becoming more sophisticated. For example, Samsung has announced a phone that will receive 40 satellite television channels. In the future, you may be able to request —and receive on the spot—a program on the proper technique for administering cardiopulmonary resuscitation, for example.
- 802.11X WiFi, the wireless standard used most widely in health care today, continues to evolve into higher capacity formats with the ability for increased encryption and security when health care information is transmitted.
- Bluetooth took a little while to get traction, but now an impressive array of peripheral devices is offered so that Bluetooth-enabled devices can communicate with each other without wires. Everything from printers to bar code readers can function wirelessly at distances up to 30 feet. Exchanging patient data,

reporting patient outcomes from home, and even communicating between our automobile and gas pump is already in place.

■ The global positioning system (GPS) may have a health care role in locating patients who suffer from debilitating conditions and dementia. A company called Wherify (www.wherifywireless.com) has developed a GPS personal locator that costs about $200—it's a digital watch you can place on a small child or a parent with Alzheimer's disease to locate them in an instant. A tiny rivet in the band prevents the watch from being removed easily.

■ 3G, short for "third-generation wireless," is a wireless format launched in Europe and Japan that is quickly being adopted in the United States because of its higher bandwidth connecting information appliances. Imagine DSL-speed connectivity between devices the size of a cell phone.

■ Voice-over-IP (VOIP) uses the Internet to move voice communication over long distances, bypassing telephone carriers like AT&T. Some health systems report saving several hundred thousands of dollars because of VOIP, which combines the Internet and specially formatted telephones or radiofrequency devices for hands-free communication between members of the health care team. The cost of installing VOIP technology has become reasonable for corporate clients in comparison with the increasingly high cost of telephone communication. Some users report that the communication quality of VOIP is not quite as good as standard telephone service but is acceptable.

■ EV-DO is the name of a new U.S. variant of the European 3G format. Offered by Verizon Wireless, EV-DO is being tested in San Diego, Washington, D.C., and 32 other cities to allow high-speed connectivity on cellular telephones and other information appliances such as notebook or tablet computers. Using this system, a home health care company could provide treatment and interact with a health system that is located all the way across the country from the patient's bedroom.

■ Short messaging system (SMS) is the transmission of short text messages to and from a cell phone or other device, with a typical limit of 135 characters. Although nearly 100% of health care providers in the audience at my presentations have cell phones, only about 50% have ever received a text message. SMS has great potential for communicating alerts, critical laboratory results, and verification requests.

■ The WiFi-enabled, hands-free communications badge developed by the Vocera Company (www.vocera.com)

is a small, wearable device with a single activation button. You simply say the name of the party you wish to communicate with or the role of the person you are seeking, such as a courier or laboratory technician, who accepts the incoming call by saying "yes." Health systems using this technology have reported faster response times for assistance and for rush medication orders.

■ The SRAM cell phone memory chip is a new type of memory chip that is 30% smaller. Just introduced by Samsung, its intended use is to allow simple, personal information management functions in cellular telephones, but eventually it could be of great use to first responders—police, firefighters, emergency medical technicians, etc. When the day arrives that people store electronic medical records on their cell phones, an injured person's record could be transmitted to a first responder's PDA with the simple press of a key—similar to how most cell phones dial 911 if you press only the 9 key.

■ Remote monitoring of patients, one of the most exciting innovations that wireless technology allows in the health care setting, is happening at high levels in only a few locations today. For example, intensivists, a relatively new type of critical care physician, can monitor as many as 90 patients in five hospitals via telemetry—transmitting or retrieving data over long-distance communication links, such as satellite or telephone. The intensivist checks displays that digitally and graphically show vital signs, laboratory data, even nursing notes. If a vital sign is significantly out of normal range, the patient's total information set is brought to the display array of nine screens. The physician can "zoom in" via telemedicine video to examine the patient and can use additional voice and video connections to coordinate on-site care.

Wearable Computers the Next Fashion

Newsweek magazine featured an article in its June 7, 2004, issue about how cell phones could become the killer of the desktop computers. With more than 1.5 billion mobile phones in the world that can take pictures, browse the Web, send and receive e-mail, and even let us talk to people, why own a computer? In Tokyo, people can watch TV, read books and magazines, and play games on their cell phones, the article said.[2] Is this the prelude to the "wearable computers" my colleagues and

A wearable computer may include a keyboard strapped to the user's forearm, but more likely it will be activated by voice input.

I have been talking about for years? I think it's only a matter of time before wearable computers become everyday appliances that process our data and our communication.

Computers of the future will be different in many ways, but will still make use of the five components that make up every computer today: inputs, outputs, storage, memory, and processors.

The most common inputs on a computer are the keyboard and mouse. A wearable computer may include a keyboard strapped to the users' forearm, but more likely it will be activated by voice input.[3] Continuous speech recognition, even with its current flaws, is already faster than the typing speed of the average computer user. The input device will probably be connected by Bluetooth and will be part of the headset the user wears.

Outputs for computers usually consist of displays, printers, and speakers. Displays for wearable computers could be incorporated into eyeglasses, with the display screen centered in the vision of one eye, and the viewing screen in the peripheral vision of one eye or in a virtual reality display for both eyes—simulating three dimensions. Large-screen plasma displays could be strategically placed around organizations for collaborative computing. Conceivably the wearable computer will transmit a screen compatible with a larger display and information displayed on the plasma screens will be touchscreen-sensitive, so you can manipulate it without a keyboard, using your fingers or verbal commands.

Wearable computers will use printers located around an organization, to which files can be forwarded wirelessly. Operating printer functions will be controlled by voice commands. In place of desktop speakers or a speaker built into your laptop you'll use an earbud or speaker in your wireless headset.

Memory and storage will be part of the computer you wear, but memory backup will occur wirelessly and seamlessly each time someone on the organization's care team needs access to your data. Although processor chips will initially be part of the wearable computer, over time more computing will be done on a network that allows less powerful devices to be carried by the end user. Being able to speak to a larger, more powerful computer may be more desirable than working with the remote wearable computer's onboard technology. Users will be able to connect wirelessly to a single database to synchronize the data in their wearable computers, so all members of the health care team have access to the same information.

Robotics Ready to Run

With robotics, tasks that humans used to do are performed mechanically. Robotics works best with tedious and repetitive tasks. For example, robotic welders on an automobile assembly line produce much more accurate welds than humans can. Robotics is already used in many areas of health care. For example, surgical robots allow a surgeon in the United States to perform a complicated procedure remotely in the United Kingdom; pharmacy dispensing robots fill bottles and vials, and patient mover robots lift and transport patients. As this book goes to press, Sony has announced the first "running robot," a 23-inch, 15-pound creature that can trot at a speed of 15 yards per minute. Sony's robot is capable of losing contact with the ground for 0.4 second—a major advance for a robot, but not quite the full second that humans' feet are off the ground during certain strides. Sony does not claim that its robot is really "useful" yet; it is more for entertainment value. Apparently it does a pretty good break dance and moonwalk.

Although robots like this do not yet exist in health care, the Pyxis Helpmate (at www.pyxis.com/prodDetails.aspx?pid=64), which looks a little like R2D2 in *Star Wars*, transports medications, lab samples, supplies, meals, medical records, and equipment. If a meal tray or stat medication is required in a patient room, the Helpmate will navigate floors and elevators while avoiding collisions with patients along the route. The Helpmate is cost-effective as long as the courier it replaces is making more than five dollars an hour.

> *i* Artificial intelligence is a branch of computer science concerned with developing machines and software that can perform activities thought to require the intelligence of a human being.

Artificial Intelligence a No Brainer

Artificial intelligence is a branch of computer science concerned with developing machines and software that can perform activities thought to require the intelligence of a human being. Artificial intelligence in health care has been around for years, such as the software from Apache (www.apache.org) that helps physicians make decisions concerning end-of-life support. It uses a complicated algorithm to give a score on the patient's likelihood of surviving or the feasibility of expending large amounts of medical resources. There are several artificial intelligence diagnostic programs, ranging from those that identify pathophysiological processes to automated EKG consults that examine waveforms produced during the procedure. Progress in artificial intelligence has been slow because human reasoning

Progress in artificial intelligence has been slow because human reasoning involves more than simple logic.

involves more than simple logic. Today's emphasis on evidence-based medicine, however, promises to build the need for artificial intelligence that matches variables from the literature to individual patient cases.[4]

Gadgets Galore

Auburn University has an industrial design department that teaches creativity through exercises—such as combining household items with animals to free designers from conventional thinking. Researchers trying to eliminate tooth decay have thought about how sharks regenerate teeth, for example. One Auburn student combined a flashlight with a giraffe and, coincidentally, a few months later, Black & Decker's "snake light" was introduced to U.S. markets, a flexible light capable of bending into whatever shape is required. As we look to the future, imagination is our only limitation. The science fiction of our childhood becomes our adult reality.

Not long ago I came across a Swiss Army knife/USB memory device that embeds all the usual knives, screwdrivers, tweezers, and scissors but it also has a flash drive memory device.[5] We are going to continue to see technological implements being combined whenever it make sense.

Eventually radio-frequency identification chips will be placed inside jewelry and could possibly be used to broadcast our medical records in emergencies. Buses and other public transportation may be equipped to let people check their e-mail during commutes—an infrastructure the airline industry is installing now. One day it will be commonplace for you to shop using devices that compare the best price on the planet to the item on the sale rack in front of you. Bring GPS into the mix and the sky's the limit. Imagine being able to monitor a sick relative remotely and get an individual broadcast of your child's soccer game while you're on a business trip.

Informatics—Part of the Routine

As health care becomes a completely digital industry, the systematic processing of data should improve so rapidly that, eventually, we can eliminate the problems associated with conjecture and human memory's limits. We'll be able to cut costs associated with such inefficient, wasteful practices as ordering redundant tests. We'll have easy ways to apply evidence-based knowledge and to collect new knowledge so we make even better health care decisions in the future.

The digital world will never be perfect, however. Unforeseen problems will emerge where technology actually produces errors. For example, during a late-night visit to a patient's bedside, a prescriber may order an injection to be administered at 8 a.m. Unfortunately, if this order is placed at one minute past midnight, the machine may not recognize the prescriber's intention for the injection to be administered in 8 hours and instead might schedule the dose for 32 hours later.

Information content and its integrity during transmission must be of the highest quality for patients to be managed successfully. Standardized language that can be applied to all populations of patients will be critical, and in both large and small organizations, strategies will need to be in place to continually improve information management. Monitoring an organization's medication error rate, for example, can determine how accurate the technologically supported processes really are. At the most basic level, every transaction in a health care organization can be captured and analyzed for continuous quality improvement.

Informatics training should be a part of routine operations in any health care organization—from how to find the on-off switch to how to use continuous speech recognition programs to document patient care. Continuing education, so important for maintaining a good informatics knowledge base, will increasingly become "just-in-time," so that knowledge is supplied at the moment it is needed to support operations and decision making.

> Informatics training should be a part of routine operations in any health care organization—from how to find the on-off switch to how to use continuous speech recognition programs to document patient care.

How To Prepare for What's Ahead

Everybody, from the physician to the nurse, pharmacist, medical coder, technician, and receptionist, uses technology at some level—but most health care workers are so busy they don't have time to step back and look at their organization from a system level. Can someone standing at a single subway stop in New York City fathom the complexity of the entire subway system? To stay on top of technology and prepare for what's ahead, system analysis should be incorporated into the job description of certain health care staff. These staff should be prepared to help with the following[6]:

Think about revolution, not just evolution. Instead of falling into the trap of focusing on ways to tweak current processes, do a little daydreaming. Ask yourself how new technology could be matched with a particular problem.

1. Develop a schematic for the information flow and data repositories in your organization so you can visualize potential problem areas and anticipate ripple effects when new technologies are introduced for various work processes. Figure 4-1 on page 78 is an example of a schematic.

2. Pinpoint important technologies that will have an impact on your operations before they are introduced to the market. In addition to mining the Internet or subscribing to technology journals, try to attend exhibitions of new products at least twice a year such as Comdex (www.medialiveinternational.com/global/comdex), one of the biggest general computing exhibitions in the world, and the annual conference and exhibition of the Healthcare Information and Management Systems Society (www.himss.org).

3. Monitor competitors to learn about their technology mix. What technologies are they using? How are they benefiting from them? If you hire anyone who used to work for a competitor, find out what he liked best about the technology in his old position.

4. Think about revolution, not just evolution. In other words, when looking at new technology, think beyond potential changes in access, quality, and cost. Instead of falling into the trap of focusing on ways to tweak current processes, do a little daydreaming. Ask yourself how new technology could be matched with a particular problem your organization is experiencing.

5. See if it's possible for innovation to become part of your organization's branding. People call facial tissue Kleenex even when it's a different brand. Choose a vision statement phrase such as "most progressive health care organization" and work it into all your institutional promotion activities; soon others will be repeating your branding phrases.

6. Procure approval from the highest administrative levels before you plan a major technology project. Efforts such as computerized prescriber order entry can fail if administrators are not on board from the start and fully prepared to weather the pain of implementation.

7. Involve clinicians in all aspects of planning, selection, and implementation when they will be affected by adopting a new technology. Identify stakeholder groups and bring in respected representatives who can communicate their group's functional requirements so that they have a sense of ownership in the final product.

8. Avoid cookie-cutter approaches. A solution in one environment probably won't work in another without modification. When possible, select products that produce data in an industry-standard format, such as XML, but that can be adapted to individual work styles and preferences.

9. Be prepared to adjust the technology strategy to cope with unforeseen changes. Markets shrink, products come and go, mergers and acquisitions take place, and natural catastrophes occur. Realize that sometimes you may have to improvise so you don't lose momentum.

In my organization, we just found a Bluetooth-connected bar code scanner for $40 that can replace an older workstation that was heavy and bulky and cost $500. Finding products that produce immediate benefits in your organization can be both fun and rewarding. Good hunting!

ACTIVITY 16-1

Emerging Technologies

You are an informatics specialist working in a progressive health system. You have been asked to survey emerging technologies that can be used to improve your organization's productivity. Do the following:

1. Look for new technologies and existing technologies with new applications that may be useful in your organization.
2. Select two or three that seem to provide greatest value and analyze these in more detail. Investigate whether your competitors are using these technologies, how they like them, and how committed they are to using them.
3. Evaluate the fit of these technologies to your organization.
4. Write a report with your opinions (backed up with facts) about which technologies are promising. An appointed committee from your organization must be able to read your report and gain a quick understanding of each technology, its maturity in the marketplace, the competition's level of commitment, the technology's potential value to your organization, and why you think a particular technology warrants further consideration.

References

1. Cove MJ. Technology Forecast Reports. www.healthtechcenter.org. Accessed July 8, 2004.

2. Margolis M, Johnson S, Itoi K, et al. The humblest digital city; only way to communicate; living the wireless lifestyle; a future with nowhere to hide (series of articles). *Newsweek International.* June 7, 2004.

3. Mann S. Keynote Address for the First International Conference on Wearable Computing, May 12-13, 1998, Fairfax, Va. http://wearcam.org/icwckeynote.html. Accessed July 13, 2004.

4. Coiera E. *Artificial Intelligence Systems in Routine Clinical Use.* www.coiera.com/ailist/list-idx.htm. Accessed July 13, 2004.

5. *Gadgets Update Report.* www.thinkgeek.com/gadgets/tools/6b3b/images/887. Accessed July 13, 2004.

6. Bauer JC. *Technology and the Future of Healthcare.* www.superiorconsultant.com/Pressroom/Articles/TGI_Bauer_TechnologyFuturePaper.pdf. Accessed July 13, 2004.

Glossary

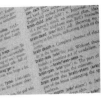

#'s

802.11X: A wireless standard that allows increased encryption and security when health care information is transmitted.

A

Aggregator: A company specializing in collecting and sharing information.

Application service providers (ASP): Third-party entities that manage and distribute software-based services from a central data center across a WAN or via the Internet.

Application software: Software programs used to solve a specific problem or carry out a specific activity. Examples in health care include physician charge capture software, nursing software for documenting patient progress notes, laboratory software for analyzing and reporting results, and pharmacy software for medication management.

Artificial intelligence (AI): Programs that enable machines to do tasks that humans perform by using intelligence and problem-solving skills.

Automated systems: Machines controlled by a computer to perform work that requires tedious repetition, tiresome movement, intense concentration, immense memory retention, or meticulous record keeping.

Automation: The technological takeover of repetitive, tedious tasks to free people for work that involves judgment, abstract thinking, and other high-level cognitive processes.

B

Background: The picture or color scheme on the computer desktop, often arbitrarily set when the operating system is installed on the computer.

Bar code medication administration (BCMA) system: Using a laptop and standard bar code scanner, this system, developed by the Veterans Health Administration, displays real-time information for each patient, such as medications that need to be administered at a certain time.

Bar code point of care (BPOC) systems: Medication administration systems designed to collect critical chart information and decrease medication errors.

Batch processing: Processing a group of transactions at once after accumulating them over a specified period.

Bit: The smallest unit of information on a computer; holds the value of 0 or 1 only.

Bluetooth: A wireless connection that enables devices to exchange information, replacing cables and infrared connections.

Boolean operators: Words such as AND, OR, and NOT that are routinely used to combine search terms.

Brick and click: A business with both a physical presence and e-commerce access.

Brick and mortar: A business that has a physical presence in the community.

Broadband: A telecommunication medium that can carry a wide range of frequencies simultaneously, such as multiple data, voice, or video channels.

Browser: Software used to display Web pages; provides a graphical interface that lets users click buttons, icons, and menu options to view and navigate.

Bus topology: A network with a central channel and many nodes connected to it, each node operating independently. A failure at one node does not affect the other nodes and new nodes are easily added. An example of a bus topology network is Ethernet.

Byte: 8 bits; holds the value of a single character. Increments include kilobyte or KB (1024 bytes), megabyte or MB (1,048,576 bytes), gigabyte or GB (1,073,741,824 bytes), and terabyte or TB (1,099,511,627,776 bytes).

C

Case-control study: A clinical study in which people with a particular disease are compared to a similar group of people without the disease to define risk factors that may have led to the disease.

Cellular phone: A handheld mobile radiotelephone that uses the air as the transmission medium between geographical locations broken into cells, each cell containing a short-range transmission tower.

Central fill: A type of integrated drug distribution in which a group of pharmacies, such as mail-order pharmacies, operates one high-volume dispensing facility. Pharmacists in one location securely transmit prescriptions over the Internet to a call center.

Central processing unit (CPU): The computer's main processing chip, the "brains" of the computer. Also known as the processor, microprocessor, chip, or central processor, the CPU executes all instructions and influences the computer's overall speed.

Clinical data repositories (CDR): Storehouses of information, paper or electronic, that contain test results, medication information, discharge summaries, progress notes, and other individual patient information.

Clinical decision support systems (CDSS): Systems designed to help practitioners make informed patient care decisions based on patient specific information as well as the latest research findings from the literature and other sources.

Clinical information systems: Combinations of hardware and software operating on a network that moves data to where clinical departments and practitioners need it.

Coaxial cable: A multichannel communication cable containing a main signal wire surrounded by another wire, either braided or a solid sheath.

Cohort study: A study that follows a population over time to see if there is a difference between groups exposed to factors of interest and groups not exposed to them.

Community health information network (CHIN): A series of Web-based connections that allows patients access to their own health care information.

Computer: A programmable machine that responds to a system of standard instructions (program) in a well-defined manner and can run, process, or carry out these programs.

Computer science: Broad area describing the study of computing systems; includes theories, methods, design issues, and implementation.

Computer viruses: Malicious programs that continuously modify data in an infected computer.

Computerized prescriber order entry (CPOE) system: A combination of hardware and software for capturing and transmitting medication orders. Intended to prevent medical errors, increase efficiency, and decrease costs.

Content provider: Any health care entity that creates and publishes information for patients or practitioners.

Critically appraised topics (CATs): An evidence-based tool for teaching and learning evidence-based medicine (EBM) that consists of a structured, one-page document that uses the five steps of EBM.

Customer relationship management: Involves capturing and tracking information about customer or patient preferences, usually with the help of software, allowing organizations to follow up and promote services that individuals may be interested in.

D

Data: A representation of facts or concepts.

Data rate: Speed that the hard drive can return data to the central processing unit (CPU). Current industry standards for data rates are between 5 and 40 MB/second.

Database: An organized collection of related information.

Data-processing systems: Systems that tabulate raw data and create spreadsheets or other documents that can be read and interpreted.

Decision science: The application of mathematical modeling and analysis to the decision-making process.

Decision support systems (DSS): A class of information systems that helps users solve unstructured roblems and make decisions.

Decisional privacy: Excluding others from decisions or restricting the dissemination of facts related to decisions made by a person and his or her group of intimates, such as health care or marital decisions.

Defragment: A system maintenance task that combines all similar data on the hard drive to avoid system delay caused by gaps in data that were stored separately.

Denial of service attack: The disabling of Web sites by viruses programmed to tell hundreds or thousands of infected computers to access a targeted Web site continuously.

Digital product delivery: Any type of product that can be downloaded or transferred electronically such as music, movies, photography, etc.

Digital subscriber lines (DSL): Technology that allows high-speed data communication over existing copper telephone lines.

Disease-oriented evidence (DOE): Studies based on pathophysiologic end points and etiology.

Disruptive technologies: Any new device or information processing breakthrough with a profound effect on technologies that preceded it.

Domain name: A name that uniquely identifies an Internet computer site and assigns that name to a specific IP address.

Domain name server (DNS): An Internet service that translates domain names into IP addresses.

Drug use review (DUR) messages: Messages received by pharmacists and prescribers during computerized order entry when clinical information systems detect potential problems in a patient's medication therapy, such as drug interactions or allergies.

E

E-commerce: Conducting business over the Internet including retail sales, wholesale networks, government interaction with businesses or consumers and consumers doing business with other consumers.

E-health: Telehealth activities over the Internet.

Electronic cash: Also called cybercash, a money transfer where the consumer's money is held in escrow by a third-party company until the buyer is satisfied with the e-commerce transaction.

Electronic check: Authorization of an electronic funds transfer directly from a consumer's bank account, usually requiring routing and bank account information from the consumer.

Electronic health record (EHR): Repository of information about a patient's health in a computer-readable format. The term is sometimes used interchangeably with electronic medical record.

Electronic medical record (EMR): A computerized version of a paper medical record, containing information about a patient's diagnoses, treatments, etc.

Electronic medication administration record (eMAR): Employs bar codes and other technology to provide health care providers with medication, administration, and dosage information for each patient.

Encoders: Translate messages from their original form into a form suitable for transmission.

Encryption: Converting plain text information into code to prevent unauthorized viewing of protected health information.

Enterprise software: Intended for a larger user base, serving individuals across a complete enterprise, such as order entry and billing applications.

Evidence-based medicine: The conscientious, explicit, and judicious use of current best evidence in making decisions about the care of individual patients, combining clinical expertise, evidence, and an intimate knowledge of the individual patient's situation, beliefs, priorities, and values.

Evidence-based practice guidelines: Incorporating the best scientific evidence available into the guideline process, stressing extensive documentation of methods and evidence used to make recommendations. Tools that help practitioners make decisions regarding diseases and treatments.

Evolution, Data Only (EV-DO): U.S. variant of European 3G format that provides high-speed connectivity on cellular telephones and other information appliances such as notebook or tablet computers.

Expert systems (ES): A type of artificial intelligence that can repetitively and accurately solve problems using human expertise, stored knowledge, and inferences.

Extensible markup language (XML): A standard for creating expandable information formats that allow both the format and the data to be transmitted and interpreted between different applications and organizations.

Extranet: Unlike an intranet, which is accessible only to people who are members of the same organization, an extranet provides various levels of accessibility to outsiders.

F

Fiber-optic cable: The fastest transmission medium; uses high-quality strands of glass and/or plastic containing the fibers, cladding (a thin coating), and jacket (a protective layer) to carry the telecommunication signal as light waves.

File management application: A component of the operating system that allows the user to access and manage files. You can also buy separate file management systems.

File transfer protocol (FTP): A standard or protocol that enables people to share documents and applications over the Internet.

Firewall: Specialized hardware or software designed to protect a computer or network from unauthorized access and external threats, such as hackers.

Five rights: A system of checks to decrease errors in medication administration.

G

Global positioning system (GPS): A system of satellites and receiving devices used to compute positions on the Earth.

Gramm-Leach-Bliley Financial Modernization Act (GLB): A 1999 Congressional act dealing with the privacy of financial information by removing barriers between financial institutions and modernized financial services regulations that apply to banks, credit unions, securities firms, and insurance companies.

Granular format: Information arranged to allow the user to jump quickly to the critical bit of information needed.

Graphical user interface (GUI): User-friendly screens with pictures and icons designed to send commands to the computer system, providing clearer presentation of information to the user.

H

Handheld portable computing devices: Small, personal electronic devices (such as PDAs) that provide personal information management as well as data capture and display capabilities.

Hardware: The physical, mechanical, and tangible parts of a computer system.

Health care informatics: The application of computer science and information technologies to advance health-related disciplines and specialties.

Health Insurance Portability & Accountability Act (HIPAA): A 1996 Congressional act providing guidelines for the flow of health care data and information.

Health plan employer data and information set (HEDIS): A set of standardized measures of health plan performance that allows patients and employers to compare quality, patient satisfaction, financial information, and other aspects of health plans.

Heuristics: Rules of thumb and decision-making shortcuts that guide you toward probable solutions to a problem.

Hypertext markup language (HTML): The coding language used to create documents for Web pages and to format other information that is viewable in a browser.

I

Identity theft: The deliberate assumption of another person's identity and the fraudulent use of such knowledge.

Information: A collection of data, presented in any medium, that has meaning.

Informational privacy: The right to determine when and to what extent information about a person can be communicated to others.

Information brokers: Companies that offer access to information in key topic categories.

Information science: The study of information in terms of its creation, use, and management.

Information systems: Computer and communications hardware, software, networks, and other components that supply information. In health care, these systems typically support clinical activities as well as scheduling and reimbursement.

Information technology: The activities and tools used to locate, manipulate, store, and disseminate information.

Information therapy: Patient education based on clear evidence and delivered at the most useful moment.

Infrared: A line-of-sight transmission method that uses air as the transmission medium and light waves to transfer data.

Input devices: Components used to enter information and data into the computer, such as mouse, keyboard, microphone, data gloves, joysticks, light pens, and styli.

Instant messaging: A form of electronic communication that involves immediate display of typed correspondence between two or more users who are all online simultaneously.

Intelligent systems: A class of data-processing systems composed of artificial intelligence and expert systems, used to supplement or replicate human decision-making functions for specific, well-defined problems.

Interactive voice response (IVR) systems: Used to route callers through menus based on the caller's response to questions.

Internet: A large global network made up of thousands of smaller networks, which is accessible by computers and handheld devices. The World Wide Web is one element of the Internet.

Internet protocol (IP) number: A unique numeric identifier that specifies hosts and networks.

Internet service provider (ISP): A company that provides Internet access services to consumers and businesses.

Internet2 Consortium: An effort led by over 180 universities working in partnership with industry and government to develop a high-speed network that facilitates data transmission for educational, research, and other applications.

Interoperability: The capability of two or more devices to freely transmit data regardless of the device manufacturers.

Intranet: A network of computers in an organization.

L

Local area network (LAN): A network consisting of nodes connected over a relatively small area, usually spanning the distance of one building or a group of buildings.

M

Management information systems (MIS): Systems (usually computer-based) used in an organization for ongoing data collection and analysis so that managers receive the information they need to plan, direct, and control activities.

Management science: The study of decision making and planning within an organizational setting.

Memory: Physical chips on which data and programs are temporarily stored; also used to manipulate data and programs during user's interaction with the computer.

MeSH (Medical Subject Headings): The National Library of Medicine's controlled vocabulary used for indexing articles.

Meta-analysis: A literature review combining many pieces of primary literature in an easy-to-understand format with summaries and conclusions. Also called a quantitative systematic review.

Metropolitan area network (MAN): A MAN is larger than a LAN, roughly the size of a city, connecting nodes dispersed across many blocks. This type of network is also a type of WAN.

Microwave transmission: Signals sent through the air (or space) between transmission stations, not using a physical component.

Mobile care: Allows practitioners to be connected to information and to each other wherever they need to render care.

Modified systematic approach: A seven-step method of responding to medication or health-related questions that improves accuracy, effectiveness, and efficiency.

Multiple user accounts: Allows each person who uses a computer system to customize features for individual needs, including the desktop, taskbar, and Start Menu.

N

Natural language processing: Use of computers to interpret and manipulate words as part of a language. Speech recognition is a form of natural language processing.

Network: An interconnected group of systems or devices, remote from one another.

Node: A device, such as a computer or printer, that is attached to a network.

Notebook computer: A compact portable computer smaller and lighter than a laptop—ideal for the mobility needed in some health care environments.

O

Online processing: Real-time or near real-time processing of transactions as they occur.

Online service provider: Internet sites that allow people to interact with professionals in a particular field outside their community.

Open standards: Data transfer standards that are not specific to a single hardware manufacturer or device.

Open systems interconnection (OSI): An internationally recognized set of standards for communication between computer systems.

Operating system (OS): Functional systems software that "controls" a computer system; considered the foundation on which all other components rest.

Output devices: Components that allow the user to see the results of interaction with the computer such as, monitors, printers, speakers, and fax machines.

P

Patient-oriented evidence that matters (POEM): Literature that addresses questions health care professionals face and has the potential to change the way a practitioner practices because it focuses on key outcomes such as morbidity, mortality, decreased hospitalizations, and quality of life.

Permanent storage devices: Hard drives, tape drives, floppy disks, CD-ROMs, DVD-ROMs, and other devices that permanently store data and software.

Personal digital assistant (PDA): A handheld computer roughly the size of a deck of cards that provides personal information management as well as data capture and display capabilities. Other names that may signify the same thing are pocket PC, palmtop, palm, or palm pilot.

Personal evaluation system (PES): Software designed to interact with the patient by clicking on images and answering questions to produce the most likely diagnosis.

Personal software: Designed for use by a single person to support individual needs, such as word processors, Web browsers, e-mail, spreadsheets, and database programs.

Pharming: The exploitation of a vulnerability in the DNS server software that allows a hacker to acquire the domain name for a site, and to redirect traffic from that Web site to another Web site, also known as DNS hijacking.

Phishing: A form of identity theft in which a scammer uses an authentic-looking e-mail to trick recipients into giving out sensitive personal information.

PICO (population, intervention, and clinical outcomes) method: A way of framing a clinical question by determining the relevant patients, necessary interventions, and patient-relevant consequences.

Picture-archiving and communication systems (PACS): A means to store, retrieve, distribute, and display digital medical images so they can be archived or viewed at diagnostic, reporting, consultation, and remote computer workstations.

Point of care: The place where providers render care to patients.

Point of care technologies: Devices such as notebook computers, desktop computers, and PDAs used to move drug knowledge, disease information, and diagnostic aids to patients instead of having to bring patients to the care.

Portal: A Web site that serves as an entry point to other Web sites.

Primary literature: Original research (clinical trials) generally published in journals representing the most current information available including details of research methodology.

Protocols: Also known as network communication standards, protocols are predefined, agreed-upon rules for the structure and function of communication across networks. These rules are used to control the flow of traffic across hardware that may or may not be similar.

Pure play: A business that operates entirely as an e-commerce entity.

Push technology: Automatically delivering information via the Internet to a preselected audience.

Q

Qualitative analysis: An approach to risk analysis that ascribes relative rank to threats and vulnerability of assets according to seriousness, then matches potential level of threat to potential asset loss to select appropriate safeguards.

Quantitative analysis: An approach to risk analysis that measures and assigns objective numeric value to assets, potential threat impacts, safeguard effectiveness, safeguard costs, uncertainty, and probability.

R

Radiofrequency identification (RFID): Small chips or electrical transponders that send out a signal. In health care, this technology is used to quickly help locate or authenticate patients, providers, and equipment.

RAM (random access memory): Temporary memory that stores programs and data while the user interacts with the computer.

Randomized controlled trial (RCT): A study in which patients are randomized to a treatment group or a placebo group and are followed forward in time to determine whether they have a particular outcome.

Receiver: The physical component within the telecommunication system that accepts the message prior to the decoding process.

Reverse auction: A type of auction where the buyer posts their needs and suppliers bid for the business.

Review article: An article that assembles, critically evaluates, and synthesizes the results of primary investigations addressing a specific topic or problem, which should include all recent and relevant studies but may or may not state its authors' criteria for including or excluding studies or methods of searching for information.

Ring topology: A network in which all data travel through all nodes with each node analyzing the data it receives and keeping only the data addressed to it. All other data are forwarded to the next node.

Robotics: Devices programmed to perform precise or tedious tasks in an effort to increase speed and accuracy.

ROM (read-only memory): Permanent in nature and cannot usually be modified by the user; normally stores the instructions used for booting up or starting a computer.

Router: Hardware that sends data traffic through computers and networks to the destination that the sender intends.

RPM (revolutions per minute): The measure of a computer hard drive's spinning speed.

Rules engine: Intelligence-based system that is based on "if-then" parameters gleaned from actual experience; identifies potential problems and suggests resolution options.

S

Satellite phone: A wireless phone that uses satellites to make calls from even the remotest mountaintop.

Search engine: A Web site whose primary function is gathering and reporting information available on the Internet or a portion of the Internet.

Secondary literature: Databases such as Medline that help health care professionals locate primary and tertiary literature.

Seek time: How long the central processing unit has to wait for data to be returned when requested from the hard drive. Current industry standards for seek times range from 10 to 20 milliseconds.

Shielded twisted-pair wire (STP): Twisted-pair wire surrounded by an additional protective layer of insulation that reduces interference.

Short messaging system (SMS): The transmission of short text messages to and from a cell phone or other device.

Signal attenuation: Loss in power of the signal between the transmitting and receiving points.

Smart phone: A cell phone with a microprocessor, memory, screen, and built-in modem. Smart phones combine some capabilities of a PC on a handset, including Internet and e-mail access.

Smart prompts: Alerts built into DSS that suggest other evidence-based actions that can be taken to optimize patient care practices.

Software: Data and instructions that control a computer.

Spam: Unsolicited or junk e-mail messages.

Spin rate: A computer hard drive's spinning speed, measured in revolutions per minute (RPM).

Spyware: Software that covertly gathers information and allows unauthorized access to the user's computer over the Internet.

Standard identifiers: Numbers used to identify health care providers, health plans, employers, and patients.

Star topology: A type of network that has a central node, known as the hub, through which all data must pass.

Start menu: Operating system feature closely related to the taskbar.

Subnotebook computers: Miniature notebook computers that are larger than PDAs but smaller than traditional notebook computers.

Systematic review: A review of systematically identified research or studies that assembles, critically evaluates, and synthesizes the results of primary investigations addressing a specific topic or problem.

Systems software: Software that controls the activity of the computer hardware and various other applications and provides a means for interacting with the computer system (user interface).

T

Tablet PC: A notebook-shaped computer that users operate with a stylus or a touch screen, so no keyboard or mouse is necessary.

Taskbar: The starting point of user interaction with a computer system; contains links to application software, controls for system maintenance, shortcuts to locations and software within the computer system, the Help feature, and other system functions.

Technology: Any tool that extends the capabilities of the user or performs tasks the user finds repetitive or tedious.

Telecommunication medium: Anything that carries an electronic signal between a source and a destination.

Telehealth: The use of electronic information and telecommunication technologies to support distance clinical health care, patient and professional health-related education, public health, and health administration.

Telemedicine: Use of telecommunications technology for medical diagnosis and patient care when the provider and client are separated by distance.

Telenursing: Use of telecommunications technology in nursing to enhance patient care.

Telepharmacy: Using telecommunications technology to expand the delivery of pharmaceutical care and practices.

Telnet: A standard Internet protocol for accessing remote systems.

Tertiary literature: Reference books, etc., offering comprehensive information in a single source including easy to use overviews and helpful background information.

Thin clients: Low-cost computing devices that access applications and data from a secure central server over a network without storing them locally on a PDA or other point of care device.

Third-generation wireless (3G): Wireless format launched in Europe and Japan with higher bandwidth connecting information appliances.

Threat: Any potential danger to the information system that exploits a vulnerability.

Topology: How individual network nodes (or devices, such as printers and computers) are physically and logically connected to other nodes on the network.

Transaction-processing systems (TPS): The lowest-level data-processing systems; used to process transactions that are part of normal business activities such as order entry, inventory control, payroll, accounts payable and receivable, and general ledger systems.

Transmission control protocol/internet protocol (TCP/IP): A set of rules that establishes the method with which data are transmitted over the Internet between two computers.

Transmitters: Device that takes an encoded message and sends it through the communication medium to the receiver.

Twisted-pair wire: Cable consisting of two independently insulated wires twisted around each other to reduce interference.

U

Uniform resource locator (URL): A Web site address.

Unshielded twisted-pair (UTP): Twisted-pair wire that does not contain a protective layer of insulation.

USENET News: Communities of Internet users with common interests who subscribe to posted news and discussion issues.

V

Videoconferencing: Allows multiple individuals in different locations to communicate over the Internet with voice, data, and video capabilities.

Viral marketing: A marketing strategy that encourages e-mail recipients to pass along messages to others in order to generate additional exposure.

Virtual private networking (VPN): A system configuration that uses firewalls, secure logon procedures, and authentication certificates to provide mobile users secure remote access to a private network.

Virtual storefront: A business that conducts transactions over the Internet that would traditionally have taken place by consumers walking into the business or calling on the telephone.

Virus: Software programs capable of reproducing themselves, which infect files and programs and spread through sharing infected files or disks; a form of electronic vandalism.

Voice-over-IP (VOIP): Communication that uses the Internet to move voice transmissions over long distances, bypassing telephone use.

Vulnerability: A software, hardware, or organizational weakness that may allow unauthorized access.

W

Webcast: Online conferences and presentations from which participants can retrieve information, audio, and slides.

Webinar: An Internet-based seminar that allows attendees to participate by receiving and sharing information and asking questions.

Web page: A document on the World Wide Web, identified by a unique URL.

Web site: A location on the World Wide Web. A Web site is the entire collection of Web pages for a specific organization, person, or interest group. The first page you see on the site is usually the home page.

Wide area network (WAN): A network that spans a large geographic area, often composed of many LANs and MANs connected together. The most extreme example of a WAN is the Internet.

WiMax: A wireless connection that enables computing stations or devices to be networked together across roughly 30 miles.

Wireless air panel: A touch-screen monitor used to remotely access the data and images on a personal computer.

Wireless fidelity (Wi-Fi): Inexpensive, user-friendly wireless network access at high speeds from any location.

Wireless local area network: A network that uses radio waves instead of physical wires to connect devices in the same office, floor, or building.

Wirelessly connected computers on wheels (COW): Workstations integrated into a moveable stand with full-sized display and extra-long battery life for use by mobile health care professionals.

Workgroup software: Provides features to assist groups of people working together on a specific task, such as chat sessions, whiteboards, videoconferencing, etc.

World Wide Web: The collection of all interconnected Web servers available on the Internet. Most Web documents are created using the hypertext markup language (html) coding system.

Worms: Malicious programs that automatically copy themselves and distribute the copies to other computer systems via e-mail attachments or direct connections.

Annotated Bibliography of Online Glossaries

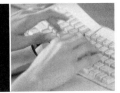

The following online glossaries are helpful sources of information, definitions, and explanations related to health care informatics, science, and other key topics.

Big Pond Glossary of PC and Internet Terminology
www.users.bigpond.com/jenkos/G.htm
At this straightforward site, you can quickly look up a term by its first letter in the alphabet or by scrolling through an index of all entries.

Health Canada eHealth Resources
www.hc-sc.gc.ca/ohih-bsi/res/gloss_e.html
This site links you to other informatics-related resources on health care informatics, telehealth, telecommunications, etc. It also contains an e-health glossary, conference calendar, and many other useful tools.

Healthcare Informatics Glossary
www.healthcare-informatics.com/issues/1998/01_98/glossary.htm
Published by the journal *Healthcare Informatics,* this glossary is displayed in a scrolling, article format. The material is readable and clear, but it was published in 1998, so beware of dating issues.

Language Automation Site
www.lai.com/glossaries.html
An inventory of online glossaries divided alphabetically by the language in which the glossary is presented, from Afrikaans to Yiddish. Some glossaries define technical terms, while others are more general. Some are translated into English while others are presented in the host language only.

Matisse Enzer's Glossary of Internet Terms
www.matisse.net/files/glossary.html
An alphabetical listing of common Internet terms you can easily scroll through for a quick primer, or select the first letter of the term you're searching for. "See also" links send you to related terms.

National Biological Information Infrastructure Glossary Listing
www.nbii.gov/datainfo/onlineref/dictionaries.html
On a single page, this site organizes access to glossaries that relate to biology, science, genomics, the environment, and agriculture.

Netdictionary
www.netdictionary.com
An alphabetical reference guide to technical, cultural, and humorous terms and acronyms related to the Internet. Different versions are offered, including Java and HTML.

NetLingo
www.netlingo.com
This commercial site sells downloadable Internet-related resources but also offers comprehensive glossaries in such categories as online business terms, online marketing, technical terms, and online jargon.

Statistics Explained
www.animatedsoftware.com/statglos/statglos.htm
This site presents two versions of a glossary explaining statistical terms: a standard HTML version and a Flash version. Although the definitions are a bit cumbersome, they are accompanied by graphics that clearly illustrate the meanings.

Webopedia
www.pcwebopedia.com
This popular site has been around for several years. It has a great search feature that takes you straight to the definitions of terms you type in, or you can browse categories, such as Computer Science or Networks. Although it does contain banner advertising, the site is well organized and packed with information.

What is by TechTarget Network
whatis.techtarget.com
Provides selected glossaries and quick reference articles on Internet topics, software, and technology.

1000 Dictionaries
www.1000dictionaries.com/medical_glossaries_1.html
Although loaded up with advertising and annoying pop-ups, this site has lots of useful glossaries, including a special medical glossary listing. It's a good idea to have a pop-up stopper in place before visiting the site.

Index

online processing, 65
online resources, 18–19, 85–88, 125, 207–227.
See also consumer health information; information
resources
evaluating, 230–236, 328
health care informatics, 18–19
telehealth, 293
online transactions, 116, 120, 122, 312. *See also*
e-commerce
HIPAA rules for, 360, 362
open standards, telecommunication, 146
Open Systems Interconnection (OSI) model, 146–147
versus TCP/IP, 148
operating system (OS), 34–36. *See also* Windows
operating system
functions of, 35–36
identification of computer specifics using, 33
information management within, 41–44
installing and removing software using, 45
relation between other components and, 35
order reconciliation, at point of care, 176
organizational culture
and diffusion of innovation, 105, 376–379, 388–389
and patient safety issues, 173
OSI model, 146–147
versus TCP/IP, 148
outcomes measurement
and evidence-based medicine, 255, 265
and point of care technology, 182–183
research design for, 249
use of, 89–90
using information systems for, 89–92
outpatient care, systems approach to, 81
output devices, 28–29, 384
overwrapping, of unit-dose medications, 98

P

Papago Indian Reservation, 282
paper-based systems, moving to electronic systems
from, 56–58, 69
parallel design, 244
patient care planning, using evidence-based medicine
software, 90, 178
Patient Care Technologies, 284, 291
patient compliance, and research results, 249
patient consent, 362
patient data, privacy of. *See* privacy
patient education, 323–340. *See also* consumer health
information
sources for, 329–334
Patient Education: The Care Notes System, Aftercare
Instruction & Drug Leaflets, 217
patient-focused care
and health care reform, 324–326

and Internet usage, 120–122
and point of care technology, 168
patient identification
in documentation systems, 95, 104
at point of care, 174
and privacy issues, 345
standards for, 362
patient participation, and telehealth initiatives, 285
patient preferences, data collection on, 81
patient profile applications, using, 41–42
patient-provider communication, 88–89, 122, 379
patient reminders, e-mail, 88–89
patient safety
and automated pharmacy systems, 102–104,
170–171, 174–176
at point of care, 173–177, 184
patient satisfaction, measurement of, 92
payment systems, e-commerce, 312, 320
payroll systems, 65, 67–68
PedsCCM and IntensiveCare.com: Resources for
Practicing Evidence-Based Medicine, 274
Penelope Surgical Instrument Server, 73
Pentium processors, 31
performance-enhancing technology, 79–80
permanent storage devices, 30, 41, 46
personal digital assistants (PDAs), 60, 167, 178–182
adoption of, 180
basic skills, 180–182
cautions with, 179
combined with cell phones, 141
information resources for, 221–223
infrared transmission from, 142
and patient safety, 173
speech recognition software with, 74
uses for, 179
personal evaluation system (PES), 333
personal software, 36
Person-To-Person sharing programs, 351
Pharmacist.com, 126
The Pharmacist's Letter, 338
pharmacy, retail
privacy issues, 346
Web sites, 290
pharmacy communication, online medication
reference systems with, 175–176
Pharmacy Informatics.com, 19
pharmacy practice
application service providers in, 159
automation in, 96–103 (*See also* automated
pharmacy systems)
bar codes used in, 79–80, 97, 100–101, 103
decision support systems in, 71–72, 170
expert systems in, 72
mail service, 99–100
online integration of, 117

R

radio frequency identification (RFID), 104, 386
RAM (random access memory), 29, 33, 44
randomized controlled trials (RCT), 243–244, 249, 258
receivers, 135
recommendation grades, in systematic reviews, 261–262
Recycle Bin, 44
reference sources
    clinical use of, 197–200
    online, 125, 175
reference systems, medication, with enhanced
  pharmacy communication, 175–176
regulatory issues
    and HIPAA administration, 359
    and security concerns, 348–349
    with telehealth, 297
reimbursement, for telehealth services, 297
RelayHealth, 307
reliability, of practice guidelines, 239
remote dispensing, 289–290
remote health services, telehealth initiatives, 286–287
remote patient monitoring, 383
removing software, 45
repackaging, of bulk medicines, 98, 100
reproducibility, of practice guidelines, 239
REPRORISK System (Micromedex), 217
research
    and adoption of new technology, 379
    sponsorship, 248
    subject selection criteria, 248
    telehealth, 297
    using Internet for, 129
research design
    and evidence-based medicine, 256, 258
    understanding, 243
resources. *See also* information resources; online resources
    health care informatics, 18–19
    patient education, 329–334
    telehealth, 293
Restore option, 44
results section, evaluating, 247, 250
reverse auctions, 304–305
reviews
    grades in, 261–262
    of practice guidelines, 240
    systematic, 224–225, 258–259
revolutions per minute (RPM), 30
Ridgeview Medical Center, 379
ring networks, 50
risk acceptance, 366
risk analysis, 364–366
risk management
    HIPAA regulations on, 364–366
    and patient safety issues, 173

and security issues, 351–358
risk transfer, 366
RoboForm, 350
robotics, 73, 98, 385
ROM (read-only memory), 29
routers (Internet), 111
rural health services, telehealth initiatives, 286–287

S

sample size, 248
Sarbanes-Oxley Act, 349
satellite Internet access, 115, 153–154
satellite phones, 381
satellite transmission, 140–141, 143
saving data, 46
scanning
    biometric, 104
    medication, 79–80
ScriptPro SP 200, 97, 103
search engines
    positioning Web sites on, 316
    using, 122–124
secondary literature, 192, 208–211
    searching, 201–204
security, 343, 351–358
    administration, 347–349, 355–357
    HIPAA rules on, 360–361, 363–366
seek time, 30
sharing programs, 351
Shaughnessy, Allen F., 265
shielded twisted-pair wire (STP), 138
Sholes, Christopher, 28
shortcuts, adding to desktop, 38–39
short messaging system (SMS), 382
signal-to-noise ratio, 135
silos, removing, 62–63
single-loss expectancy (SLE), 365
Slawson, David C., 265
smart phones, 60, 141
smart prompts, 172
software, 27, 34–36. *See also specific type*
    antispyware, 350
    antivirus, 350, 354, 357
    backup utility, 46
    for blood transfusion checks, 177
    choosing and integrating, 82
    classification of, 36
    computerized prescriber order entry, 171–172
    customer relationship management, 81, 316–317, 321
    decision support, 94, 169, 170, 385
    distribution, 158–159
    documentation, 93–94
    health care examples of, 36
    installing and removing, 45

telehealth, 117, 122, 133, 162, 277–299
    definition of, 279–280
    and e-commerce, 307
    examples of, 281–283
    goals for, 280, 283
    history of, 280–281
    implementation of, 295–298, 299
    online resources, 293
    reimbursement for, 297
    trends in, 278, 283–284, 383
telemedicine, 286–288, 383
    and e-commerce, 307
Telemedicine Information Exchange (TIE), 296
telenursing, 291–292
telepharmacy, 288–290
telephones, 133, 136, 138
    cellular, 141–142, 383
    satellite, 381
    smart, 60
telepsychiatry, 288
telesurgery, 286
TELNET, 112
tertiary literature, 192, 212–218
    evaluating, 197–200
theft, 353
therapeutic outcomes, measurement of, 90–91
thesauri, 201
thin clients, 172
third-generation wireless (3G), 382
third-party payers
    and management information systems, 69
    privacy regulations, 366–368
    transaction processing with, 68
TOMES System, 217
topology, network, 48–50
touch screens, 92, 167
ToxPoints System, 218
transaction(s), online, 116, 120, 122, 312. See also
e-commerce
    HIPAA rules for, 360, 362
transaction-processing systems (TPS), 65, 67–68
transfusions, blood, safety checks for, 177
transmission capacity, 137
Transmission Control Protocol/Internet Protocol
    (TCP/IP), 111–112, 147
    versus OSI model, 148
transmitters, 135
tree networks, 50
TRIP database, 268–269
Trissel's Tables of Physical Compatibility, 216
Trojan Horse, 353
twisted-pair wire, 138, 143, 144

U

UK Health Informatics Society, 13
uniform resource locator (URL), 111, 118
uninstalling software, 45
unique identifiers standards, 362
unit-dose medication dispensers, 15, 98, 100
United States
    government networking protocol, 111–112, 147
    health care informatics education programs in,
        20–22
United States High-Performance Computing Act, 110
universities, with health care informatics programs,
    20–22
University of California Davis Medical Center, 287
unshielded twisted-pair wire (UTP), 138, 144
upgrading (computer), 33–34
URAC, 234–235
urban health services, telehealth initiatives, 287
USB flash memory, 357
USCF Stanford Health Care System, 117
USENET News, 112
user accounts, multiple, 40–41
user authentication and verification, 41
user preferences, for data-processing systems,
    identifying, 59
The Users' Guides to the Medical Literature: A Manual
    for Evidence-Based Clinical Practice, 241–242
Users' Guides to the Medical Literature (AMA), 261, 269
USP DI Drug Reference Guides, 216, 218
UWB (ultra wideband), 61

V

validity, of practice guidelines, 239–240
Veterans Affairs (VA) system, 99, 187–188
videoconferencing, 159–160
    in telemedicine, 287, 290
viral marketing, 315–316
virtual privacy network (VPN), 179, 352
virtual storefronts, 304
virtual visits, 307
viruses, computer, 110, 353–354
    protection against, 350, 354, 357
Vocera Company, 382
voice-over-IP (VOIP), 382
voice response systems, interactive, 72–73

W

Wagner, Gustav, 4
Walgreens, 117
wardriving, 353
Warren, Samuel, 344
wayfinding, 306
wearable computers, 383–384